Simplified Approach to Orthopedic Physiotherapy
Rationale and Rehabilitation

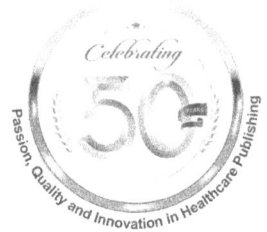

Simplified Approach to Orthopedic Physiotherapy
Rationale and Rehabilitation

Mukesh Sharma
BPT MPT (Musculoskeletal Disorders) MIAP

Assistant Professor
TDTR DAV Institute of Physiotherapy and Rehabilitation
Yamunanagar, Haryana, India

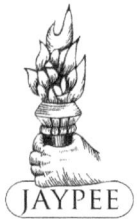

JAYPEE BROTHERS MEDICAL PUBLISHERS
The Health Sciences Publisher
New Delhi | London

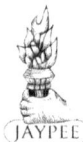 **Jaypee Brothers Medical Publishers (P) Ltd**

Headquarters
Jaypee Brothers Medical Publishers (P) Ltd
4838/24, Ansari Road, Daryaganj
New Delhi 110 002, India
Phone: +91-11-43574357
Fax: +91-11-43574314
Email: jaypee@jaypeebrothers.com

Overseas Office
J.P. Medical Ltd
83 Victoria Street, London
SW1H 0HW (UK)
Phone: +44 20 3170 8910
Fax: +44 (0)20 3008 6180
Email: info@jpmedpub.com

© 2020, Jaypee Brothers Medical Publishers

The views and opinions expressed in this book are solely those of the original contributor(s)/author(s) and do not necessarily represent those of editor(s) of the book.

All rights reserved. No part of this publication may be reproduced, stored or transmitted in any form or by any means, electronic, mechanical, photocopying, recording or otherwise, without the prior permission in writing of the publishers.

All brand names and product names used in this book are trade names, service marks, trademarks or registered trademarks of their respective owners. The publisher is not associated with any product or vendor mentioned in this book.

Medical knowledge and practice change constantly. This book is designed to provide accurate, authoritative information about the subject matter in question. However, readers are advised to check the most current information available on procedures included and check information from the manufacturer of each product to be administered, to verify the recommended dose, formula, method and duration of administration, adverse effects and contraindications. It is the responsibility of the practitioner to take all appropriate safety precautions. Neither the publisher nor the author(s)/editor(s) assume any liability for any injury and/or damage to persons or property arising from or related to use of material in this book.

This book is sold on the understanding that the publisher is not engaged in providing professional medical services. If such advice or services are required, the services of a competent medical professional should be sought.

Every effort has been made where necessary to contact holders of copyright to obtain permission to reproduce copyright material. If any have been inadvertently overlooked, the publisher will be pleased to make the necessary arrangements at the first opportunity. The **CD/DVD-ROM** (if any) provided in the sealed envelope with this book is complimentary and free of cost. **Not meant for sale.**

Inquiries for bulk sales may be solicited at: jaypee@jaypeebrothers.com

Simplified Approach to Orthopedic Physiotherapy: Rationale and Rehabilitation

First Edition: **2020**

ISBN: **978-93-5270-961-8**

Dedicated to

God, my family and my friends

Preface

Physiotherapy is a health care system that is solicited with improving the quality of life by preventing, assessing and diagnosing any ailment and managing it conservatively with therapeutic interventions and rehabilitation.

The scope and technology of orthopedic physiotherapy continue to evolve and require new techniques and approaches. As physiotherapy forms the mainstay of conservative treatment, hence it plays an integral role in the management of musculoskeletal conditions and trauma. As a physiotherapist strongly contributes to the improvement of daily life activities, one should have good skill base and knowledge.

Nonetheless, the core knowledge of different orthopedic conditions, clinical examination, objective assessment and diagnosis of the condition and its management are essential to physiotherapy practice. Physiotherapy is a profession where there is a relationship of trust between the patient and the therapist, and the therapist is recognized to have comprehensive knowledge and skills relevant to physiotherapy practice. Therefore understanding established and recent physiotherapy approaches is imperative.

This book reflects the need for integral approach to physiotherapy. It is a book which can be used as a reference by the physiotherapy undergraduate and postgraduate students, researchers, academicians and clinical physiotherapists. This book aims at developing clinical reasoning and problem solving approach in treating various orthopedic conditions as well as providing theoretic base along.

This book also seeks to teach the fundamental approach to physiotherapy practice so that the diagnosis and physiotherapy treatment are merged into established pattern. It elaborates the detailed information of all the possible musculoskeletal conditions with their pathophysiology, symptoms, epidemiology, assessment and diagnosis along with their surgical and nonsurgical management based on current rationale. This book includes the most accepted established exercise protocol which is an important way to provide evidence-based practice.

Nevertheless, the content and presentation of book is designed with an assortment of text with required figures, images, tables, and flowcharts to make it more comprehensible for the readers. This book tries to cover all the possible musculoskeletal conditions and trauma like soft tissue injuries of different regions of body, various joint deformities, different types of arthritis, peripheral nerve injuries, amputation and detailed orthopedic physiotherapy assessment.

I hope that this text will be beneficial for upgrading your knowledge regarding musculoskeletal conditions and their physiotherapy management. It will surely meet the need of all orthopedic physiotherapists.

Mukesh Sharma

Acknowledgments

It is my esteemed pleasure to present this book and I first thank God and my beloved mother Smt Krishna Devi whose heavenly blessings have helped me to sail very easily through adversities of life.

It is an ineffable feeling to express my heartiest regards to my father Shri DV Apherya for his constant love, enthusiasm and never ending encouragement during the whole period of this project. The cordial and encouraging support given by him always made me dream higher and work harder to upgrade my knowledge and move my career forward. This book is the result of his best intentions coupled with my hard work manifested practically. He is literally a source of motivation to improve myself not just professionally but personally.

My heartfelt regards also goes to my mother in law Smt Chander Lekha Sharma for her incessant love, blessings and appreciation. I owe an infinite gratitude to my husband Dr Vinay Sharma for showering his unbound affection, assistance and great understanding with utmost zeal. Words cannot express my feelings towards my gifted son Aarav who bestows me with his innocent love and sweet gestures.

Words are not adequate enough to express my gratitude and deep sense of indebtedness to my colleague Dr Pooja Attrey for providing incessant and altruistic help, moral support, proper rectifications of the problems encountered during this project. I would like to thank her for contributing a chapter "Approach to Orthopedic Physiotherapy Assessment" in this book.

I should be failing in my duties if I do not acknowledge the cooperation and acceptance provided by my family and my students. This gave me confidence and laid the first stepping milestone for this project.

Last but not the least, I wish to express my thanks to M/s Jaypee Brothers Medical Publishers (P) Ltd, New Delhi, India for giving me this valuable chance to publish my work with them.

Contents

1. **Soft Tissue Injuries**   1

    General Introduction to Soft Tissue Injury *1;*   **Shoulder Injuries** *4;*
    Rotator Cuff Injury *4;*   Frozen Shoulder *10;*   Subacromial Bursitis *14;*
    Elbow Injuries *18;*   Tennis Elbow *18;*   Golfer's Elbow *22;*
    Volkmann's Ischemic Contracture *25;*   Olecranon Bursitis *29;*
    Hand and Wrist Injuries *31;*   Dupuytren's Contracture *31;*
    De Quervain's Tenosynovitis *34;*   Ganglion *37;*   **Knee Injuries** *39;*
    Meniscal Injury *39;*   Anterior Cruciate Ligament Injury *43;*
    Posterior Cruciate Ligament Injury *47;*   Osgood-Schlatter Disease *51;*
    Knee Bursitis *54;*   **Ankle and Foot Injuries** *56;*   Ankle Sprain *56;*
    Plantar Fasciitis *60;*   Retrocalcaneal Bursitis *63*

2. **Fractures and Dislocations**   66

    General Introduction of Fracture *66;*   Classification of Fractures *66;*
    Complications of Fracture *70;*   Stages of Fracture Healing *71;*
    Upper Limb Fractures *74;*   Clavicle Fracture *74;*   Scapular Fracture *76;*
    Proximal Humeral Fracture *78;*   Humeral Shaft Fracture *81;*
    Distal Humeral Fracture *82;*   Ulnar Olecranon Fracture *85;*
    Radial Head Fracture *86;*   Forearm Fractures *88;*
    Wrist Fracture/Distal Radius Fractures *91;*   Colles' Fracture *91;*
    Smith's Fracture *91;*   Barton's Fracture *92;*   Chauffeur Fracture *92;*
    Die Punch Fracture *92;*   Carpal Fracture *94;*   Scaphoid Fracture *94;*
    Triquentrum Fracture *96;*   Trepezium Fracture *96;*   Lunate Fracture *97;*
    Capitate Fracture *97;*   Hamate Fracture *97;*   Metacarpal Fracture *98;*
    Lower Limb Fractures *100;*   Pelvic Fracture *100;*   Proximal Femoral Fracture *103;*
    Femoral Shaft Fracture *107;*   Distal Femoral Fracture *109;*
    Supracondylar Fracture *109;*   Patellar Fracture *111;*   Proximal Tibial Fracture *113;*
    Tibial Shaft Fracture *115;*   Distal Tibial Fracture/Tibial Plafond Fracture *117;*
    Tarsal Fracture *119;*   Metatarsal Fracture *123;*   **Vertebral Fracture** *125;*
    Atlas Fracture (Jafferson Fracture) *125;*   Axis Fracture *127;*
    Lower Cervical Vertebrae Fracture *129;*   Thoracolumbar Vertebrae Fracture *130;*
    Management of Unstable Vertebral Fractures *134;*   **Fractures Nomenclature** *137;*
    Dislocations *139;*   Shoulder Dislocation *139;*   Elbow Dislocation *142;*
    Hip Dislocation *144;*   Patellar Dislocation *146*

3. **Deformities**   150

    Hip Deformities *150;*   Coxa Vara *150;*   Coxa Valga *153;*   **Knee Deformities** *154;*
    Genu Varum *154;*   Genu Valgum *157;*   **Foot Deformities** *159;*   Pes Cavus *159;*
    Pes Planus *162;*   **Spinal Deformities** *165;*   Scoliosis *165;*   Kyphosis *172;*
    Lordosis *176*

4. Peripheral Nerve Lesion — 180

General Introduction of Peripheral Nerve Lesion *180*; Mononeuropathy *181*; **Upper Limb Nerve Lesions** *188*; Radial Nerve Injury *188*; Median Nerve Injury *189*; Ulnar Nerve Injury *193*; **Lower Limb Nerve Lesions** *197*; Sciatic Nerve *197*; Tibial Nerve *197*; Common Peroneal Nerve *198*; Femoral Nerve *199*; **Entrapment Neuropathy** *199*; Pathogenesis *199*; Thoracic Outlet Syndrome *200*; Carpal Tunnel Syndrome *210*; Piriformis Syndrome *214*; Tarsal Tunnel Syndrome *217*

5. Spinal Disorders — 220

Spondylosis *220*; Spondylolisthesis *222*; Ankylosing Spondylitis *227*; Prolapsed Intervertebral Disease *234*; TB Spine (Pott's Spine) *241*

6. Arthritis — 246

Osteoarthritis *246*; Rheumatoid Arthritis *251*; Gouty Arthritis *258*

7. Metabolic Bone Diseases — 262

Osteoporosis *262*; Rickets and Osteomalacia *267*

8. Arthroplasty — 272

Total Knee Replacement *273*; Total Hip Replacement *275*

9. Arthrodesis — 278

Shoulder Arthrodesis *278*; Elbow Arthrodesis *279*; Wrist Arthrodesis *279*; Hip Arthrodesis *280*; Knee Arthrodesis *280*; Ankle Arthrodesis *280*

10. Amputation — 282

Level of Amputation *282*; Characteristics of ideal stump *283*; Stump Management *285*; Postoperative Physiotherapy Management *287*

11. Legg-Calvé-Perthes Disease — 298

12. Edema — 302

13. Complex Regional Pain Syndrome — 306

14. Fibromyalgia — 312

15. Approach to Orthopedic Physiotherapy Assessment — 316

Subjective Assessment *316*; Pain Assessment *316*; Objective Assessment *316*

Index — 323

Abbreviations

- **AAROM:** Active-assisted range of motion
- **Abds:** Abdominals
- **AC joint:** Acromioclavicular joint
- **ACL:** Anterior cruciate ligament
- **ADLs:** Activity of daily lifes
- **AROM:** Active range of motion
- **BOS:** Base of support
- **CKCE:** Close kinetic chain exercises
- **CMC joint:** Carpometacarpal joint
- **CoG:** Center of gravity
- **CRPS:** Complex regional pain syndrome
- **CVA:** Cerebrovascular accident
- **DIP joint:** Distal interphalangeal joint
- **ER:** External rotation
- **FOOSH:** Fall on outstretched hand
- **FWB:** Full weight-bearing
- **FWBAT:** Full weight-bearing as tolerance
- **Hams:** Hamstring
- **IFT:** Interferential therapy
- **IR:** Internal rotation
- **LE:** Lower extremity
- **MCP joint:** Metacarpophalangeal joint
- **MMT:** Manual muscle testing
- **MVA:** Motor vehicle accident
- **NSAIDs:** Nonsteroidal anti-inflammatory drugs
- **NWB:** Nonweight-bearing
- **OA:** Osteoarthritis
- **OKCE:** Open kinetic chain exercises
- **ORIF:** Open reduction and internal fixation
- **PCL:** Posterior cruciate ligament
- **PIP:** Proximal interphalangeal joint
- **PNF:** Proprioceptive neuromuscular facilitation
- **PROM:** Passive range of motion
- **PWB:** Partial weight-bearing
- **Quads:** Quadriceps
- **RA:** Rheumatoid arthritis
- **RD:** Radial deviation
- **ROM:** Range of motion
- **SLR:** Straight leg raising
- **TENS:** Transcutaneous electrical nerve stimulation
- **TL:** Thoracolumbar
- **TOS:** Thoracic outlet syndrome
- **TTWB:** Toe touch weight-bearing
- **UD:** Ulnar deviation
- **UE:** Upper extremity
- **US:** Ultrasound
- **VIC:** Volkmann ischemic contracture
- **WB:** Weight-bearing
- **WBAT:** Weight-bearing as tolerance

CHAPTER 1

Soft Tissue Injuries

■ GENERAL INTRODUCTION TO SOFT TISSUE INJURY

Soft tissue injuries (STI) refer to injury to the soft tissues like ligaments, muscles, bursae or tendons that commonly presents with pain, tenderness and swelling. Various types of soft tissue injuries are contusions, sprains, strains, tendonitis and bursitis.

Etiology

There are two fundamental types of soft tissue injuries:
1. **Acute injuries:** These are caused by a sudden injury or trauma, such as direct blow or fall on the area, e.g. sprains, strains, and contusions.
2. **Overuse injuries:** These are caused by repeated activities and occur progressively with time when injured area does not get enough time for healing between the episodes of injuries, e.g. tendinitis and bursitis.

Types of Soft Tissue Injury

Acute Soft Tissue Injuries

- **Sprains:** A sprain is a sudden stretch or tear of one or more ligaments (a band of connective tissue that attaches the distal end of two bones and helps to stabilize and support the joints) due to direct blow, twist or fall on the area, e.g. medial collateral ligament sprain of knee, ankle sprain, etc. Sprains are classified on basis of the degree of severity (Fig. 1):
  - **Grade 1 sprain (mild):** Mild damage to the ligament.
  - **Grade 2 sprain (moderate):** Partial tear of the ligament. It causes increased laxity of ligament.
  - **Grade 3 sprain (severe):** Complete tear of the ligament. It causes marked instability of joint.
- **Strains:** A strain is stretched or torn muscle (moves the different parts of body) or tendons (a fibrous band that connects the

Grade I
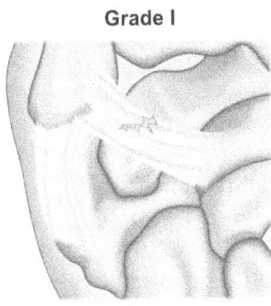
Ligaments stretched or slightly torn

Grade II
Ligaments partially torn

Grade III
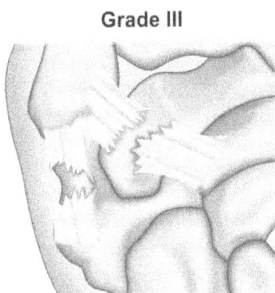
Ligaments completely torn

Fig. 1: Classification of sprains.

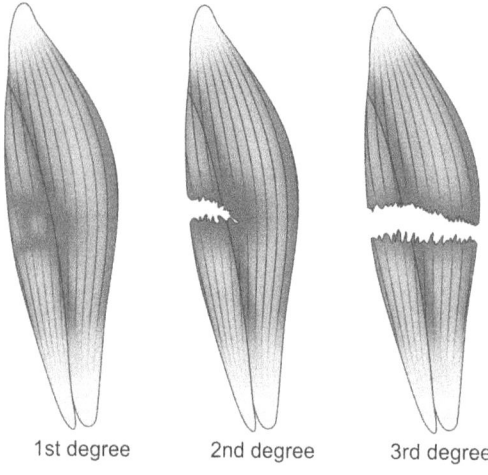

Fig. 2: Classification of strain.

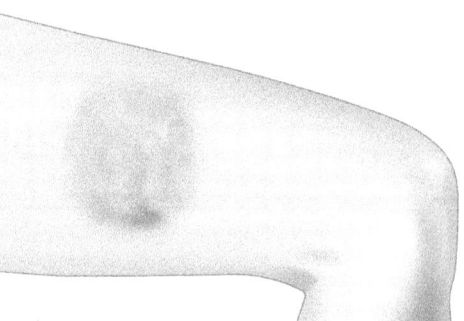

Fig. 3: Muscle contusions or bruises.

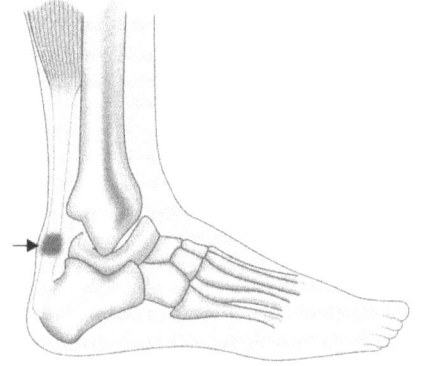

Fig. 4: Tendinitis (arrow).

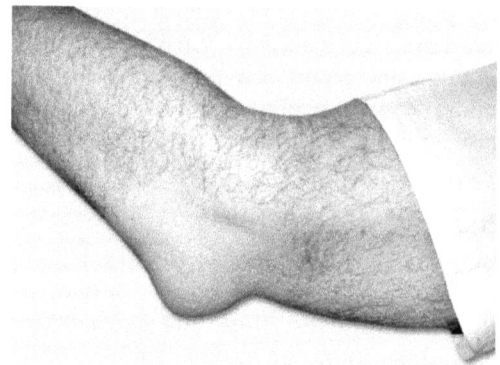

Fig. 5: Bursitis.

muscles to the bone), e.g. biceps strains, calf strain, etc (Fig. 2).
- **First degree:** Mild damage to muscles/tendons.
- **Second degree:** Partial tear of muscle/tendon.
- **Third degree:** Complete tear of muscle/tendon.

- **Contusions (bruises) (Fig. 3):** A contusion is a bruise or hematoma which refers to discoloration of the skin due to collection of blood outside the blood vessels underneath the skin. It is commonly caused by direct blow or fall on the hard surface.

Common Overuse Soft Tissue Injuries
- **Tendinitis (Fig. 4):** It refers to inflammation of tendon (a fibrous band that connects muscles to bone) or tendon sheath (covering of tendon). It is usually caused by overuse of tendon in the course of work, athletics or daily activities. It is most often associated with repetitive movements. It is characterized by pain and swelling that aggravates with activity, e.g. supraspinatus tendinitis, achilles tendinitis, etc.
- **Bursitis (Fig. 5):** It refers to inflammation of a bursa (a small fluid filled sacs present between the soft tissues and bone that helps to counter friction between them during movement of joint). It is usually caused by repeated movement of area. Commonly associated with tendinitis, e.g. prepatellar bursitis, subacromial bursitis, etc.

Clinical Presentation
Soft tissue injuries present with acute symptoms like:
- Pain that worsen with activity of affected area.
- Swelling, tenderness and bruising present over affected and surrounding area.
- Redness and warmth of area.
- Instability of adjacent joints that gradually leads to weakness of surrounding muscles.
- Severe injuries may lead to loss of function.

Management
There are principally three stages of treatment:

Stage One: Acute Phase (Protection Phase)
In initial 24-72 hours, before getting a reliable diagnosis, therapist should protect the injured area and begins with **PRICE** regime.

PRICE Regime (Fig. 6)
- **Protect:** Injured area should be protected by reducing the activity or by immobilizing the affected part temporarily with splint or braces as activity can further damaged the injured tissue.
- **Rest:** Relative rest to injured area is needed to reduce pain, swelling and further damage. Use of assistive devices, such as sling for upper limb and crutches, for lower limb to take off the weight from an injured limb aid in healing process.
- **Ice:** Cold application is used to reduce pain and inflammation. It should be applied for 10-15 minutes after every 2-3 hours.
- **Compression:** Compression is used to support injury and minimize swelling. Bandaging an area can be used for compression. Compression bandage should not be too tight that may reduce normal circulation to the area.
- **Elevation:** Injured part should be elevated above the heart level to reduce pain and swelling for short periods of time.

Mild injuries can be treated conservatively without medicine. Moderate to severe injuries require medical or surgical treatment.

HARM factors should be avoided in initial 48 to 72 hours after injury (Fig. 7).
- **Heat:** Heat application (e.g. hot fomentation, hot shower, hot rubs), etc. should be avoided as it may further worsen the condition by increasing inflammation and blood flow to the area.
- **Alcohol:** Avoid alcohol consumption as it has an effect of vasodilatation that may increase inflammation and bleeding.
- **Running or exercise:** Intensive activity may increase pain, swelling and blood flow to the area.

P	R	I	C	E
Protect injury from further damage	Rest the injury site for few days to ease pain	Ice the area that has pain	Compress the area with bandage to limit swelling	Elevate the injured part preferably above heart level

Fig. 6: PRICE regime.

H	A	R	M
Heat can increase blood flow which may increase swelling, so do not take hot bath or use a hot pack	Alcohol drinking can increase bleeding and swelling in injured area	Running or other forms of exercises can cause further damage	Massaging the injured area can cause further damage or swelling

Fig. 7: HARM factors.

- **Massage:** Direct massage over injured area will stimulate blood flow to the area and may additionally damage the injured tissues.

Stage Two: Subacute Phase (Repair Phase)

In this phase, swelling and joint stiffness gradually diminishes and start to regain normal ROM.
- **Pain relieving modalities:** Modalities, such as ultrasound/TENS/EMS/IFT are used to reduce pain, inflammation and muscle spasm.
- **Massage:** Gentle massage could be helpful in drainage of inflammatory products. It has to perform proximal to the site of injury and not directly over the injured area.
- **Mobility exercises:** It helps to improve circulation, stimulate tonically depressed joint mechanoreceptors and also facilitate the movement of synovial fluid. Mobility exercises should be gradually progress from PROM to AAROM to AROM exercises with in pain free ROM.
- **Strengthening exercises:** Initially isometric exercise of affected area should be given to maintain muscle strength and to prevent muscle atrophy. Strengthening exercises of area proximal to affected area is given to restore functional ability of patient.
- **Joint mobilization (Grades I and II):** It helps to accelerate the movement of accumulated fluid, to break adhesion and to restore mobility between joint surfaces.

Stage Three: Last Stage (Remodeling Phase)

At 6 weeks post-soft tissue injury: In this phase patient retrieve his normal functional activities.
- Free mobility exercises in complete range
- Strengthening exercises of affected area also
- Joint mobilization (Grades III and IV)
- Stretching
- Proprioceptive exercises
- Plyometrics
- Functional exercises.

SHOULDER INJURIES

ROTATOR CUFF INJURY (FIG. 8)

This is common sports injury in which one or more of the rotator cuff muscles or their tendons are injured. Rotator cuff is a group of four muscles (i.e. supraspinatus, infraspinatus, teres minor and subscapularis muscles) that helps to move and stabilize the shoulder joint.

Supraspinatus is the most commonly injured muscle.

Etiology

Acute/Traumatic Cause
- Abrupt and strenuous activity or an impact
- Fall on outstretched arm
- Heavy lift with a jerky motion
- Associated with shoulder injury, e.g. clavicle fracture, shoulder dislocation, etc.

Chronic/Degenerative Cause
- Overuse in combination with muscle imbalance or poor biomechanics.
- Repetitive stress, e.g. overhead throwing, rowing or weight lifting.
- With increasing age—blood circulation to rotator cuff muscles gradually diminishes that impair the natural ability to repair.

Types of Rotator Cuff Tears

1. **Partial thickness tear:** In this, the tear is partial that does not completely split the attachment of injured tendon to bone.
2. **Complete/full thickness tear:** In this, the tear goes all way long the tendon.

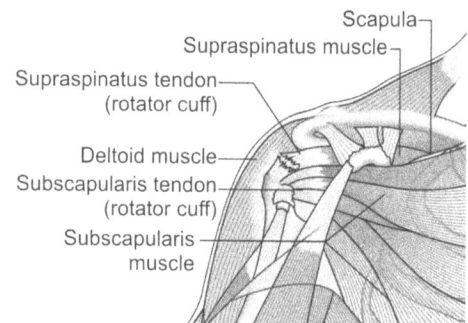

Fig 8: Rotator cuff tear.

Soft Tissue Injuries

Table 1: Rotator cuff muscles.

Muscle	Origin	Insertion	Action		Nerve
Supraspinatus	Supraspinous fossa	Greater tubercle	Abduct		Suprascapular
Infraspinatus	Infraspinous fossa	Greater tubercle	Lateral rotate	Horizontal abduct	Suprascapular
Teres minor	Superior half of axillary border	Greater tubercle	Lateral rotate	Horizontal abduct	Axillary
Subscapularis	Subscapular fossa	Lesser tubercle	Adduct	Medial rotate	Subscapular

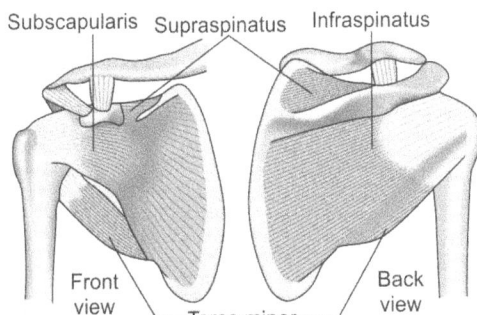

Fig. 9: Rotator cuff muscles.

Anatomy

Four muscles of rotator cuff are supraspinatus, infraspinatus, teres minor and subscapularis muscles (Table 1 and Fig. 9).

Clinical Presentation (Fig. 10)

- **Acute injury:** Intense pain radiates through the arm.
  - Limited ROM (especially shoulder abduction).
- **Chronic injury:** Pain on anterior and lateral aspect of shoulder.
  - Inability to do overhead activities.
  - Pain increases at night while reclining directly on affected shoulder.
  - Pain on reaching forward, i.e. inability to hold up a glass of water from kitchen slab.
  - Inability to lift or rotate the arm.
  - Progressive loss of motion and muscle weakness.
  - Crepitus or cracking sensation on moving the shoulder in certain positions.

Diagnosis

- **Imaging tests:**
  - **X-ray:** X-ray is used to exclude other possible conditions, although the findings are normal in rotator cuff tear.
  - **MRI scan or ultrasound:** These scans are needed to confirm the presence, location of injury and severity of condition.

Physical Examination

Patient History

Includes chief complains (e.g. pain, weakness, instability, limited ROM), how the problem started, sudden or gradual onset, aggravating factors, previous episodes of similar symptoms, any previous shoulder injury.

Examination of Specific Muscle

- **Supraspinatus tendinitis**
  - **Action:** It performs initial 0–15° of shoulder and helps deltoid muscle to abduct shoulder beyond 90°.
  - **Palpation:** It is palpated one finger width below anteromedial aspect of acromion.
  - **Special test: Empty can test (Fig. 11):** Patient is seated or standing with arm raised in scapular plane to 90° with shoulder internal rotation, elbow extension and forearm, i.e. in thumbs-down position. Therapist applies a downwardly directed force proximal to wrist and patient tries to resist this motion. This test is considered to be positive if it elicits pain or weakness.

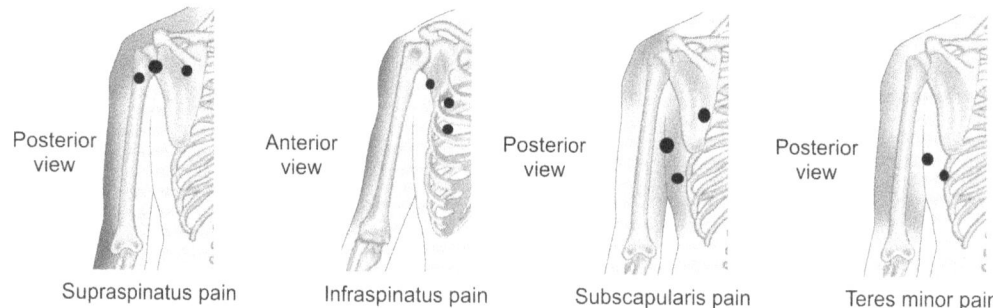

Fig. 10: Pain pattern of rotator cuff tear.

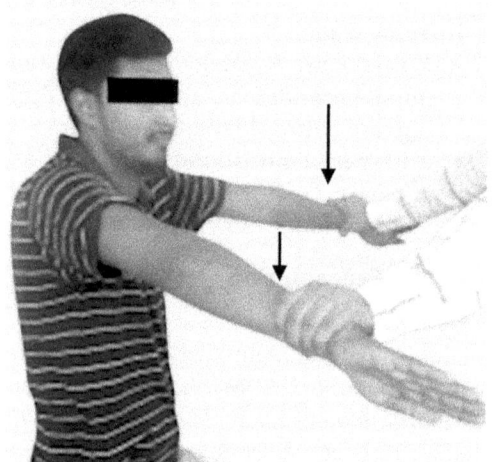

Fig. 11: Empty can test.

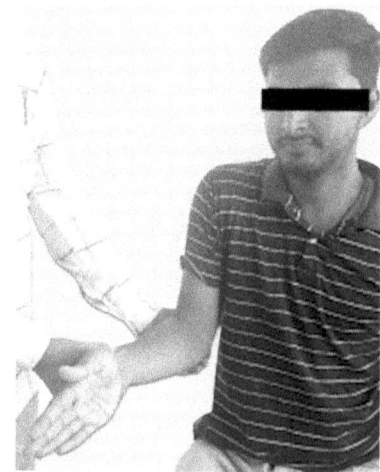

Fig. 12: Resisted lateral rotation.

- **Infraspinatus tendinitis and teres minor:**
  - **Action:** It performs lateral rotation of arm.
  - **Palpation:** It is palpated on posterior aspect of greater tubercle with slight shoulder flexion and lateral rotation.
  - **Special test: Resisted lateral rotation (Fig. 12):** Patient in sitting position with arm at side and elbow at 90° flexion. Therapist applies the force towards medial direction and the patient tries to resist movement at forearm. The test is considered to be positive if it elicits pain or weakness.
- **Subscapularis:**
  - **Action:** It performs the internal rotation of arm.
  - **Palpation:** Along inner edge of intertubercular sulcus, one inch inferior and lateral from coracoids.
  - **Special test: Lift off test/Gerber's test (Fig. 13):** Patient in standing with arm in internal rotation and hand placed behind the back in mid-lumbar region of spine. Dorsum of the hand is placed against spine. Patient attempts to raise hand off the back by extending and further internal rotating the arm at shoulder. Test is considered to be positive if patient is unable to raise hand away from back.

Soft Tissue Injuries

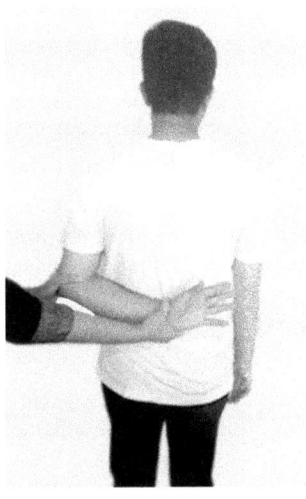

Fig. 13: Lift off test/Gerber's test.

Management

Physiotherapy Treatment Protocol

Phase I	Weeks 0–4
Precautions	Avoid provocative exercises that causes discomfort
	Patient may have an underlying coracoacromion bursitis therefore, ROM and muscle strengthening exercises should begin with arm in <90° of abduction
	Avoid abduction with rotation that create impingement maneuver
	Avoid empty can exercises
Immobilization	Sling immobilization for short period only 3–6 days
Pain control	Medications: NSAIDs
	Subacromion/intra-articular injection of corticosteroids or local anesthetic
	Therapeutic modalities: • Ice, US, HVGS • Moist heat before exercises and ice at the end of session

Contd...

Contd...

Phase I	Weeks 0–4
Shoulder movements	
Goals	Internal and external rotation equal to contralateral side with arm positioned in <90° abduction
Exercises	Begin with Codman exercises
	Passive ROM exercises: • Forward flexion and extension • Internal and external rotation • Capsular stretching for anterior, posterior and inferior capsule
	Avoid assisted motion exercises
	Progress to AROM exercises: • Finger ladder
Elbow movements	Passive to active movements • Flexion/extension 0–130° • Pronation to supination as tolerated
Muscle strengthening	Grip strengthening
	Use of arm for ADLs below shoulder level
Criteria for progression to phase II	
	Minimal pain and tenderness
	Improvement of PROM
	Return to functional ROM

Phase II	Weeks 4–8
Goals	Improve shoulder complex strength, power and endurance
Restrictions	Avoid provocative maneuvers or exercises that causes discomfort
Immobilization	Not needed
Pain control	Same as before
Shoulder movements	Equal to contralateral shoulder in all planes of movements

Contd...

Contd...

Phase II	Weeks 4–8
Exercises	Passive ROM
	Capsular stretching
	Active assisted motion exercises
	AROM exercises
Elbow movements	Passive to active movements • Flexion/extension 0–130° • Pronation and supination as tolerated
Muscle strengthening	Strengthening of remaining rotator cuff muscles
	Begin closed chain isometric strengthening • Internal and external rotation • Abduction
	Progress to open chain strengthening exercise with very low weight dumbbells • Exercises performed with elbow 90° flexion • Starting with shoulder in neutral position of 0° forward flexion, abduction and external rotation
	• Exercises done through an arc of 45° in each of 5 planes of motion
	Strengthening of deltoid

	Strengthening of scapular stabilizers
	• Closed chain exercises
	  – Scapular retraction and protraction
	  – Scapular depression and elevation
	• Progress to open chain exercises, scapular stabilizer strengthening exercises

Criteria for progression to phase III	
	Painless and complete ROM
	No pain and tenderness with strengthening exercises

Contd...

Contd...

Phase III	Weeks 8–12
Goals	Improve neuromuscular control and shoulder proprioception
	Prepare for gradual return to ADLs
	Home exercise program including strengthening and stretching exercises
Functional strengthening	Plyometric exercises
	Maximal improvement is expected by 4–6 months

Surgical Treatment

Indications

- When symptoms lasted for 6–12 months.
- When tear size is more than 3 cm
- Significant weakness and loss of shoulder function.

Surgical Interventions

Open repair or arthroscopic repair of injured structures.

Postsurgical rehabilitation protocol

Phase I	Immediate postsurgical phase (day 1–10)
Goals	Maintain integrity of the repair
	Gradually increase in PROM
	Diminish pain and inflammation
	Prevent muscular inhibition
Day 1–6	Sling or abduction brace
	Shoulder passive supine ROM • Shoulder flexion to tolerance: 0–140° • ER: 0–40°
	Scapular depression and retraction
	Active elbow/wrist/hand (E/W/H) gripping and ROM exercises
	Stretching of neck and upper quarter

Contd...

Soft Tissue Injuries

Contd...

Phase I	Immediate postsurgical phase (day 1–10)
	Cryotherapy (15–20 minutes every hour) for pain and inflammation
	Night sling or brace
Day 7–10	Continue use of sling
	Progress PROM to tolerance • Shoulder flexion to at least 140° supine • ER/IR in scapular plane to 35–45°
	Continue active E/W/H and ROM exercises
	Stretching of neck and upper quarter
	Initiate submaximal isometric exercises
	Continue use of ice for pain control
	Night brace
Precautions	Avoid lifting objects
	Avoid excessive shoulder extension
	Avoid excessive stretching exercises
	Avoid supporting of body weight by hands
	Keep incision clean and dry
Phase II	Protection phase (day 11–week 6)
Goals	Allow soft tissue healing
	Regain dynamic shoulder stability
	Decrease pain and inflammation
Day 11–14	Continue use of sling
	PROM to tolerance in supine • Shoulder flexion: 0–170° • ER/IR at least 45° in scapular plane
	Continue all isometric exercises
	Overhead pulleys

Contd...

Contd...

Phase II	Protection phase (day 11–week 6)
	Continue use of cryotherapy as needed
	Continue all precautions
Week 3–4	Patient should have full PROM
	Continue scapular stabilization exercises and initiate scapular strengthening exercises
	Initiate resisted scapular retraction
	Initiate active ER supine in scapular plane using wand to stretch at terminal range
	Initiate isotonic elbow flexion
	Initiate self-capsular stretches
	Continue use of ice as needed
	May use heat prior to ROM exercises
	Continue sling
Week 5–6	Discontinue use of sling
	May use heat prior to exercise
	Initiate AAROM and stretching exercises: • AA flexion with active extension to neutral and AA abduction with active adduction
	Initiate AROM exercises: • Shoulder flexion in scapular plane • Shoulder abduction • ER/IR side lying • Prone rowing • Prone horizontal abduction
	Biceps curls
	Start upper body ergometer below 90° elevation
Precautions	Avoid lifting heavy objects
	Avoid excessive behind the back movements
	Avoid supporting of body weight by hands and arms
	Avoid sudden jerking motions

Contd...

Contd...

Phase III	Intermediate phase (week 7-14)
Goals	Full AROM (week 8-10)
	Dynamic shoulder stability
	Gradual restoration of shoulder strength and power
	Gradual return of functional activities
Weeks 7	Continue stretching and PROM
	Continue dynamic stabilization drills
	Initiate isotonic strengthening program pain-free • ER/IR supine • Prone rowing • Prone horizontal abduction • Prone extension • Elbow flexion/extension
	Patient must be able to elevate arm without shoulder or scapular hiking before initiating isotonic, if unable, continue humeral head/scapular stabilization exercises
Week 8-13	Continue all exercise listed above
	ER side lying
	Lateral raises
	Full can in scapular plane
	Initiate light functional activities
Week 14	Continue all exercises listed above
	Progress to fundamental shoulder exercises
Phase IV	Advanced strengthening phase (week 15-22)
Goals	Maintain full nonpainful ROM
	Enhance functional use of upper limb
	Improve muscular strength and power
	Gradual return to functional activities
Week 15	Continue ROM and stretching to maintain full ROM
	Continue shoulder strengthening to fundamental shoulder exercises
	Initiate plyometrics exercises

■ FROZEN SHOULDER

Frozen shoulder is characterized by progressive pain, stiffness and limited active and passive range of motion of shoulder joint. It is also known as adhesive capsulitis (Figs. 14A and B).

Epidemiology

- Incidence appears higher in patients with diabetes and thyroid disease.
- This condition is more common in 40-60 years.
- Females are more affected than males.

Etiology

- **Primary (idiopathic) adhesive capsulitis:** Idiopathic adhesive capsulitis has no underlying etiology or cause.
- **Secondary adhesive capsulitis:** Secondary adhesive capsulitis develops from a known cause or after some traumatic or surgical events. The three major categories of the causative factors for secondary adhesive capsulitis are:
  - **Intrinsic factors:** Bicep tendinitis, rotator cuff tendinitis, rotator cuff tears, acromioclavicular arthritis, etc.
  - **Extrinsic factors:** Cardiopulmonary disease, CVA, cervical disc, humeral fracture, etc.
  - **Systemic factors:** Diabetes mellitus, hyperthyroidism, hypoadrenalism, etc.

Pathophysiology

Exact pathophysiology of adhesive capsulitis is unknown. Many authors argue that adhesive capsulitis is a chronic fibrosing condition; whereas others contend that it is inflammatory in nature. A histological study suggested that it occurs because of the proliferation of fibroblast that lay down collagen in thick bands. These bands are similar to the bands that are present in Dupuytren's disease.

However, recent studies suggests that adhesive capsulitis is both an inflammatory and a fibrosing condition. It develops as a result of

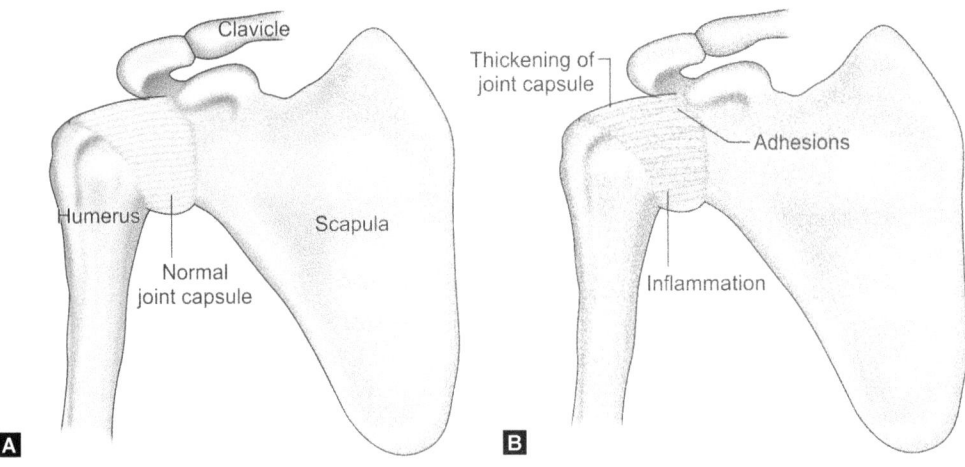

Figs. 14A and B: Normal shoulder and frozen shoulder (adhesive capsulitis).

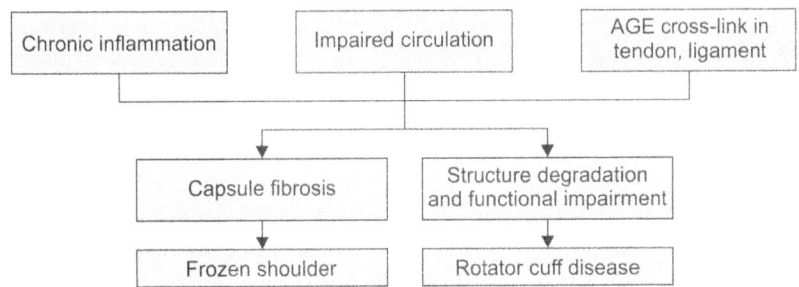

Fig. 15: Potential mechanism of frozen shoulder development related to diabetes.
(AGE: advanced glycosylation end-product)

perivascular inflammation and fibroblastic proliferation followed by capsular fibrosis and contracture.

Risk Factors

- **Diabetes mellitus:** Exact mechanism that links diabetes and adhesive capsulitis has not been identified. However, two mechanisms caused by hyperglycemia may facilitate the occurrence of frozen shoulder. First, hyperglycemia forms glycosylation products that increases the cross-linking in collagen, tendons and ligaments that makes them stiffer, weaker and progressive leads to inflammation. Secondly, hyperglycemia results in unfavorable microvascular environment around the shoulder that impairs circulation and tissue hypoxia. This collective damage may lead to joint destruction and enhancement of degenerative changes (Fig. 15).
- **Thyroid disease:** Patients have an underlying diagnosis of hyperthyroidism are at greater risk of developing adhesive capsulitis. It may be because of hyperthyroidism induced cytokines and fibroblast proliferation.
- **Prior history of adhesive capsulitis:** Patients having a prior history are at major risk of disease in contralateral shoulder.
- **Shoulder pain and immobization:** Patient having history of trauma or prolonged periods of shoulder immobilization often develop adhesive capsulitis.

- **Previous shoulder surgery:** Especially shoulder repair procedure (rotator cuff, fracture fixation, instability repairs) are associated with postoperative stiffness.
- **Females:** Women are twice as likely to develop adhesive capsulitis as men.

Clinical Presentation

It occurs in 3 stages:
1. **Freezing phase/painful stage:** Last for 3–6 months.
   - Characterized by shooting pain in shoulder that radiates down the arm.
   - Pain aggravates with activity.
   - Night pain is more pronounced.
2. **Frozen phase/adhesive stage:** Last for 3–18 months.
   - Characterized by progressive stiffness.
   - During this stage pain gradually decreases.
   - Restricted shoulder ROM in all planes.
   - Night pain progressively decreases.
   - ADLs become severely restricted.
3. **Thawing/resolution/recovery phase:** Last for 3–6 months.
   - Characterized by slow recovery of motion.
   - Pain gradually diminished.

Diagnosis

- **X-ray:** Finding is absolutely normal but it can be used to exclude other possible conditions. Abnormal findings need to be investigated further to eliminate other shoulder pathologies, such as dislocations of the shoulder, particularly locked posterior dislocations.
- **Arthrography (Figs. 16A and B):** Demonstrate marked contracture of joint capsule and obliteration of axillary fold. About 50% reduction in joint fluid volume. It remains only 5–10 mL (normal joint fluid volume is 20–30 mL).
- **MRI** to rule out any anatomical deviations or soft tissue injuries. It shows absence of axillary recess, tight and thickened capsule (Figs. 17A and B).

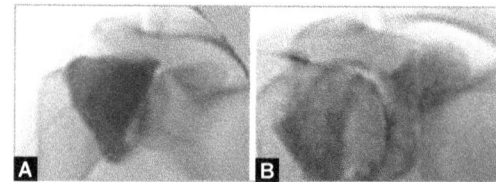

Figs. 16A and B: Arthrography. A. Normal shoulder; B. Frozen shoulder.

Examination

Patient History

Risk factors: These are strongly related with the occurrence of adhesive capsulitis include a history of trauma or surgery to affected shoulder, age: 40–60 years, past history of adhesive capsulitis and underlying diabetes mellitus.

- **Site of pain:** Lateral and anterior aspect of shoulder radiating down the arm.
- **Nature of pain:** Persistent dull aching pain that aggravates with activities. Patient often complain disturbed sleep due to increased night pain especially while rolling on to the affected shoulder.
- **Progressive loss of shoulder movement.**
- **Common complaints are:**
  - Difficulty in combing hair
  - Difficulty in reaching the back pocket of pants
  - Difficulty in fastening of hook of bra
  - Difficulty in scratching back

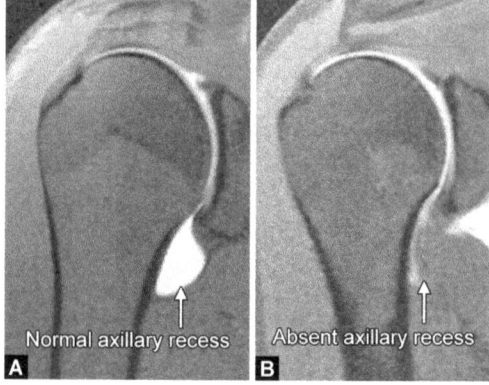

Figs. 17A and B: MRI. A. Normal shoulder; B. Frozen shoulder.

- Pain with lying on affected shoulder
- Inability to do overhead activities.

Physical Examination
- **Hallmark sign:** Global loss of active and passive range of motion of affected shoulder.
- **Limitation of PROM shows a capsular pattern**, i.e. substantial restriction of external rotation (ER) than abduction and then internal rotation (IR).
- **Empty end feel:** Present at the end ROM of shoulder joint.
- **Positive coracoid pain test:** In this test, pain is elicited by applying direct pressure on coracoid process. Many recent studies considered it to be a highly sensitive and specific clinical examination finding for adhesive capsulitis.

Management

It is "self-limiting" process.

Conservative Treatment
- **Activity modification:** Patients should avoid exacerbating activities in order to interfere with the cycle of ongoing inflammation. This may necessitate significant time off work or away from activities.
- **Oral analgesics:** NSAIDs and salicylates are used to decrease pain and inflammation in the initial phases.
- **Oral steroids:** To decrease pain and inflammation if not responding to NSAIDs.
- **Intra-articular steroid injection:** Followed by local analgesics and gentle active movement in freezing stage is also a preferred treatment.

Physiotherapy Treatment
- **To control pain:** Therapeutic modalities
  - **Ultrasound:** It decrease pain, inflammation and maintain elasticity of tissue.
  - **Moist heat/SWD:** Before mobilization, heating modalities helps to relax and supple the thick and contracted capsule.
  - **TENS/IFT/HVGPS:** Helps to reduce pain and muscle spasm.
- **To restore ROM:**
  - **ROM exercise:** ROM exercises should gradually increase from AROM to AAROM to PROM exercise of all shoulder movements especially external rotation, abduction and forward flexion.
  - **Capsular stretching:** Anterior, posterior and inferior capsular stretching. It helps to improve normal extensibility of shoulder capsule and stretch tight soft tissue and contracted para-articular structures.
  - **Joint mobilization:** It decreases pain due to neurophysiologic effects on the stimulation of peripheral mechanoreceptors and inhibition of nociceptors, it break up the adhesions and realign collagen, facilitatory effect on blood and synovial fluid circulation which reduce edema, inflammation and fibrosis. In initial painful stage, slow, gentle oscillatory movements should be given to avoid the induction of pain and muscle spasm.
  - **Active exercise program includes (Fig. 18):**
    - **Codman's pendular exercises:** This technique uses the effect of gravity to distract joint. It helps to relieve pain through traction and oscillation and provide the movement of synovial fluid. Codman's pendular exercises are performed in a forward bending position, with one hand resting on table for support and swing the other arm like a pendulum.
    - **Shoulder elevation exercises:** Patient perform shoulder elevation with the assistance of unaffected hand.
    - **Wand exercises:** Patient perform flexion and extension of shoulder by

14 Simplified Approach to Orthopedic Physiotherapy

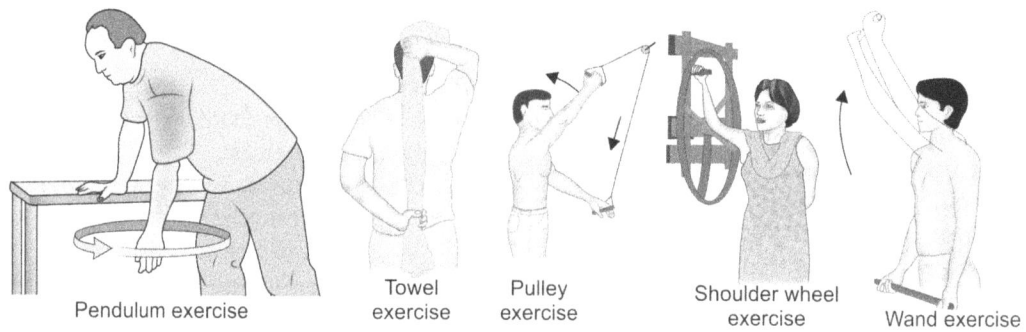

Fig. 18: Active shoulder exercises.

holding either end of wand by each hand.
- **Shoulder wheel exercises:** Patient perform active flexion and extension of shoulder by using shoulder wheel.
- **Pulley exercises:** By using pulley patient perform active shoulder movements.

- **To improve the strength and endurance of rotator cuff and scapular stabilizers in late stages:**
  - Closed kinematic chain exercises
  - Open kinematic chain exercises
  - Strengthening of scapular stabilizers
  - Deltoid strengthening.

Manipulation under anesthesia: Closed manipulation of shoulder under general anesthesia is given to break adhesive and fibrotic tissues to regain complete ROM. Significant improvement is seen in around 70% of patients. Although early manipulation is found to be more effective than manipulation given later in the disease course.

Indications
When patient failed to gain ROM after every possible conservative treatment.

Complications
- Traction nerve injuries
- Fracture dislocation
- Shoulder dislocation

- Rotator cuff ruptures
- Proximal humeral fractures.

Surgical Treatment
Indicated when patient fails to recover even after 4 months of conservative treatment.

Surgical Interventions
Arthroscopic lysis/release or open release: In surgery, adhesions, scar tissues and other possible structure that may be interfering with shoulder movement are removed.

■ SUBACROMIAL BURSITIS

It is a condition caused by inflammation of subacromial bursa. Subacromial bursa is present between supraspinatus tendon and coracoacromial ligament, acromial and coracoid process (Fig. 19).

Function of subacromial bursa: The bursa acts as a cushion and reduces friction

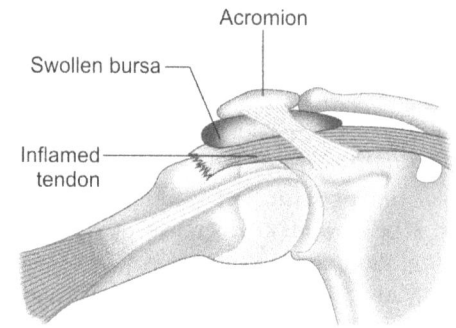

Fig. 19: Subacromial bursitis.

between supraspinatus tendon and overlying structures that helps to provide smooth motion of supraspinatus tendon.

Etiology

Following are the causative factors of sub-acromial bursitis:
- Muscle weakness of upper limb
- Calcium deposition
- Crystal deposition disorder as in gout
- Supraspinatus tendonitis
- Rotator cuff injury
- Glenohumeral instability
- Degeneration of AC joint

Predisposing Factors

- Acute trauma or overuse injury to shoulder
- Repeated overhead lifting/activity
- Repeated vigorous pulling.

Clinical Presentation (Fig. 20)

- Pain along the front and lateral side of shoulder.
- Burning or intermittent dull aching pain.
- Localized tenderness, located in anterior and superior aspect of upper third of arm.
- Nocturnal pain especially while sleeping on affected side.
- Weakness and stiffness of shoulder.
- Loss of active movements at shoulder joint.
- Restricted passive abduction of arm.

Diagnosis

- **Imaging Studies:**
  - **X-rays:** To rule out the presence of any other causative factor for pain, such as presence of any bony spur, shape of acromion, arthritis of AC joint and calcific deposits in adjacent areas.
  - **MRI:** Might be helpful to demonstrate the extension of fluid filled sac but that may not be represents the presence of bursitis as it may also be present in case of rotator cuff injury and many other pathologies.
  - **Impingement test:** In this test, some anesthetic (lidocaine) is injected adjacent to the subacromion bursa. If symptoms improve then the test is considered to be positive for subacromion bursitis.

Physical Examination

- **On Palpation (Fig. 21):**
  - Tenderness and warmth of skin that covers subacromion bursa, i.e. about 1 cm under posterior border of acromion process, just medial to posterior corner.
  - Painful "catch" at midrange when lowering from full abduction.
  - Resisted abduction is painful due to the compression of bursa under contracted deltoid muscle.

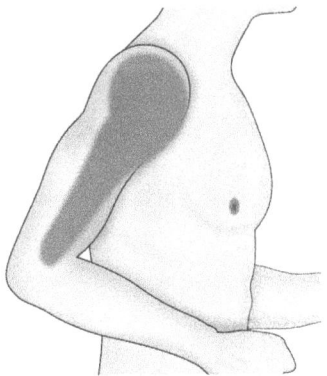

Fig. 20: Subacromion bursitis pain pattern.

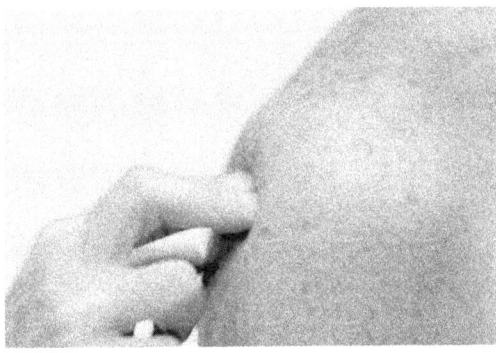

Fig. 21: Palpating subacromial space.

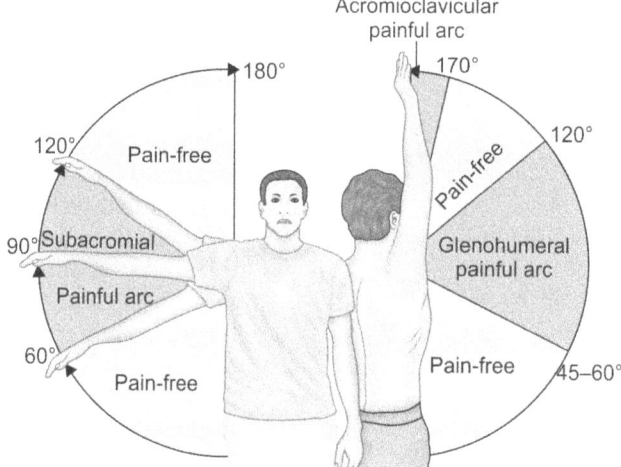

Fig. 22: Painful arc sign.

Special Test

- **Painful arc sign (Fig. 22):** Active arm abduction produce painful arc between 60–120° due to impingement of supraspinatus tendon or subacromial bursa between arch of acromion and head of humerus.
- **Speed's test (Fig. 23):** Patient performs an isometric flexion contraction against resistance of examiner. When the examiner's resistance is removed, a sudden jerking motion results and latent pain indicates a positive test for bursitis.
- **Neer's test (Fig. 24):** Therapist passively abducts arm completely with external rotation and then repeats the same movement with internal rotation. If pain produces with internal rotation, then it is indicative of supraspinatus tendinitis but is also sensitive for subacromial bursitis.

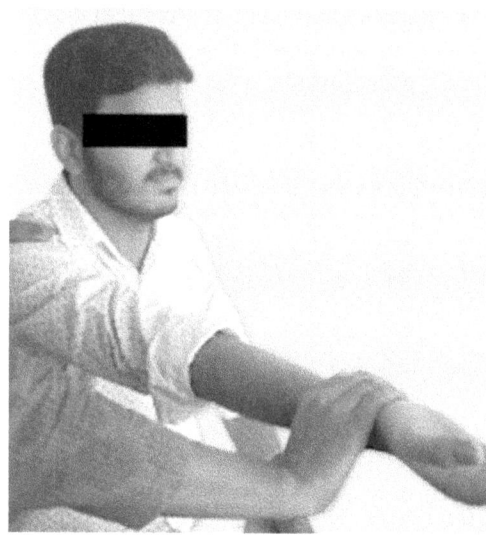

Fig. 23: Speed test.

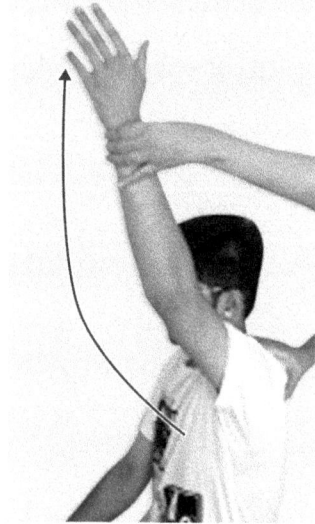

Fig. 24: Neer's test.

Soft Tissue Injuries

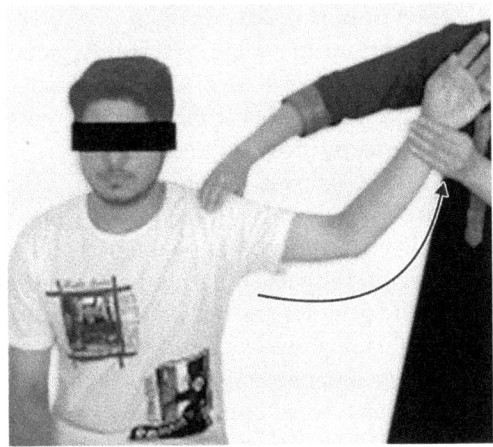

Fig. 25: Dawbarn's sign test.

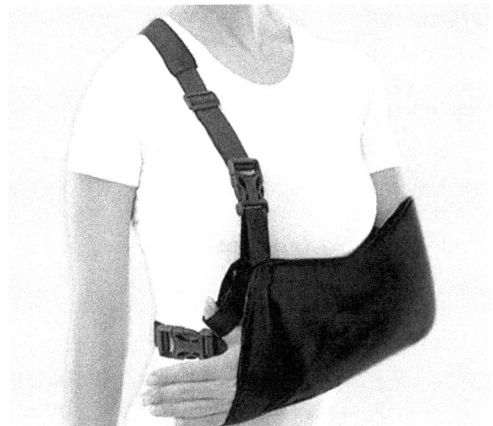

Fig. 26: Immobilizing arm in sling.

- **Dawbarn's sign test (Fig. 25):** Patient in seating position, examiner palpates anterior to acromion and passively abducts arm. When positive pain on palpation pain disappears with increasing abduction this addresses subacromion bursitis.

Management
Conservative Treatment
- **To relieve acute pain:**
  - Cryotherapy: To decrease associated pain and inflammation.
  - Relative rest by immobilizing arm in sling (Fig. 26).
- **Oral medication:** Nonsteroidal anti-inflammatory drugs help to reduce pain and inflammation.
- **Intrabursal steroid injection:** Steroid injection helps to reduce pain and inflammation when the patient is not responding to anti-inflammatory drug.

Physiotherapy Treatment
- **Rest:** Rest should be given to affected area and painful activities should be avoided as these can delay healing process.
- **Glenohumeral joint mobilization:** Joint mobilization has neurophysiological effect that helps in reducing pain and improving synovial fluid flow that aid in healing process.
- **Soft tissue massage:** Massage helps to lengthen tight muscle and reduces associated muscle spasm.
- **Proprioceptive neuromuscular facilitation (PNF):** It helps to facilitate motor control and improve the ROM of shoulder joint.
- **Therapeutic exercise:**
  - **Gentle pendulum ROM exercises:** For the prevention of adhesive capsulitis.
  - **Scapular exercises:** To improve muscular control and scapular coordination.
  - **Rotator cuff strengthening exercises:** To improve stability of shoulder.
- **Stretching exercises:** Stretching of pectoralis major, subscapularis, levator scapula, upper trapezius and pectoralis major.
- **Electrotherapeutic modalities:**
  - **Ice:** To decrease pain and inflammation.
  - **Ultrasound:** To accelerate the healing process.
- **Proprioception exercises:** These exercises improve proprioception that has a crucial role in reducing the chances of reinjury.

Surgical Treatment
Surgery is indicated when the pathology do not responds to conservative treatment and gradually impairs functional ability of patient.

Surgical Interventions

- **Bursectomy:** In this surgery affected bursa is removed either by open surgery or arthroscopic bursectomy surgery.
- **Tendon and muscle repair:** Surgical repair of damaged muscle or tendon is performed when subacromion bursitis occurs due to injury of rotator cuff muscle or tendon.
- **Subacromial decompression:** It is also known as acromioplasty. In this surgery a part of acromion is removed to generate more space for soft tissues and reduce the chances of their impingement under acromion arch. It is commonly done with bursectomy.

ELBOW INJURIES

■ TENNIS ELBOW

Also known as lateral epicondylitis, Hooter's elbow or Archer's elbow (Fig. 27).

It is a pathological condition of wrist extensor muscle at their origin on lateral epicondyle of humerus. Extensor carpi radialis brevis (ECRB) is the key muscle that is affected.

Etiology

- **Overuse or repetitive trauma of forearm muscles:** Repeated actions, such as wringing clothes or twisting movements (using screw driver), etc.
- **Direct impact** or fall on elbow.
- **Occupation:** That requires repetitive activities and extensive use of forearm muscles, e.g. plumbers, blacksmiths carpenters, autoworkers, cook, painters, etc.
- **In racket sports:** Repetitive poor hand stroke, using racket that is too tightly strung or too short, hitting the ball off the center on the racket, hitting heavy or wet ball and gripping the racket too tightly. All these factors puts a lot of stress on forearm muscles and tendons and causes their progressive wear and tear. It commonly occurs in tennis players therefore the condition is also known as "tennis elbow".

Clinical Presentation

- Pain and tenderness on lateral aspect of elbow that may also radiate into upper and lower arm (Fig. 28).
- Pain aggravates on lifting, make a fist or grip an object, twisting forearm, open a door, shake hand, raise the hand or straighten the wrist.
- Pain usually last for between 6–12 weeks.
- Pain and stiffness on full extension of forearm.

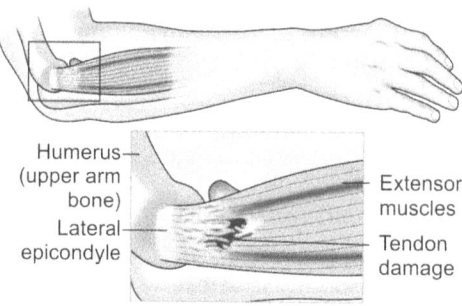

Fig. 27: Tennis elbow.

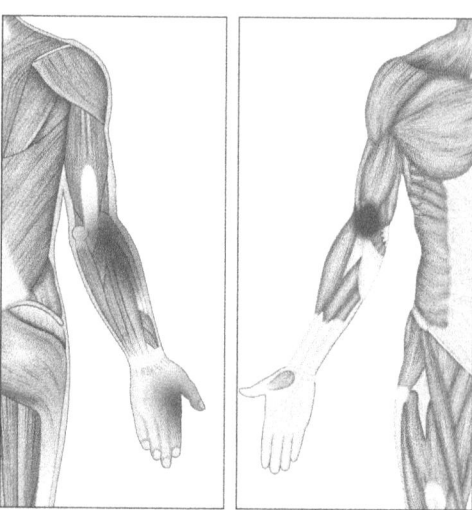

Fig. 28: Tennis elbow pain pattern.

Soft Tissue Injuries

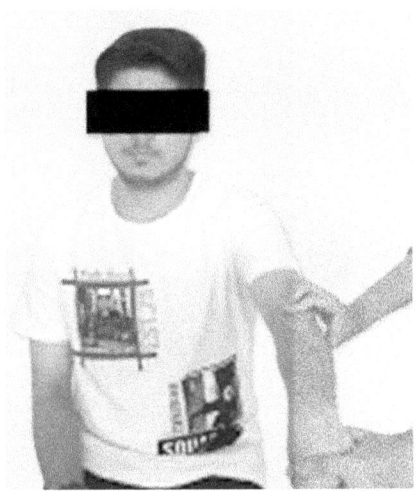

Fig. 29: Mill's test.

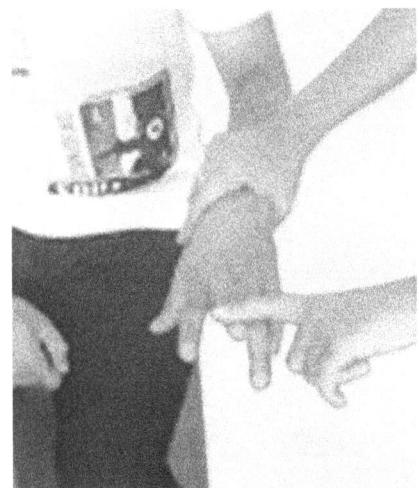

Fig. 30: Maudsley's test.

Diagnosis
- **Imaging studies:**
  - **X-ray:** X-ray findings help to rule out other pathology. It also assist to find out the possible causes that may predispose the condition like calcium deposits on lateral epicondyle or degenerative changes in elbow joint.
  - **MRI or ultrasound:** Shows the degree of tendon damage and to diagnose any other soft tissue injury or any other pathology near elbow.

Physical Examination
- **Observation:** Presence of mild swelling and ecchymosis near lateral epicondyle or over dorsal forearm.
- **Palpation:**
  - Tenderness: Point tenderness is present near, i.e. anterior and distal to lateral epicondyle of humerus (bony attachment of common extensor tendon) and tenderness over muscle of dorsal forearm may also be present.
  - Pain increases by wrist extension against resistance with forearm pronation.
  - Elbow extension may be limited.

- **Mill's test (Fig. 29):** Therapist palpates lateral condyle with one hand and passively pronates forearm, flexes wrist and extend elbow with other hand. Test is considered to be positive if it elicits pain.
- **Maudsley's test (Fig. 30):** Therapist resists extension of middle finger. Test is considered to be positive if it elicits pain over lateral epicondyle.
- **Cozen's test (Fig. 31):** Therapist stabilize elbow and palpate lateral epicondyle with one hand and ask patient to make fist, pronate forearm, radially deviate and extend the wrist. With other hand therapist applies a resistance on patient hand against wrist extension. The test is considered to be positive if it elicits pain over lateral epicondyle.

Management
Conservative Treatment
- **Activity restriction:** Elimination of painful activities, e.g. repetitive pronation/supination and lifting heavy weight.
  - Avoidance of grasping in pronation.
  - Lifting should be done with forearm in supination and with both upper extremity.

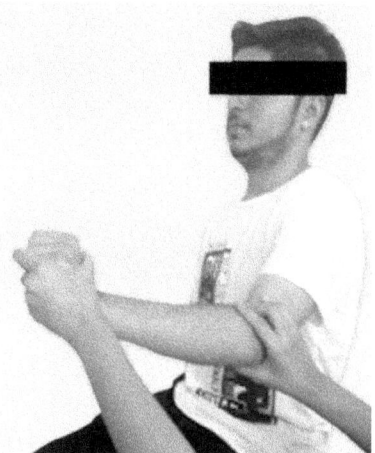

Fig. 31: Cozen's test.

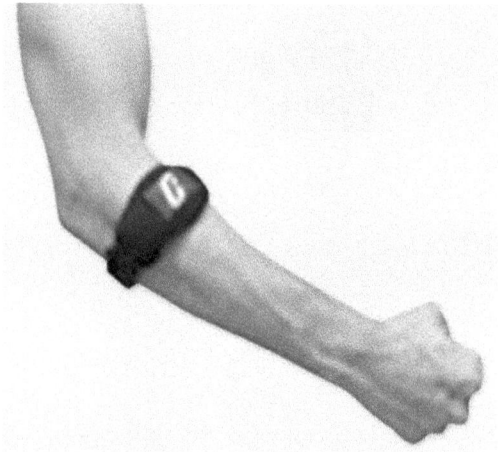

Fig. 32: Elbow brace for tennis elbow.

- **Correction of mechanics:**
  - Racket players should avoid too tight grip and poor back hand stroke.
  - While typing, support the forearm by placing elbow on stacked towel to avoid pain.
- **Analgesics and NSAIDs** are used to decrease pain and inflammation.
- **Counterforce bracing (Fig. 32):**
  - Elbow bracing is used only during aggravating activity.
  - It provides support and protection.
  - It minimizes the undue stress on forearm muscles and tendons.
  - It is 5–6 cm wide and should be worn 2 fingerbreadths distal to painful area of lateral epicondyle.
  - **Side effect:** Prolonged use of brace could lead to weakening of tendon and can actually worsen the problem.
- **Wrist splint:** Wrist in 45° dorsiflexion for 6 to 8 weeks.
  - It may ease pain by helping to rest muscles that pull on elbow.
- **Glyceryl trinitrate:** A patch applied over painful area opens up blood vessels and improves outcomes in initial 6 months. It is of 5 mm width and should be change in every 24 hours. Sometimes these patches cause headache as their side effect.
- **Autologous blood injection:** Platelet rich plasma is injected in the affected area that helps to heal the involved tendon.
- **Cortisone injection:** These are used to decrease pain and inflammation. 3 injections in a year and after every 3 months to avoid possible tendon rupture. It is used when patient is not responding to other conservative treatment.

Physiotherapy Treatment

For short-term, i.e. within first 6 weeks steroid injections are good in relieving pain but for long-term relief, physiotherapy has best results.

- **Cryotherapy:** It helps to reduce pain and inflammation. It is applied for 10–15 minutes, 4–6 times daily.
- **Therapeutic modalities:** To reduce pain and inflammation and to accelerate healing process. Modalities, such as LASER therapy, ultrasound, phonophoresis, iontophoresis, whirlpool, HVGS, shock wave therapy can be used.
- **Soft tissue massage (deep friction massage and kneading):** It is given over affected area and should be applied

Soft Tissue Injuries

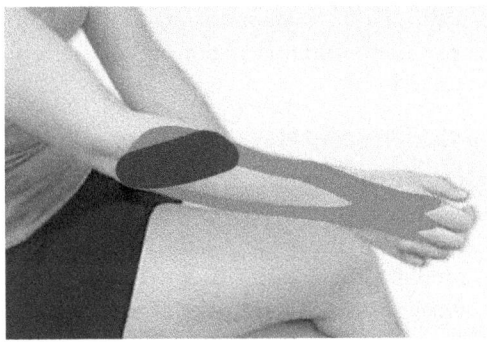

Fig. 33: Taping in tennis elbow.

transverse to the direction of fibers. Friction massage aids in regeneration of connective tissue and prevents adhesion formation and ruptures the unwanted adhesions. It is also known to decrease pain after few minutes of application.

- **Tennis elbow taping (Fig. 33):** Taping helps to avoid or minimize undue stress on forearm extensors and to support elbow during activity.
- **ROM exercises:** Along with ROM exercise emphasization should be given on end range and passive stretching to maintain mobility of joint.
- **Stretching exercises (Fig. 34A):** Passive stretch of forearm extensors is given with wrist in flexion, ulnar deviation (UD) and elbow in complete extension.
- **Strengthening exercises (Fig. 34B):** Gentle progressive resistance exercises for strengthening of grip, wrist flexors and extensors, forearm supinators and pronators biceps, triceps and rotator cuff.
- **Ball squeeze:** Squeeze ball for 3 seconds then relax.
- **Forearm supination and pronation:** Holding small dumbbell in the hand of affected arm.
- **Hammer biceps curl:** Stand with your feet kept apart. Hold a light dumbbell in the hand of affected elbow. Keep the arm closer to the body with fingers turning inward. Bend elbow until arm is at 90° angle.
- **Darts:** Lie on stomach with arm at the sides and palm facing down. Squeeze the shoulder blades together and slowly lift the arm and chest off the ground.
- **Joint mobilization:** Mobilization helps to relax tense muscles, break up scar tissues and reduce fluid buildup in tissue.

Surgical Treatment

Indications
When symptoms do not resolve with nonsurgical treatment.

Surgical Interventions
- **Tendon debridement surgery:** In tendon debridement, unhealthy muscle is removed and healthy muscle is again reconnected to bone.
- **Tendon release:** Lateral epicondyle release. In this surgery, extensor tendon of forearm is separated from its attachment at lateral epicondyle. Surgeon splits the tendon and removes the adhesions, scar tissue or any bone spur if may present then the tendon is sutured again to near by soft tissue.

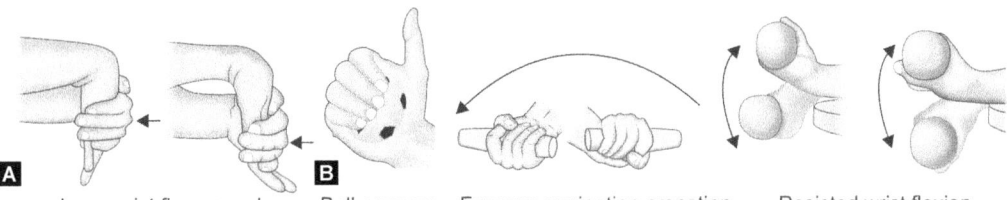

A. Long wrist flexors and extensors stretch B. Ball squeeze Forearm supination pronation Resisted wrist flexion and extension

Figs. 34A and B: A. Stretching exercises; B. Strengthening exercises.

GOLFER'S ELBOW

It is chronic inflammation of flexors muscles of forearm as a result of repetitive or unusual stress. It is also known as medial epicondylitis, suitcase elbow, baseball elbow and forehand tennis elbow (Fig. 35).

Etiology

- **Muscle weakness:** Muscle weakness of hand and forearm muscles.
- **Activities:** Throwing, chopping wood with an axe, using many hand tools.
- **Overuse:** Playing or working excessively with repetitive movement at wrist.
- **Improper equipments:** Using inappropriate tools having incorrect weight and grip size.
- **Poor playing techniques (Fig. 36):** Such as excessive wrist movement, bumpy strokes, etc.
- **Repetitive stress or overuse of forearm flexor pronator musculature:** Chronic repetitive concentric and eccentric contraction of flexor pronator group of forearm leads to degenerative changes in musculotendinous region of medial epicondyle.

Clinical Presentation (Fig. 37)

- Pain and tenderness on inner side of elbow.
- Pain may radiate down the forearm from medial epicondyle.
- Weakness in hand or wrist of affected arm.
- Numbness or tingling sensation in 4th and 5th fingers.
- Pain on gripping or twisting things.
- Pain on wrist flexion.

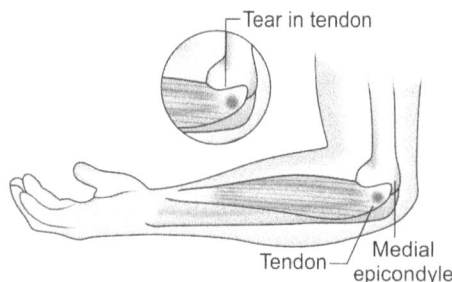

Fig. 35: Golfer's elbow.

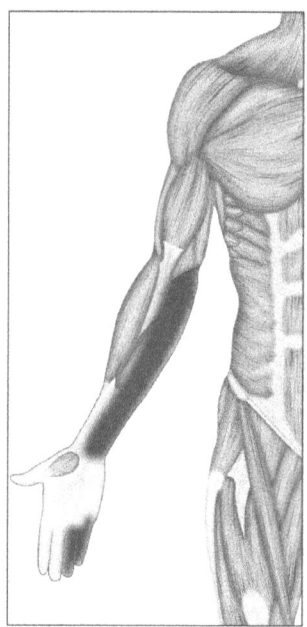

Fig. 37: Golfer's elbow pain pattern.

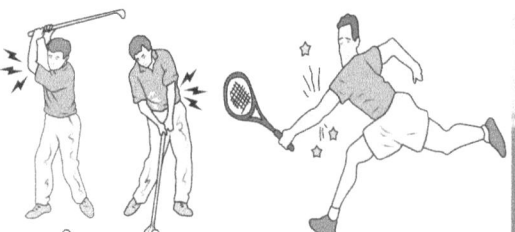

Fig. 36: Poor playing techniques.

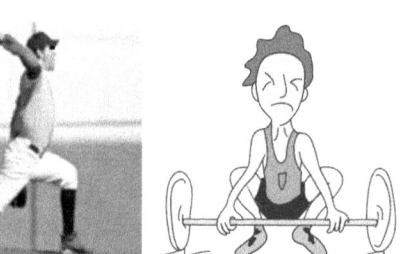

Soft Tissue Injuries

Diagnosis
- **Imaging studies:**
  - **X-ray:** The X-ray findings help to rule out other possible pathology. It also assist to find out the possible causes that may predispose the condition like calcium deposits on medial epicondyle or degenerative changes in elbow joint
  - **MRI or ultrasound:** To find out the location of tendon injury and diagnose the presence of any other soft tissue injury or any other pathology near elbow.

Physical Examination
- **Observation:** Presence of local swelling and warmth.
- **Palpation:**
  - Tenderness over medial aspect of elbow.
  - Gradual limitation of ROM that gradually leads to flexion contracture.
  - Pain increases by wrist flexion against resistance with forearm pronation.
  - Pain with passive stretching of wrist flexors.
- **Special test:**
  - **Golfer's elbow test (Fig. 38):** Examiner supports and palpates medial epicondyle elbow with one hand and supinates forearm and extends the wrist and elbow with other hand. Reproduction of pain around medial epicondyle shows the presence of medial epicondylitis.
  - **Reverse Cozen's test (Fig. 39):** Patient seated with elbow kept at 120° of flexion, forearm supinated with wrist slightly flexed towards the ulna. Examiner puts pressure on the palm using one hand. He stabilizes the elbow and palpates medial epicondyle using his other hand. The test is considered positive if pain is reproduced in the area of medial epicondyle.
  - **Resisted forearm pronation and wrist flexion (Fig. 40):** Therapist palpates on the medial epicondyle of patient and ask the patient to perform wrist flexion and forearm pronation against resistance. Reproduction of pain around medial epicondyle indicates the presence of medial epicondylitis.

Management
Conservative Treatment
- **Ice:** Icing is given for reducing pain and inflammation.

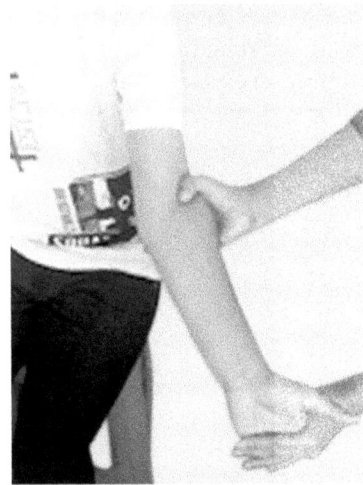

Fig. 38: Golfer's elbow test.

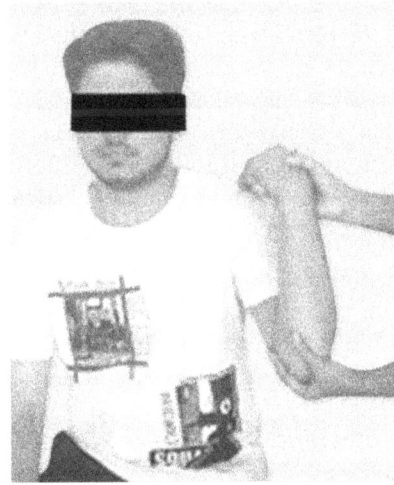

Fig. 39: Reverse Cozen's test.

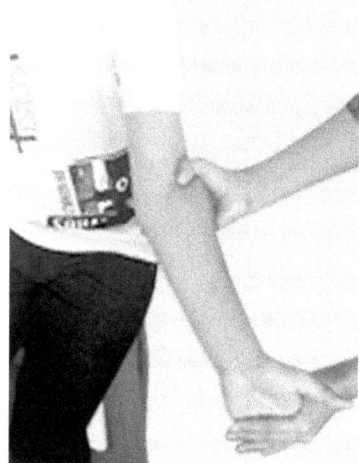

Fig. 40: Reverse Mill's test.

- **NSAIDs:** Helps to reduce pain and inflammation.
- **Stretching exercises**: Stretching of involved forearm flexors muscles is given for reducing strain on inflamed tendons.
- **Counterforce bracing (Fig. 41):** Bracing should be worn 1 to 2 inch below the elbow.
  - Elbow bracing is used only during aggravating activity.
  - It provides support and protection.
  - Reduces strain from elbow tendon.
- **Platelet rich plasma (PRP):** "Blood spinning" therapy heals the tendon by injecting the platelet rich plasma in the affected area.
- **Cortisone injections:** In severe cases, when the patient is not responding to other conservative therapies. Cortisone injection is recommended to reduce pain and inflammation.

Physiotherapy Treatment

For short-term effect, i.e. within first 6 weeks steroid injections are good in relieving pain but for long-term relief physiotherapy has best results.
- **Cryotherapy:** Cryo application for 10–15 minutes, 4–6 times per day to reduce pain and inflammation.

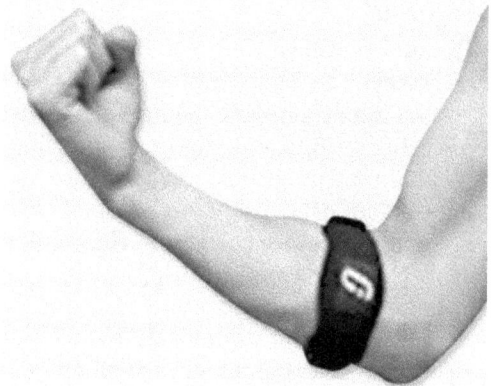

Fig. 41: Elbow brace for golfer's elbow.

- **Therapeutic modalities:** Modalities such as laser therapy, ultrasound, phonophoresis, iontophoresis, whirlpool, HVGS, shock wave therapy have an integral role in reducing pain and inflammation and accelerating the healing process.
- **Soft tissue massage (deep friction massage and kneading):** Massage helps to reduce the pain and to prevent adhesion formation. It also breaks unwanted adhesions and improves connective tissue regeneration.
- **Taping (Fig. 42):** Taping helps to avoid or minimize undue stress on forearm flexors and to support elbow during activity.
- **Range of motion (ROM) exercises:** During ROM exercises emphasization should be given on end range and passive stretching.
- **Stretching exercises:** Stretching of wrist extensor and flexors muscles.

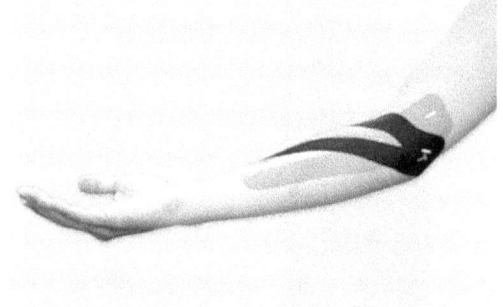

Fig. 42: Taping for golfer's elbow.

- **Neural stretch:** A neural stretch of ulnar nerve may be beneficial to release trapped nerve in scar tissue as it runs very close to medial epicondyle.
- **Strengthening exercises:** Exercises should be initiated as soon as pain allows:
  - **Isometric wrist flexion:** Initiate with isometric exercises. Exercises should be pain-free and repeated twice a day.
  - **Dynamic exercises:** Gradually progress to isotonic exercises initially without resistance and gradually progress to resistance exercises using a light weight of about 1 kg or a resistance band.
  - **Wrist extension:** Should be performed with palm facing down to ensure that these are pain-free.
  - Gentle PRE for grip strength, forearm supinators, pronators, biceps, triceps and rotator cuff strengthening.

Surgical Treatment

Indications
- When symptoms do not resolve with non-surgical treatment.
- Rarely required to correct chronic or recurrent tendinitis.

Surgical Interventions
- **Tendon debridement surgery:** In tendon debridement technique, diseased muscle is removed and reattaches the healthy muscle back to bone.
- **Medial epicondylectomy and ulnar nerve release:** Medial epicondyle is resected to remove pressure on the compressed ulnar nerve. It helps in smooth gliding of nerve during elbow movements.
- **Medial epicondyle release:** Goal of surgery is to take off the tension from flexor tendon. Surgeon splits flexor tendon from its attachment at medial epicondyle and removes any scar tissue or bony spur if present. In certain surgery the distal free end of flexor tendon is stapled with adjacent fascial tissue.

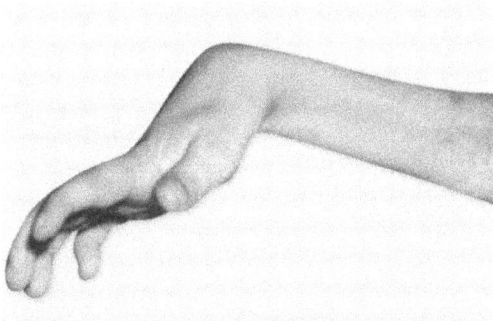

Fig. 43: Volkmann's ischemic contracture.

■ VOLKMANN'S ISCHEMIC CONTRACTURE

Volkmann's ischemic contracture (VIC) refers to the permanent shortening and fibrosis of forearm muscles following any forearm injury causing claw like deformity of wrist and hand (Fig. 43).

Etiology

Compartment syndrome refers to the condition where blood flow is compromised in a concised compartment due to elevation of pressure inside the compartment that further leads to necrosis of soft tissue, such as nerves, muscles or skin. The pressure inside the compartment increases because of uncontrolled swelling. VIC occurs as a consequence of inappropriate treatment of compartment syndrome where necrosed soft tissues gradually changes into fibrosed tissues.

Predisposing Factors

- Crush injuries, fracture or any trauma of upper extremity
- Prolonged external compression, e.g. by poor fitted splint or plaster cast
- Bleeding disorders, e.g. hemophilia
- Animal bites
- Injection of medicines in forearm
- Abrupt extensive exercises.

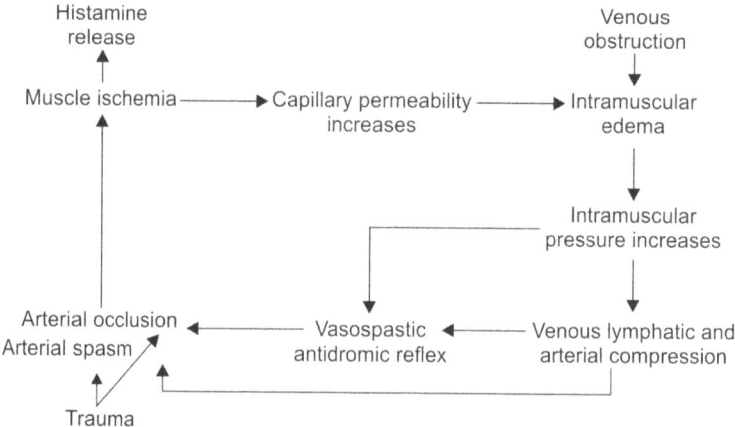

Fig. 44: Ischemia-edema cycle in Volkmann ischemic contracture given by Eaton and Green.

Pathophysiology (Fig. 44)

Condition that reduce the size of compartment (like direct trauma, crush injury, etc.) or increase in compartment pressure (like edema, internal bleeding, etc.) can cause compartment syndrome. With increase in intracompartment pressure, blood flow of area is compromised that affect the viability of tissues. When interstial pressure overrides the intravascular pressure of capillaries, walls of capillaries collapses and blood flow to the area is completely obstructed. This results in necrosis of soft tissues present in the compartment. This local tissue necrosis further leads to local edema which in turn further elevates the intracompartmental pressure. Different types of tissues have different tolerance to prolonged ischemia. Nerve tissue have less tolerance to ischemia and found to have abnormal function after 30 minutes and complete functional loss after 12–24 hours whereas muscle tissue shows functional impairment after 2–4 hours and complete functional loss after 4–12 hours.

Classification

Mild VIC (Fig. 45)
- Involves superficial volar group of muscles.
- Flexion contracture of 2–3 fingers due to partial ischemia of muscles.
- Minimal sensory changes.
- Intrinsic muscles are not affected.

Moderate VIC (Fig. 46)
- Deep flexors muscles and intrinsic muscles are affected.

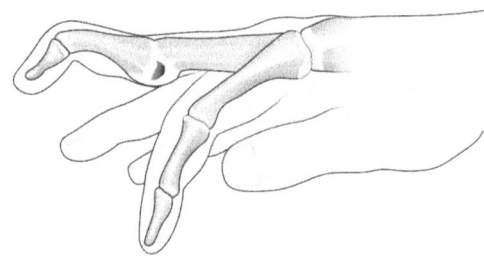

Fig. 45: Mild VIC.

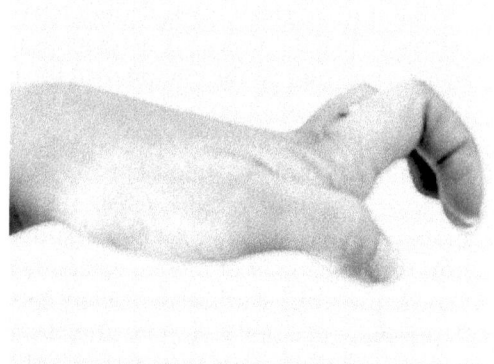

Fig. 46: Moderate VIC.

Soft Tissue Injuries

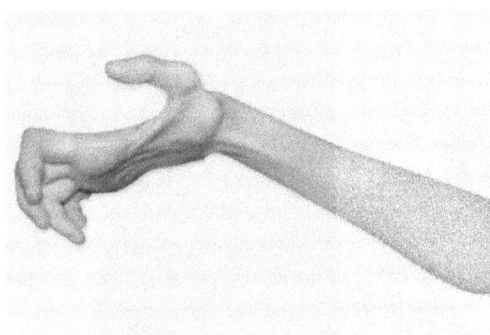

Fig. 47: Severe VIC.

- Median and ulnar nerve are involved.
- Severe flexion deformity and contracture of fingers and thumb.

Severe VIC (Fig. 47)
- Flexor and extensor forearm muscles are affected.
- Impaired sensory and motor feedback.
- Severe deformity and wasting of hand and forearm.
- Severely dry and wrinkled skin with ulceration.

Clinical Presentation
- If local compression is the cause, then 5 Ps:
  - **Pain:** Stretch pain
  - Pink color
  - Pulse intact (good capillary refilling)
  - Paresthesia (commonly in median nerve zone)
  - Paresis.
- If arterial injury is the cause, then 5 Ps
  - **Pain:** Stretch pain
  - Pallor (cyanosis)
  - Pulselessness
  - Paresthesia
  - Paralysis.

Diagnosis
Measurement of intracompartmental pressure (ICP) using Wick or slit catheter technique, simple needle manometer system, infusion techniques, pressure transducers or a hand-held manometer (e.g. stryker device). Surgical intervention is necessary if ICP is greater than 30 mm Hg.

Physical Examination
- **Observation:**
  - Forearm may be swollen and shiny.
  - Paleness of skin.
- **Palpation:**
  - **Early sign:** Altered skin sensation.
  - Pain on passive movements of fingers.
  - Pain is disproportionate to injury.
  - **Late sign:** Tenderness caused by edema.
  - Absence of capillary refill in nail bed.
  - Tissue firmness.

Management
Immediate Measures
- Removal of tight occlusive dressing
- Split plaster cast
- Elevation of limb
- Analgesics
- Emergency fasciotomy to prevent progression of Volkmann's contracture.

Treatment after the occurrence of contracture is determined by the severity of contracture:
- **Mild VIC:** Managed with physiotherapy, dynamic splinting and surgical procedures, such as tendon lengthening and tendon slide.
- **Moderate VIC:** Managed with surgical procedure like neurolysis of median and ulnar nerve, tendon transfer of extensors and tendon slide.
- **Severe VIC:** Managed with debridement surgeries, partial or radical along with scar tissue release and salvaging techniques.

Physiotherapy Treatment in Mild Type of VIC
Goals
- To maintain PROM
- To maintain and improve strength of available muscles
- To correct deformity
- Sensory reeducation
- Muscle reeducation.

Treatment

In early stage: After the relief of intrinsic pressure, no time should be lost in gradual extension of involved muscles.
- **To maintain ROM and to reduce edema:** Heat, massage, active ROM of uninvolved joints, stretching of involved joints till pain eviction.

Treatment when deformity has been present for days or weeks:
- Heat and massage helps to maintain ROM and to reduce edema if present.
- Gradual and continued stretching of contracted tissues in acute conditions which lasts for about week.
- According to Sir Robert Jones method (Fig. 48):
  - Initially wrist is passively flexed to allow the fingers to extend by means of small gutter splint or ordinary tongue depressors.
  - Thereafter the therapist attempts to extent MCP which is contracted.
  - After few days, longer splint which extends the wrist is applied.
  - After that the wrist is then extended further each day.

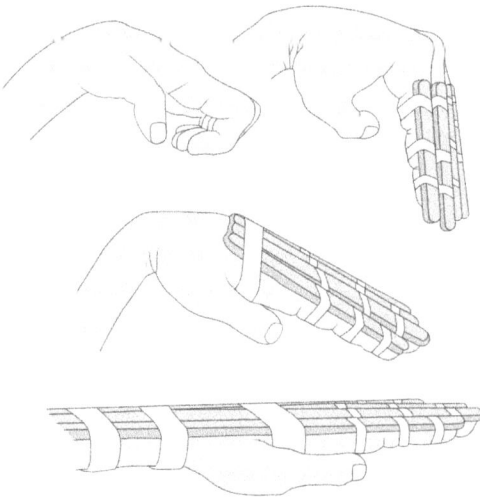

Fig. 48: Sir Robert Jones method.

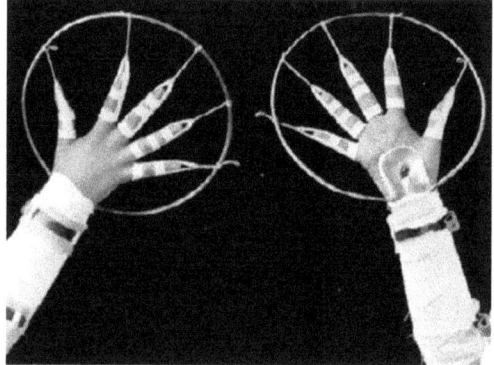

Fig. 49: Banjo splints.

- Once fingers and MCP joints are straightened, molded palmar and forearm splint with a hinge at wrist to assist dorsiflexion at wrist may be used.
- **Banjo splints (Fig. 49):** This splint is used with rubber band fastened to adhesive tape on the fingers. To be exercised all the times is more beneficiary.
- **Splinting:** It should always be combined with radiant heat, whirlpool bath, contrast bath, gentle massage and in some instances electrical stimulation of muscles.
- **Heat:** Heating has relaxing action on musculature. It can be given by using IRR or immersion method for half an hour in whirlpool bath at temperature 110° that produces peripheral hyperemia.
- **Massage:** Starting with light effleurage, progressing to deeper petrissage (kneading) to friction (a circular rolling motion to loosen scar and adhesion).
- **Electrical stimulation:** Sinusoidal current produce rhythmic contractions to combat atrophy, and produce deep massage and improved circulation. It should always be given (for 5 minutes) within the limits of fatigue.
- **Passive ROM exercises:** ROM exercises are given to maintain suppleness of soft tissue and to prevent adhesion and contracture formation.

Soft Tissue Injuries

- **Stretching exercises:** Stretching helps to loosen contracted ligaments, muscles and adhesions in stiff joint. It should be slow, steady and gradually increasing. In case of aggravated pain, swelling and decrease in ROM, the intensity of stretching should be reduced in the coming treatment sessions.

◼ OLECRANON BURSITIS

Inflammation of bursa present on posterior aspect of elbow over olecranon process. Olecranon bursa is the most superficial bursa in human body that is present on the dorsal aspect of olecranon. Due to its location, olecranon bursa is frequently affected by bursitis. It is also known as Student's elbow, Barfly elbow, Plumber's elbow or Miner's elbow (Fig. 50).

Etiology
- **Direct injury:** Such as direct hit or fall on elbow.
- **Prolonged pressure:** Leaning on elbow against a hard surface over a long time can irritate bursa due to friction or too much pressure.
- **Infection:** Bursa can be infected from a cut, scrape, or insect bite.
- **Arthritis:** Bursa may become inflamed as part of a generalized arthritis.
- **Idiopathic:** Many cases occur for no apparent reason.

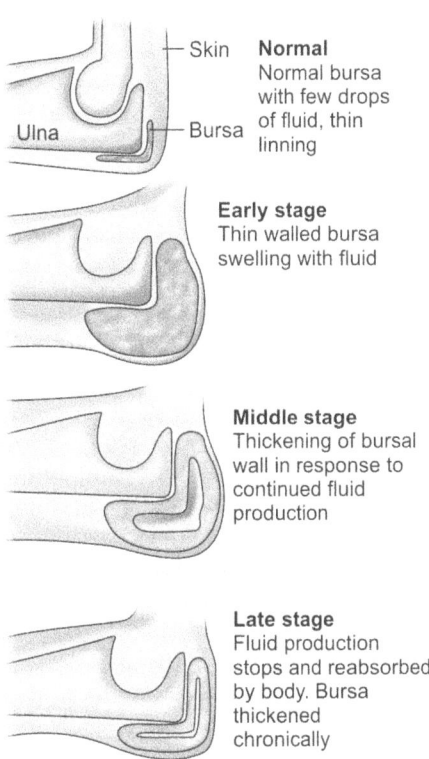

Fig. 51: Stages of bursitis.

Stages of Bursitis (Fig. 51)
- **Early stage:** The bursa becomes swelled due to any of the above mentioned causes.
- **Middle stage:** Gradually the lining of bursa thickened in response to continued production of fluid inside the bursa.
- **Late stage:** Finally production of fluid stops and bursal lining will remain thickened chronically.

Types of Olecranon Bursitis
- **Infectious (septic):** Approximately 20% bursitis cases are septic. Most of septic bursitis are caused by bacterial infections and rarely by fungi and algae.
- **Traumatic (aseptic):** It is the most common variety of olecranon bursitis. It is caused by traumatic insult that results in intrabursal bleeding, release of inflammatory mediators, and subsequent swelling.

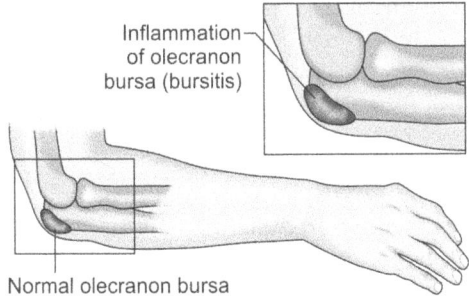

Fig. 50: Olecranon bursitis.

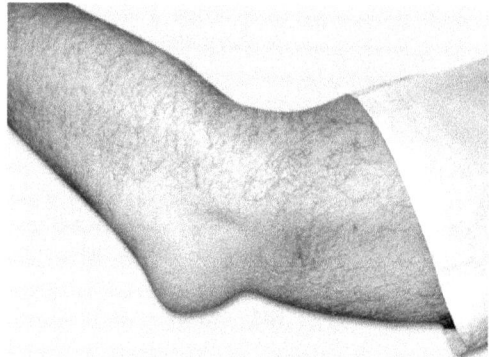

Fig. 52: Olecrenon bursitis (swelling).

- **Inflammatory:** Various inflammatory causes of olecranon bursitis are rheumatoid arthritis, gout, systemic lupus erythematosus, pigmented villonodular synovitis (PVNS), and pseudogout.

Clinical Presentation

- **Swelling:** A tender bump present over olecranon process. This is usually the first symptom (Fig. 52).
- **Pain:** Olecranon bursitis is usually painless but may be painful with elbow movement or pressure on elbow.
- **Redness or warmth:** Caused by infection in bursa.
- **Tenderness:** Another sign is sensitivity in and around the elbow.
- **Pus:** In infected bursitis, a yellow or white, thick, cloudy fluid draining from the bursa.

Diagnosis

- **Imaging studies:**
  - **X-ray:** Radiography may be used to determine the cause of bursitis, such as a broken bone or a piece of bony growth (called a bone spur) or arthritis. Bone spurs on olecranon could repeatedly cause elbow bursitis.
  - **Ultrasound:** It may be used to identify loose bodies, rheumatoid nodules, or tophaceous gout as underlying causes of the bursitis.
  - **MRI scan:** MRI may be used for additional assessment in presence of severe symptomatology and concern for osteomyelitis or abscess.
- **Laboratory test:**
  - **Blood test:** Blood test is used to check an infection, but this is not usually very helpful.
  - Sample of fluid from bursa using a needle is taken to lab for further testing. Presence of pus indicates that the bursa is infected.

Physical Examination

- **Patient history:** A thorough history is needed to rule out secondary causes of olecranon bursitis which can include rheumatoid arthritis, gout, systemic lupus erythematosus, and pseudogout.
- **Observation:**
  - A unilateral distended bursa can be 5-6 cm long and 2.5 cm wide overlying the proximal ulna.
  - Erythema is more commonly present in septic bursitis than aseptic cases.
  - Appearance of very prominent olecranon.
- **Palpation:**
  - Acute aseptic olecranon bursitis is heralded by a nontender fluctuant mass over proximal olecranon in more than 80% of cases.
  - In septic olecranon bursitis, affected bursa is warm, tender and erythematous.
  - Elbow ROM restriction depends on the extent of disease and degree of tenderness associated with bursal inflammation.
  - Severe cases of bursitis can have an associated joint effusion that further restricts range of motion.

Management

Conservative Treatments

Aseptic Bursitis

- **Observation:** No treatment may be needed. A small painless thickening or

Soft Tissue Injuries

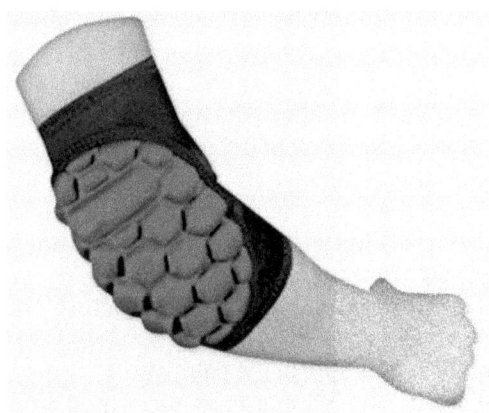

Fig. 53: Elbow pad.

swelling is often clear by itself with time. Only observation is required to check the progression of bursitis.
- **Protection of elbow:** Wearing elbow pads (Fig. 53) or a wrap to cushion the elbow. It helps to protect elbow from excessive friction.
- **RICE therapy:**
  - **Rest and activity modification:** Avoid activities that put direct pressure on affected elbow and can increase or cause the inflammation of bursa, e.g. inclining over the elbow.
  - **Ice:** Cold pack application for 10–15 minutes, twice or thrice a day to decrease the pain and inflammation.
  - **Compression:** Application of elastic compression bandage over the elbow joint to reduce swelling.
  - **Elevation:** Keep elbow above the heart level to reduce swelling.
- **Electrotherapy modalities:** Ultrasound (phonophoresis) and pain relieving modalities (electrical stimulation/TENS/IFT) helps to reduce pain swelling and accelerate healing process.
- **Nonsteroidal anti-inflammatory drugs:** To reduce pain and inflammation.
- **Steroid injection:** To reduce pain and inflammation but because of its potential side effects it is commonly used for troublesome cases that are not managed with other possible conservative treatments.
- **Aspiration of fluid:** In this, fluid from inflamed bursa is aspirated with the help of syringe to decrease pressure.
- **Therapeutic exercises:** After ablation of bursitis symptoms, strengthening and stretching should be initiated to maintain and improve the strength and flexibility of muscles.

Surgical Treatment
Septic Olecranon Bursitis
- **Antibiotics:** Use of antibiotics depends on the type of microorganism causing infection (often *Staphylococcus aureus*).
- **Surgery:**
  Indications:
  - Failure of nonsurgical management
  - Cases of recurrent chronic bursitis not responding to nonsurgical management.
  - Persistent or worsening cellulitis after 24–28 hours of antibiotic treatment.
  - Presence of skin necrosis, fistula, abscess or phlegmon.
  - Worsening systemic signs, such as fever, tachycardia, low blood pressure, chills.
- **Surgical techniques:**
  - Irrigation or open bursectomy
  - Arthroscopic bursectomy.

HAND AND WRIST INJURIES
■ DUPUYTREN'S CONTRACTURE

Dupuytren's contracture refers to flexion deformity of hand due to progressive thickening and tightness of palmar fascia (Fig. 54).

Etiology
Cause is unknown, there are however some risk factors which are linked to the condition:
- **Hereditary:** 60–70% cases have genetic predisposition.
- **Age:** More prevalent in middle age, i.e. after 40.

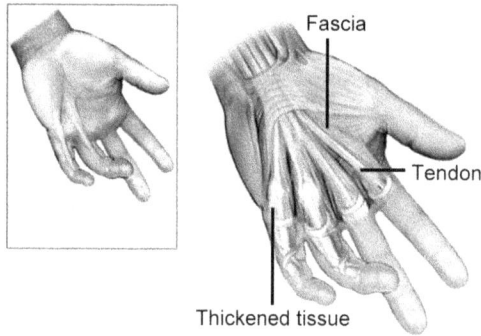

Fig. 54: Dupuytren's contracture.

- **Alcohol abuse and smokers:** Alcoholics especially those having cirrhosis of liver are at higher risk of developing Dupuytren's contracture.
- **Gender:** Males are ten times more likely to develop this condition in comparison to females.
- **Associated diseases:** Diabetics, HIV, cancer and epileptic patients are at higher risk of developing this condition.

Pathophysiology

It occurs in 3 phases:
1. **Proliferative phase:** In this stage there is proliferation of fibroblast and eruption of nodule takes place.
2. **Involutional phase:** In involutional phase, proliferated myofibroblast are oriented along the tension line in nodule that gradually results in the nodular thickening and contracture of palmar fascia.
3. **Residual phase:** In residual phase, diffuse thickening and contracture of palmar fascia progressively result in the contracture of joint.

Stages of Dupuytren's contracture on clinical basis (Fig. 55)

Stage 1: A nodule in the palm.
Stage 2: The fibrous cord developed from nodule that crosses the MCP joint and develops contracture.
Stage 3: The fibrous cord crosses the PIP joint resulting in the flexion deformity of the finger.

Clinical Presentation (Fig. 56)

- Painless nodule in palm that develops into a cord like band.
- Difficulty in extending fingers.
- Curling up of 4th and 5th fingers and are unable to be easily straightened.
- Thickening of lines in palm of hands.

Diagnosis

Imaging studies: MRI or ultrasound helps to validate the diagnosis.

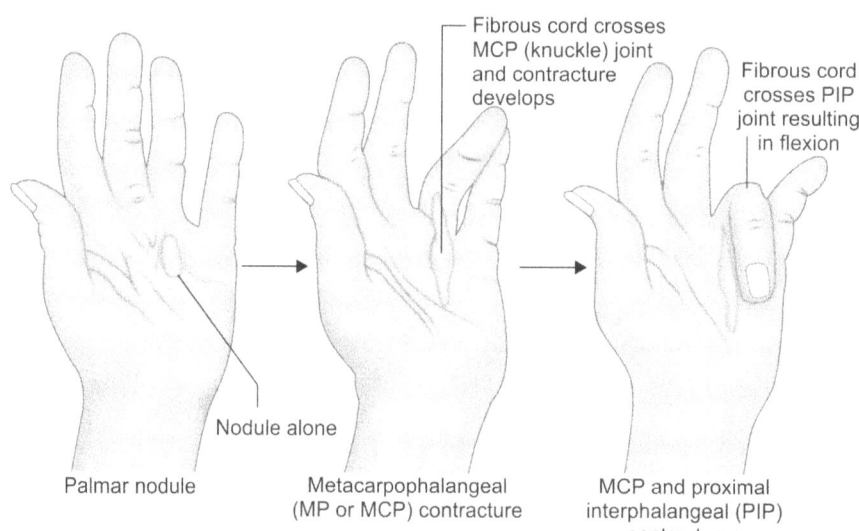

Fig. 55: Stages of Dupuytren's contracture.

Soft Tissue Injuries

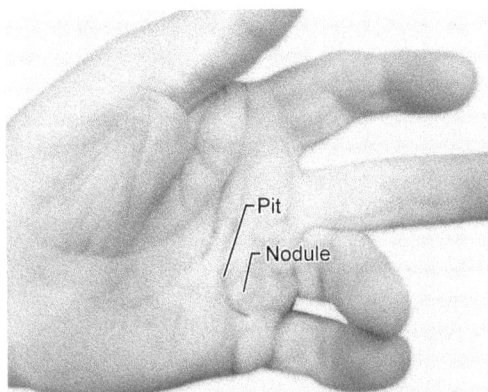

Fig. 56: Painless nodule in the palm.

Physical Examination
Palpation
- Firm nodules that may be tender.
- Painless cord proximal to nodule.
- Blanching of skin on finger extension
- Pits or indentation in the skin of palm.
- Presence of MCP and PIP joint contracture.

Special Test
Hueston tabletop test (Fig. 57): Patient is asked to place palm flat on the table. Test is considered to be positive if patient is not able to touch the palm to table.

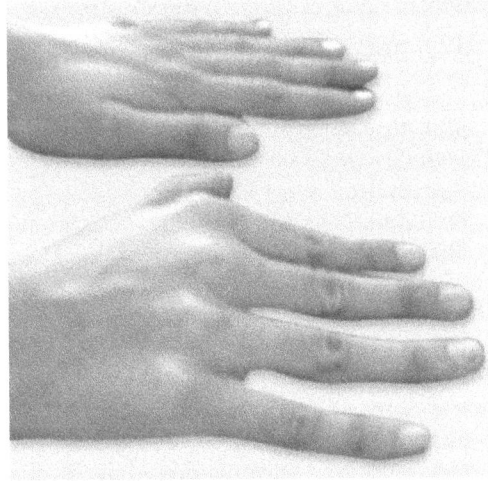

Fig. 57: Hueston tabletop test.

Management
Conservative Treatment
- **Corticosteroid injection:** It relieves local inflammation, pain and decrease the size of nodules.
- **XIAFLEX** (Collagenase *Clostridium histolyticum*): Injection into cord may result in enzymatic disruption of cord.

Physiotherapy Treatment
- **Heating through hot pack or wax therapy:** To control pain and slow the progression of contracture and to make the tissue supple and relaxed before stretching.
- **Ultrasound:** To decrease pain and inflammation and to soften the nodule and break down its adherence with underlying tissues.
- **Gentle stretching exercises:** Gentle pain free stretching with 15 second hold and 10 times repetition. Vigorous stretching can cause microtrauma to fascia which can aggravate the condition.
- **Tissue mobilization technique:** Kneading should be given to free the adherence of cord to underlying tissue.
- **Massaging** the palm of hand and forearm to decrease the tension of palmar fascia and make it more supple.
- **Splinting (Fig. 58):** In severe case splinting assist in straightening of fingers. Usually worn at night.
- **Tendon glide exercises:** These exercises cause isolated movement of superficial and deep tendons of flexor muscles. These are performed by making a variety of fists, e.g. straight fist, hook fist, duck fist and full fist (Fig. 59).
- **Range of motion exercises:** ROM exercises helps to increase and maintain the mobility of wrist and hand joints.

Surgical Treatment
Indications
- MCP joint contracture >30°
- Any degree of PIP contracture

34   Simplified Approach to Orthopedic Physiotherapy

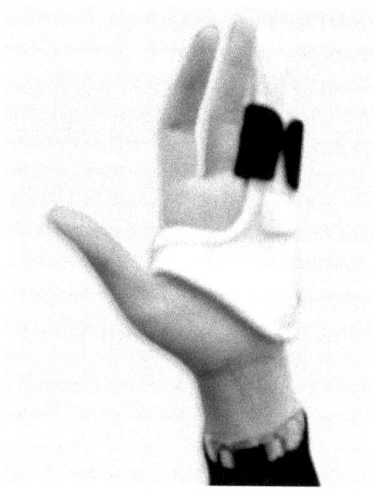

Fig. 58: Splinting.

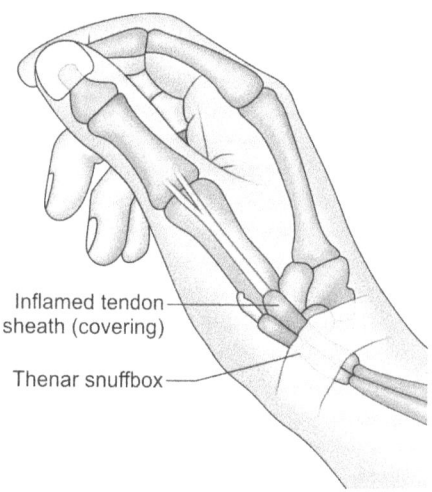

Fig. 60: De Quervain's tenosynovitis.

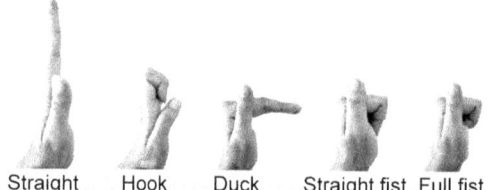

Fig. 59: Tendon glide exercises.

- Functional disability
- In bilateral cases, initially dominant hand is operated followed by the next hand.

Surgical Interventions
- **Fasciectomy:** In fasciectomy, only the diseased dupuytren's tissue is excised. In radical fasciectomy all the palmar fascia is resected.
- **Dermofasciectomy:** In dermofasciectomy, the fascia along with the skin is excised as a block of tissue.
- **Fasciotomy:** Fasciotomy involves cutting of cord without any removal of the tissues.

■ DE QUERVAIN'S TENOSYNOVITIS

De Quervain tenosynovitis is an inflammation of tendons enclosed in first dorsal compartment (which includes abductor pollicis longus and extensor pollicis brevis) at wrist (Fig. 60).

It is also known as Gamer's thumb as it is more commonly present in extensive users of mobile phones.

Etiology
First dorsal compartment is around 2 cm wide and present over styloid process. Tendons of the abductor pollicis longus and extensor pollicis brevis pass through it. These two tendons are held tightly by overlying extensor retinaculum (Fig. 61). Any inflammation or thickening of tendon impairs the smooth gliding of tendons through the sheath.

Epidemiology
- It occur most oftenly in age between 30 and 50 years.
- Females are six times more oftenly affected than males.
- Dominant hand is more commonly affected.

Predisposing Factors
- Direct injury/trauma on wrist.
- **Pregnancy:** Hormonal alterations in pregnancy may affect the integrity of all small joints.
- **Occupations:** Occupations that involve repeated hand movements like carpenter,

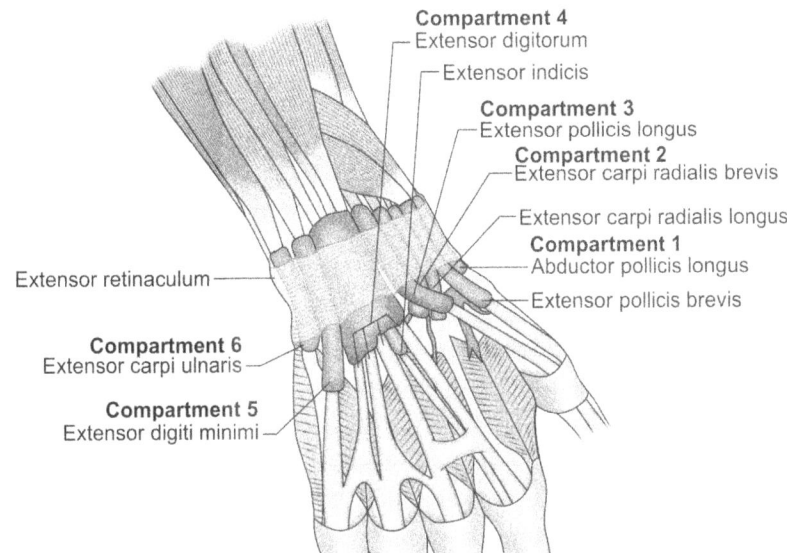

Fig. 61: Extensor retinaculum of hand.

plumber, gardener and sports activities like tennis, golf and badminton are at more risk of developing de Quervain's disease.
- Activities that include overwork of thumb and wrist movement especially radial and ulnar deviation, such as: wringing out wet clothes, long use of computer mouse, use of scissors, surgical tongs, texting, hammering, knitting, etc.
- **Inflammatory arthritis:** Such as rheumatoid arthritis.

Clinical Presentation
- **Pain:** Constant aching, burning, pulling sensation on lateral aspect of wrist.
- Swelling over the radial styloid (in the anatomical snuff box).
- Pain aggravates on grasping and raising objects with wrist.
- **Tenderness:** At the tip of radial styloid.
- Weakness and paresthesia in hand especially thumb.
- Catching or snapping sensation in thumb during movement.
- Numbness or tingling that might radiate to upper part of the forearm.
- Painful thumb movement, particularly when pinching or grasping things.

Diagnosis
Radiographs findings: X-rays are not usually needed for conventional diagnosis. It may be helpful to rule out other conditions like osteoarthritis at thumb, i.e. of first CMC joint.

Physical Examination
Palpation
- Tenderness at the base of thumb.
- Crepitus during the movement of thumb.
- Swelling around dorsal aspect of the base of thumb and/or near the radial styloid process.
- Tendon sheath may feel thick and hard.

Examination of ROM
- Painful resisted radial deviation.
- Decreased and painful CMC joint movement of 1st digit.

Measurement of Resisted Muscle Strength
- Fist grip strength
- Pinch strength (pinch gauge)

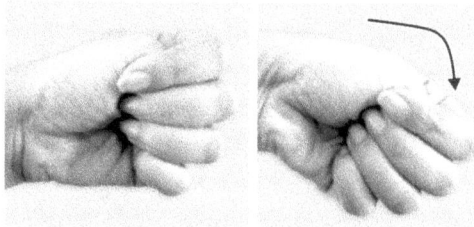

Fig. 62: Finkelstein test.

Special Test
- **Finkelstein test (Fig. 62):** Subject makes a fist around a thumb and performs active or active assisted flexion of thumb along with ulnar deviation of wrist. A positive test indicates the production of pain at base of the thumb due to stretching of muscles.
- **Eichhoff maneuver:** Subject makes a fist around the thumb and performs ulnar deviation of wrist. Test is considered to be positive if it elicits pain which is relieved by the extension of thumb while maintaining the wrist in ulnar deviation.

Management
Conservative Treatment
- NSAIDs is used to decrease pain and inflammation.
- **Rest:** Avoidance of activity that precipitate the symptoms.
- **Thumb spica splint (Fig. 63):** It is used to immobilize the thumb that helps to accelerate the healing process.
- **Corticosteroid injection:** Corticosteroid injection is injected in first dorsal compartment to reduce pain and inflammation in acute cases.

Physiotherapy Treatment
- **Cold compression:** Cryo application for 10 to 12 minutes over the inflamed area to decrease pain and inflammation in acute cases.
- **Hot pack:** In chronic condition, hot pack is given to relax and loosen tight musculature.
- **Ultrasonic therapy:** Ultrasonography is used to decrease pain, inflammation,

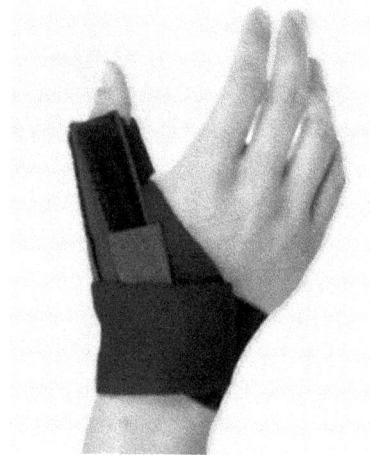

Fig. 63: Thumb spica splint.

break down adhesions and accelerate healing process.
- **Phonophoresis:** Ultrasound with 10% hydrocortisone. To reduce pain and inflammation and to aid in healing process.
- **Cold laser:** For reducing localized swelling of tendon.
- **Massage:** Deep friction massage technique is used to relax tight tissues. It also prevents adhesion formation and ruptures unwanted adhesions.
- **Gentle active and passive motion of thumb and wrist:** To maintain and improve joint mobility and prevent contracture and deformity of joint.
- **Strengthening exercises:** Strengthening of intrinsic hand muscles, wrist and forearm muscles to improve grip and pinch strength.
- **Stretching exercises:** Stretching should be started after the initial pain subsides—stretching of thenar muscles is necessary to improve the flexibility of tight muscles.

Surgical Treatment
Indication
- Severe pain
- Persistence of symptoms after conservative interventions.
- Functional disability due to pain.

Surgical Technique
Surgical release of 1st dorsal compartment: This surgical release technique helps to relieve pressure of tendons and restore free tendon gliding by splitting first dorsal compartment.

▪ GANGLION

A ganglion is a noncancerous sac containing thick clear jelly like fluid present near the distal joints (Fig. 64).

It develops from the sheath around tendon or joint capsule.

Epidemiology
Ganglions are mostly present in females. The prevalence ratio of female to male is 3:1. It usually occurs between 20-40 years. Approximately 70% ganglions are dorsal ganglion, while the remainders are volar wrist ganglions. It most oftenly originate within the wrist joint, but occasionally may arise from the tendon sheath.

Etiology
- **Mild sprains or other repeated injuries (wear or tear, on repeated use):** Repeated injuries leads to progressive wear and tear of tendon sheath. A ganglion is formed by fluid that escaped from the injured tendon sheath.
- **Post-traumatic:** Ganglion may develop after any trauma to the affected area.

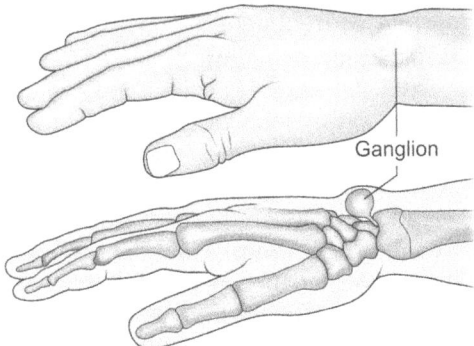

Fig. 64: Ganglion.

- Occupation that requires repeated or continuous wrist bending, such as welder, boilermaker.

Predisposing Factors
- **Gender and age:** Although it may occur in anyone at any age but they usually develops in females commonly between 20-30 years.
- **Arthritis:** Arthritis of DIP joints adjacent to the degenerated joint are at great risk of developing ganglion.
- **Tendon injury:** Patients having the history of tendon injury are at great risk of developing ganglion in coming years.
- **Scapholunate instability:** Injury of scapholunate interosseous ligament could be the cause of dorsal cyst formation.

Pathophysiology
Ganglion is a disc like cyst/lump filled with synovial fluid. They are usually smaller of around 1-3 cm but occasionally larger ganglion (up to 8 cm) has been reported. The fluid is harmless and not cancerous. Macroscopically, they tend to be smooth, white, and firm with an underlying stalk connection to the joint surface. They are mobile, nonadherent to underlying tissue, compressible, and not usually directly painful on palpation. Cysts may compress surrounding neurovascular structures due to which patients may experience wrist pain, paresthesia, intrinsic muscle paralysis, and/or coolness of the hand or fingers as a result.

Common Sites of Ganglion (Fig. 65)
- **Around the wrist:**
  - **Dorsal carpal (70%):** A lump that grows over the dorsal aspect of the wrist. It is located near and distal to lister tubercle and originates from scapholunate articulation.
  - **Volar carpal (20%):** Ganglion found on the volar aspect of the wrist between the thumb and radial pulse point and emerges from radiocarpal or scaphotrapeziotrapezoidal joint.

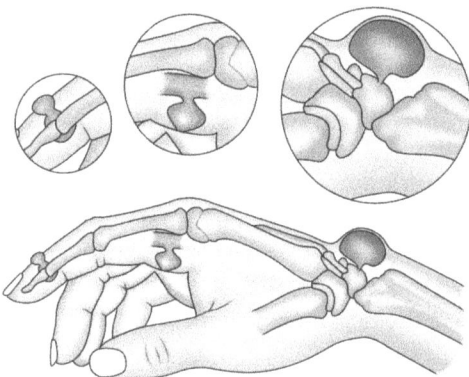

Fig. 65: Sites of ganglion.

- **Volar retinacular (10%):** It is found on the volar aspect of wrist and emerges from the ruptured tendon sheath fluid.
- **Over DIP joint:** It develops on the dorsal aspect of fingertip just below the cuticle, where they are called mucous cysts.
- Base of fingers (in the palm).
- Upper surface of foot.

Clinical Presentation

- Ganglions are commonly oval or circular that may be boggy or rigid.
- Size of ganglion can vary, i.e. from pea size to about 8 cm. But average size is about 1 cm.
- The size of ganglions often increases temporarily with strenuous activity of the involved extremity but it return to normal size during the periods of rest.
- Most ganglion are either painless or causes little discomfort unless they overlying any neurological structures.
- When present over the neurological structure it may cause pain and tingling sensation.
- Constant pain that worsen with activity.
- Ganglion may cause muscle weakness when present over the tendon of that muscle.

Diagnosis

Imaging Studies

- **X-ray:** To investigate the associated problems, such as arthritic joints or bony spurs.
- **MRI:** MRI plays an important role in diagnosing the condition when the ganglion is pain-free and not apparent outside.
- **Examining the aspirated fluid:** Fluid is aspirated from the cyst and evaluated for the presence of any infection.

Physical Examination

- **Observation:**
  - Location of lump.
  - Clinical appearance.
  - Transillumination (light will pass through these lumps).
- **Palpation:**
  - A well-confined bump may be palpated.
  - Ganglion is often fixed to deep tissue but not to overlying skin.
- **Sensory examination:**
  - Dorsal ganglia may compress the superficial radial nerve causing reduced sensation on the dorsum of hand.
  - Volar ganglia may compress the ulnar nerve causing reduced sensation of the small and ring fingers.
  - Volar ganglia may also compress the median nerve mimicking carpal tunnel syndrome.

Management

As ganglions are noncancerous, 50% of ganglions may disappear with time. Non-symptomatic ganglion can be managed without any treatment and only observation is required to check any unusual changes.

Conservative Treatment

- **Wrist brace or splint:** Activity often increases the size of ganglion and can also cause pain by increasing the pressure on nerve. Splint or brace is used for immobilization that helps to reduce the size of ganglion and associated symptoms.
- **Needle aspiration:** Fluid is aspirated using a syringe then an anti-inflammatory or steroid is injected into the cyst that will make it disappear. After this, wrist brace is worn constantly for 4 weeks to prevent

its recurrence. This procedure has <50% success rate and the chances of recurrence are also very high. Because it fails to eliminate the 'root' connection of the ganglion to the joint or tendon the chances of recurrence are high.

Physiotherapy Treatment
- **Ultrasound:** To reduce swelling and inflammation
- **Deep friction massage:** It may help to move the fluid out of the sac.
- **Strengthening exercises** are useful for improving hand strength, flexibility, and coordination.

Surgical Treatment
Excision or removal of cyst: In the surgery, the ganglion is removed with the involved tendon sheath and joint capsule.

KNEE INJURIES

■ MENISCAL INJURY

Meniscal tear is one of the most common knee injury (Fig. 66). Meniscus is a crescent shaped disc that act as a shock absorbers or cushion between tibia and distal femur. Each knee has two menisci: medial and lateral meniscus.

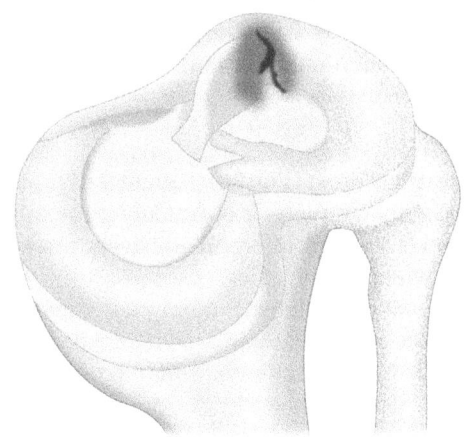

Fig. 66: Meniscal tear.

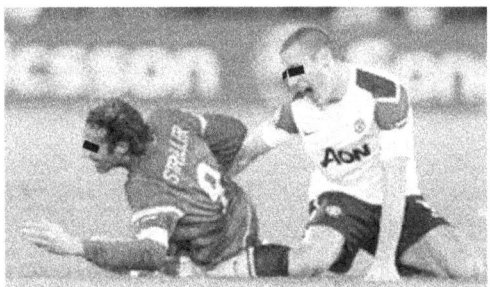

Fig. 67: Compression force coupled with rotational forces.

Function of Menisci
- Meniscus helps in load transmission and shock absorption.
- It protects underlying articular cartilage by lowering the load carried by articular cartilage and by increasing the actual contact area between femur and tibia.

Mechanism of Injury
- Compression force coupled with rotational forces to a flexed knee (Fig. 67).
- Bending of knee suddenly and extremely, e.g. fall on the ground because of missed step.
- Lifting heavy weight: On lifting heavy weight, pressure on the menisci increases up to five times the actual weight.
- Lateral meniscal tear is usually caused by application of valgus force on flexed knee with foot on the ground and femur ER.
- Medial meniscal tear is usually caused by application of varus force on flexed knee with foot on the ground and femur IR.

Clinical Presentation
- Pain on joint line, i.e. localized to meniscus.
- Swelling: Mild swelling occurs on next day with stiffness and limping.
- Sometimes locking of knee occurs in knee flexion.
- Sensation of "giving way".
- Popping, catching, grinding or clicking feeling during knee movement.

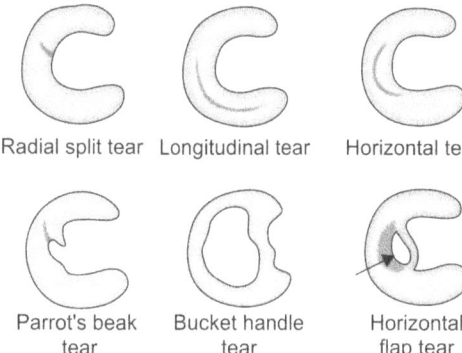

Fig. 68: Classification of meniscal tear according to anatomical location and displaced tears.

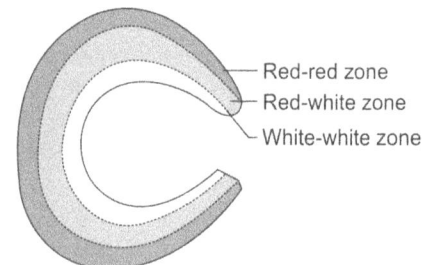

Fig. 69: Zones of meniscal blood supply.

Classification
On the basis of anatomical location and proximity to shapes, meniscal injuries are classified as (Fig. 68):
- **Longitudinal tear:** It occurs along the longitudinal axis of meniscus that split it into medial and lateral part.
- **Horizontal tear:** It splits the meniscus into upper and lower part.
- **Radial tear:** It occurs perpendicular to the longitudinal axis of meniscus that splits the meniscus into anterior and posterior part.

Displaced tears are classified as:
- **Bucket handle tear:** Displaced longitudinal tear is known as bucket handle tear.
- **Flap tear:** Displaced horizontal tear is known as flap tear.
- **Parrot beak tear:** Displaced radial tear is known as parrot beak tear.

Classification according to proximity to blood supply (Fig. 69):
- **Red-red zone:** Tear in the outermost edge of meniscus that receives most of the blood supply.
- **Red-white zone:** Tear in the middle one-third junctions between vascular and avascular portion of meniscus.
- **White-white zone:** Tear in the innermost aspect of meniscus which is the avascular portion of the meniscus.

Diagnosis
Imaging Studies
- **MRI scan or ultrasound:** It helps to evaluate the location and severity of the injury.
- **Arthroscopy:** It may be needed to study the knee when the therapist is unable to determine the cause of knee pain through these techniques.

Physical Examination
- **Patient history:** Detailed history about the cause of injury, any previous injury of knee, functional limitation and symptoms are critical to determine the tear and its optimal treatment.
- **Observation:** Therapist should observe the joint for swelling, bruising and deformity.
- **Palpation:**
  - Therapist palpate around the joint for areas of tenderness, warmth, swelling, etc.
  - Joint line palpation: Palpation along tibiofemoral joint line with the knee in 90° flexion.

Special Test
McMurray's test (Fig. 70): Patient is in supine lying with complete flexion at knee. Therapist palpates at joint line and passively extends knee with rotation of leg.

To examine lateral meniscus, therapist palpates posterolateral aspect of knee and extends knee with medial rotation of leg and a varus stress at knee.

To examine medial meniscus, therapist palpates posteromedial aspect of knee and

Soft Tissue Injuries

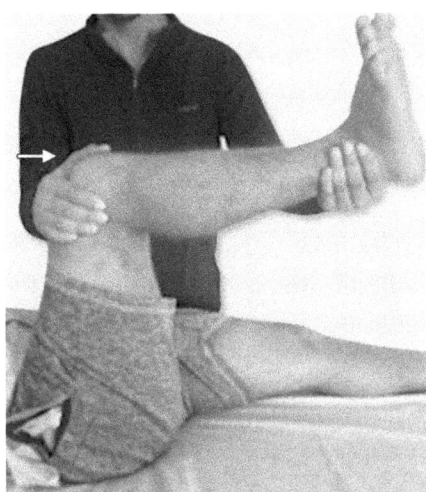

Fig. 70: McMurray's test.

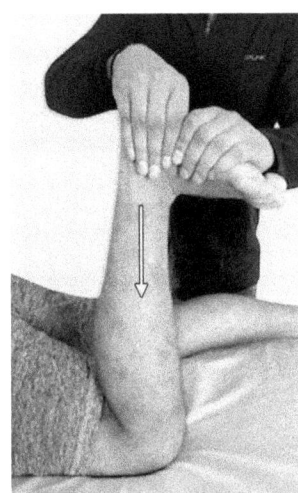

Fig. 71: Apley's compression test.

extends knee with lateral rotation of leg and a valgus stress at knee.

Test is considered positive if pain elicits or a click is felt by patient or therapist.

Apley's compression test (Fig. 71): Place the patient in prone position while keeping knee in 90° of flexion. Therapist pushes patient's foot downwards towards examining table followed by rotation of the leg.

To examine lateral meniscus, therapist rotates the leg laterally.

To examine medial meniscus, therapist rotates the leg medially.

Test is considered to be positive if patient complains of pain on lateral or medial joint line.

Management

Indications of Conservative Treatment
- Asymptomatic tear
- Tear smaller than 1 cm
- Tear located in red-red zone
- Partial thickness tear
- Degenerative tear in older patient without any mechanical symptoms
- Low demand or older patient.

Conservative Treatment
- **RICE therapy:** It is used to decrease pain and swelling.
- **NSAIDs and corticosteroid injection:** They are used to reduce pain and inflammation.
- **Knee braces and orthotics:** Braces are needed for stabilization of joint, to reduce pain and to aid in early healing.
- **Avoid aggravating activities** like jumping, running, etc. These activities may increase stress on meniscus and delays the healing process.

Maximal meniscal healing time is around 6–8 weeks.

Nonoperative physiotherapy protocol

Phase I	Week 0–1
Aim	To reduce swelling
	Maintain ability to extend the knee
	Knee flexion over 90°
Cryotherapy	For 15 minutes after every couple of hours to reduce the swelling
Compression bandage/knee support	To reduce swelling to be worn for 24 hours/day. • In initial 1–2 days during complete rest a simple elastic knee sleeve is used • Later on hinged knee brace is used to protect the medial knee ligaments and cartilage while initiating walking

Contd...

Contd...

Phase I	Week 0–1
Electrotherapy modalities	To reduce the pain and inflammation, e.g. ultrasound, TENS, IFT
Exercises	Gentle ROM exercises within limits of pain
	Isometric or static quadriceps exercises
	Double leg calf raises, hip abduction and extension
	Resistance band hamstring exercises
	Static cycling to maintain aerobic fitness

Phase II	Week 1–2
Aims	To eliminate knee swelling
	Achieve full knee ROM
Continue cryotherapy, knee support and electrotherapy modalities	
Exercises	Same as above
	Closed chain exercises for lower limb • Squats and lunges if pain allows • Leg press initially bilaterally and gradually unilaterally • Step up • Hip bridges
	Proprioceptive exercises: Wobble board balance drill

Phase III	Week 2–3
AIMS	Regain full knee ROM
	Regain normal muscle strength
	Return to ADLs
Knee support	Discontinue/not needed
Exercises	Same as above
	Running, swimming, road cycling
	Plyometrics
	Backward running, jumping, hopping and kicking

Surgical Treatment

Meniscal Repair

Indications

Presence of O'Donoghue's triad (also known as unhappy triad): Combined injury of anterior cruciate ligament, medial collateral ligament and medial meniscus.

- Acute longitudinal tear >1 cm
- Reducible tear located in white-white zone or red-white zone
- Tear in young patients < 40 years
- Tear in high demand patients
- Complex and recurrent tear.

Menisectomy

Indications

Symptomatic tears not amenable to repair.

Postoperative rehabilitation protocol

Phase I	Maximum protection phase: Week 1–6
Stage 1	Immediate postoperative: Day 1–Week 3
	RICE therapy
	Electrical muscle stimulation
	Brace locked at 0°
ROM exercises	ROM (0–90°) • Motion limited for first 7–21 days • Gradual increase in flexion, ROM as per pain allows
Mobilization	Patellar mobilization
	Scar tissue mobilization
Strengthening exercises	Quadriceps isometrics
	Hamstring isometrics (when posterior horn is repaired, then no hamstring exercise for 6 weeks)
	Hip abduction and adduction
Weight bearing	WBAT with crutches and brace locked at 0°
Proprioceptive exercises	

Contd...

Soft Tissue Injuries

Contd...

Stage 2	Weeks 4–6
	Progressive resistance exercises
	Limited range knee extension
	Toe raises
	Mini-squats
	Cycling
	Flexibility exercises
Phase II	**Moderate protection phase: Weeks 6–10**
Goals	To increase strength, power and endurance
	To regain full ROM of knee
Exercises	Same as above
	Lateral step-ups
Endurance exercises	Swimming, cycling, stair climbing
Coordination exercises	Balance board
	Backward walking
Plyometrics	
Phase III	**Advance phase: Weeks 11–15**
Goals	Increase power and endurance
	Return to ADLs
Exercises	Same as above
	Full ROM exercises
	Initiate running programs

Treatment options and their rehabilitation

Treatment option	Recommended guidelines
Nonoperative	• No brace • Crutches PWB to FWB as tolerated 0–1 week
Partial menisectomy	• No brace • Crutches PWB to FWB as tolerated 0–2 weeks
Meniscal repair	• Rehabilitation brace: 0–6 weeks • AROM: 0°–90° in first 6 weeks • PROM: Full range after 6 weeks • Crutches PWB 0–2 weeks • Crutches to advance FWB 2–6 weeks

Contd...

Contd...

Treatment option	Recommended guidelines
Meniscal allograft	• Rehabilitation brace: 0–8 weeks • AROM 0°–90° in first 6 weeks • PROM: Full range after 6 weeks • Crutches touch WB: 0–4 weeks • Crutches PWB: 4–6 weeks • FWB after 6 weeks

■ ANTERIOR CRUCIATE LIGAMENT INJURY

It is the most common knee injury in athletes engaging in sports activities like football, soccer, etc. (Fig. 72).

Functions of Anterior Cruciate Ligament

Primary function: It prevents excessive medial rotation of tibia.

Secondary function: It prevents excessive valgus/varus and prevents excessive anterior subluxation of tibia.

Anatomy (Fig. 73)

Anterior cruciate ligament (ACL) attaches to the medial and anterior aspect of tibial plateau, passes under transverse ligament and extends superiorly, laterally and posterior to attach to backward portion of the inner aspect of lateral femoral condyle.

Mechanism of Injury (Figs. 74A and B)

- **Forced hyperextension of knee:**
  - Any impact on anterior aspect of knee
  - Forced sudden contraction of quadriceps.
- **Forced hyperflexion of knee:** Sudden anterior translation of tibia.
- Following sudden change in direction.
- Quick deceleration.
- Incorrect landing from jump.

Clinical presentation

- Excessive knee pain after injury.
- Acute and excessive knee swelling within initial hours of injury.

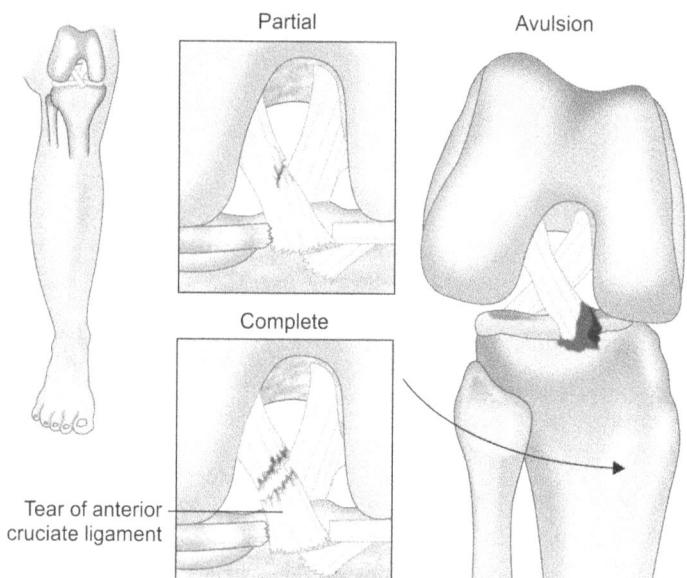

Fig. 72: Anterior cruciate ligament injury.

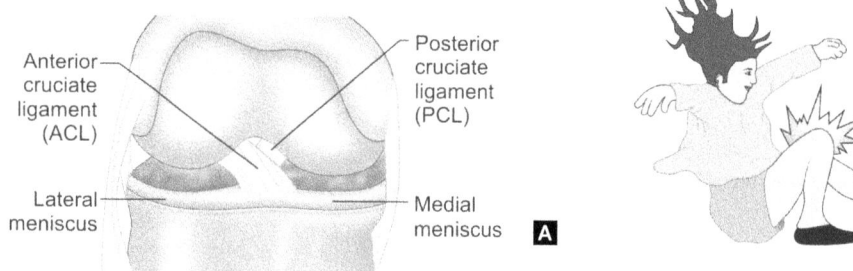

Fig. 73: Anatomy of ACL.

- At the time of injury there may be an audible 'POP', 'CRACK' or feeling of 'something giving out'.
- Primary joint instability that concealed later on by excessive swelling.
- Tenderness on medial joint line of knee joint.
- Occurrence of "giving way" particularly on twisting movements.
- Restricted knee movement.

Diagnosis

Imaging Studies

Arthroscopy, MRI scan or ultrasound: To determine the intensity, location and other analogous injuries. Rarely ACL injury occurs in isolation. Most common associated injuries are:
- Meniscal injuries
- Medial collateral ligament
- Bone bruise

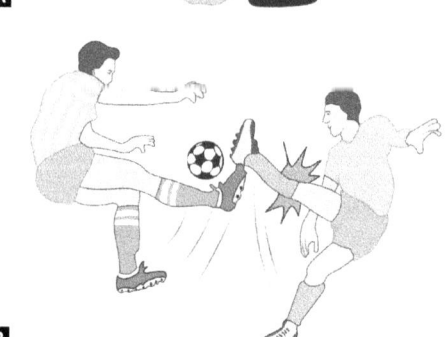

Figs. 74A and B: (A) Hyperflexion injury; (B) Hyperextension injury.

Soft Tissue Injuries

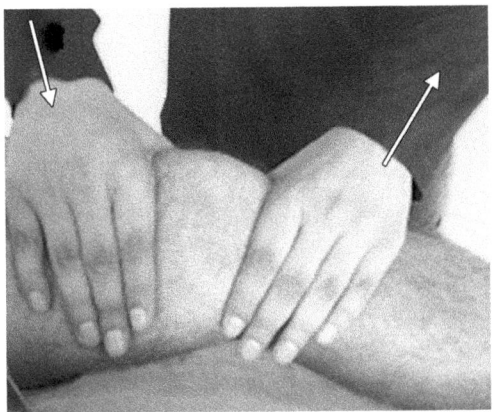

Fig. 75: Lachman anterior test.

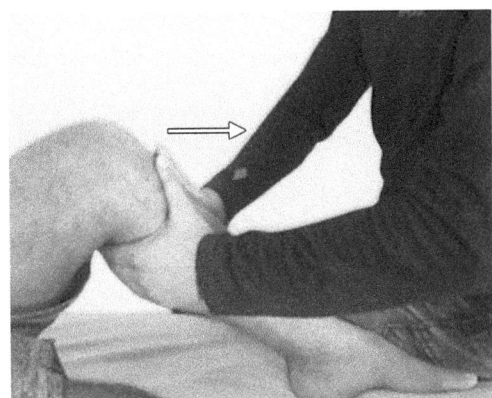

Fig. 76: Anterior drawer test.

- Osteochondral fracture
- Segond fracture
- Distal femur fracture.

Physical Examination
- **Patient history:** Detailed history about cause of injury, any previous injury of knee, functional limitation and symptoms are critical to determine the tear and its optimal treatment.
  - Commonly ACL tear occurs in non-contact twisting injuries associated with acute pain, swelling and audible "pop".
- **Observation:** Therapist observe the joint for swelling, bruising and deformity
- **Palpation:** Swelling, tenderness along with medial joint line, possible widespread mild periarticular tenderness, painful knee movements.

Special Test
- **Lachman anterior test (Fig. 75):** Place the patient in supine position while keeping knee in 15° of flexion. Therapist stabilizes distal end of femur with one hand and pulls the proximal part of tibia anteriorly with other hand. A positive test represents the feeling of soft end feel on the movement of tibia.
- **Anterior drawer test (Fig. 76):** Place the patient in supine position while keeping the knee in 90° of flexion. Therapist stabilizes the foot by siting on it and grasps the proximal tibia with both hands by placing thumb on anterior aspect of tibia. Then the therapist pulls the tibia anteriorly. A positive test represents the feeling of soft end feel on the movement of tibia.

Management

Conservative Treatment
Indications
- Age: >35 years age
- No or minimal anterior tibial subluxation.
- Not associated with any intra-articular injury
- When the patient's lifestyle is not highly active lifestyle.

Physiotherapy protocol for nonoperative ACL injury

Phase I	Motion and protection
Goals	To decrease pain and edema
	To increase strength of muscles
	To maintain ROM
	To improve patellar mobility
	Independent ambulation
To reduce pain and swelling	RICE therapy i.e. rest, ice, compression and elevation
	US, TENS, IFT or EMS
	Ankle pumps

Contd...

Contd...

Phase I	Motion and protection
Strengthening exercises	Isometric of quadriceps, hamstring, hip abductors, adductors, abdominals and quadratus lumborum
	Electrical stimulation to VMO and quadriceps
ROM	Patellar mobilization
	PROM/AROM
Stretching	Stretching of quadriceps, hamstring, hip flexors, ITB, calf muscles
CCE	Light close kinematic chain exercise, e.g. mini-squats
Proprioceptive exercise	Initiate neuromuscular control and proprioceptive exercise
Phase II	**Motion and control**
Exercises	Same as above
	Wear brace for functional activities
CKCE	Progress CCE: Step-ups, leg press, theraband kicks
OKCE	Initiate open kinematic chain exercise with precaution as it may cause excessive anterior translation of tibia on femur
Phase III	**Strength and proprioception**
Goals	Pain-free and complete AROM
	Normal strength of VMO
	Less than 20% quadriceps deficit
Treatment	Same as above
	Eccentric exercises of quadriceps and hamstring muscles
	Progress proprioceptive exercises
	Balance and coordination exercises
Phase IV	**Strength, function and endurance**
Goals	Less than 10% strength deficit and proper hamstring/quadriceps ratio

Contd...

Phase IV	Strength, function and endurance
Treatment	Same as above
	Progressive resistance exercises
	Light plyometrics
	Forward and backward step over

Surgical Treatment

Indications

- Age: <25 years
- Marked anterior tibial subluxation.
- If patient suffer from persistent knee pain.
- ACL injury causes the knee to buckle during routine activities, such as walking
- Associated intra-articular damage, e.g. avulsion fracture.
- Highly active lifestyle.

ACL reconstruction surgeries are done to repair the ACL tear and to restore knee stability and strength after the ligament has been torn. ACL tears are not usually repaired using suture to sew it back together because repaired ACLs have generally been shown to fail overtime. Therefore, the torn ACL is generally replaced by a substitute graft made of tendon. The grafts commonly used to replace ACL include:

- **Autograft, i.e. of patient himself:** Patellar tendon, hamstring tendon, or quadriceps tendon autograft
- **Allograft (taken from another person):** Patellar tendon, Achilles tendon, semi-tendinosus, gracilis, or posterior tibialis tendon.

Postsurgical rehabilitation protocol

Phase I	Week 0–2
Goals	Protect graft fixation
	Reduce pain and inflammation
	Achieve full knee extension and 0–90° knee flexion
Brace	Drop lock brace locked in extension for ambulation and sleeping

Contd...

Contd...

Phase I	Week 0–2
WB	WBAT with 2 crutches
	Discontinue crutches as tolerated after 7 days
Exercises	RICE therapy
	Heel slides, wall slides
	Quadriceps and hamstring sets
	Patellar mobilization
	NWB gastrocnemius and hamstring stretch
	SLR with brace in full extension until quadriceps strength is sufficient to prevent extensor lag
	Prone leg hangs
Phase II	Week 2–6
Goals	Restore normal gait
	Restore full ROM
	Protect graft fixation
	Improve strength, endurance and proprioception
Brace	Discontinue after 4 weeks
WB	Patellar tendon graft: Continue ambulation with brace locked in extension, may unlock for sitting and remove brace for ROM exercises
	Hamstring graft: May discontinue the brace as quadriceps control is achieved
Exercises	Mini-squats: 0–30°
	Stationary bike
	CKCE: Leg press: 0–30°
	Toe raises
	Continue stretches and prone hangs
Phase III	Weeks 6–8
Goals	Avoid overstressing of graft fixation
	Protect patellofemoral joint
	Progress strength and proprioception
Exercises	Patellar mobilization
	CKCE: One leg squat, Leg press: 0–60°
	Stair climbing: Step-up and down

Contd...

Contd...

Phase III	Weeks 6–8
	Plyometrics
	Proprioceptive exercises: Trampoline, wobble board balance
Phase IV	Week 8–12
Goals	Return to ADLs
Exercises	Continue and progress strength and flexibility program
	Proprioceptive exercises
	Plyometrics
	Lunges
	Crossover walking—agility drills

■ POSTERIOR CRUCIATE LIGAMENT INJURY

Posterior cruciate ligament (PCL) is not injured in isolation commonly because it is double stronger and thicker than the ACL. Usually it is injured in association with avulsion fracture and multiple ligaments injury (Fig. 77).

Functions of Posterior Cruciate Ligament
- **Primary function:** It prevents excessive posterior translation of tibia.
- **Secondary function:** It prevents excessive lateral rotation of tibia.
  - It prevents hyperextension and excessive valgus and varus of knee.

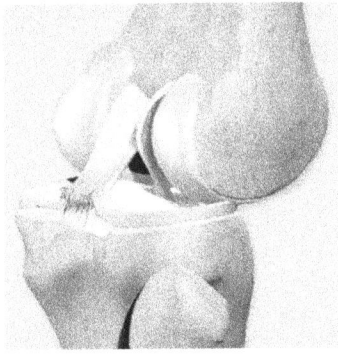

Fig. 77: Posterior cruciate ligament tear.

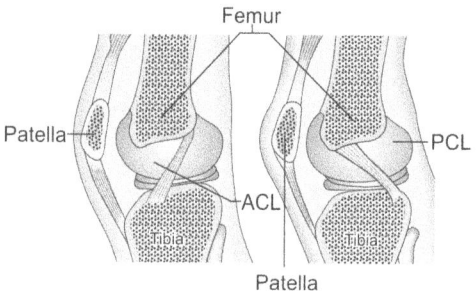

Fig. 78: Anatomy of PCL.

Anatomy (Fig. 78)

PCL attaches to posterior intercondylar area and passes anterosuperiorly to insert into the lateral surface of medial femoral condyle.

Mechanism of Injury (Figs. 79A and B)

- Direct posterior impact over anterior aspect of upper shin in flexed knee, e.g. dashboard injury.
- Fall on flexed knee with plantar flexed feet when tibial tubercle strikes against the ground causing a posterior force to the proximal tibia.
- Hyperextension of knee with combined rotational, varus or valgus stress.

Clinical Presentation

- **In acute cases:**
  - Usually minimal pain, swelling (PCL is an extrasynovial structure), instability with full ROM in isolated injury of PCL.
  - Poorly defined pain on posterior aspect of knee that sometimes involves calf.
  - Joint instability while walking on uneven surface.
- **In chronic cases:**
  - Difficulty in walking on a semiflexed knee like ascending or descending stairs, squatting, etc.
  - Prolonged walking may induce pain, instability, moderate swelling and stiffness in knee.

Diagnosis

Imaging Studies

- **Arthroscopy, MRI scan or ultrasound:** To determine the location, severity of the tear and associated injuries. Rarely PCL injury occurs in isolation. Most common associated injuries are:
  - Meniscal injuries
  - Ligamentous injuries like lateral or medial collateral ligament, anterior cruciate ligament.
  - Injury of anterior lateral femoral condyle and anterior tibial plateau.

Physical Examination

- **Patient history:** Detailed history about cause of injury, any previous injury of knee, functional limitation and symptoms are critical to determine the tear and its optimal treatment.
- **Observation:** Therapist observes joint for swelling, bruising and deformity.

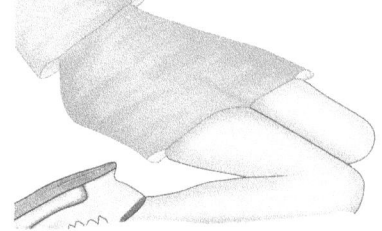
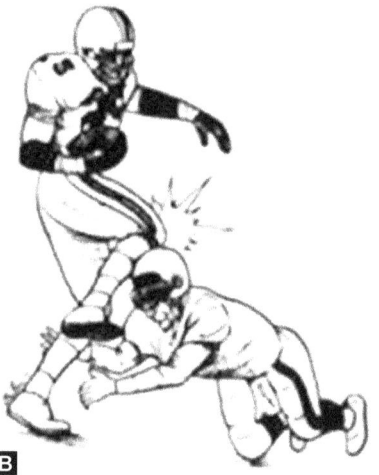

Figs. 79A and B: (A) Fall on flexed knee with foot plantar flexed; (B) Posterior blow on upper shin.

Soft Tissue Injuries

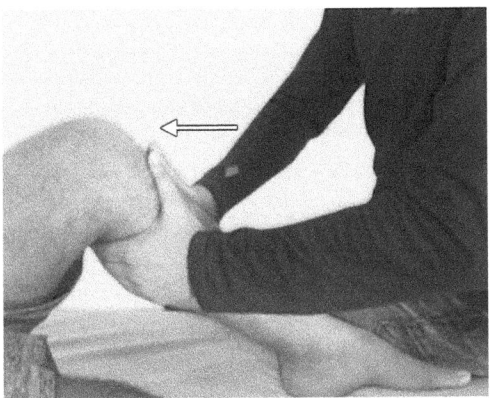

Fig. 80: Posterior drawer test.

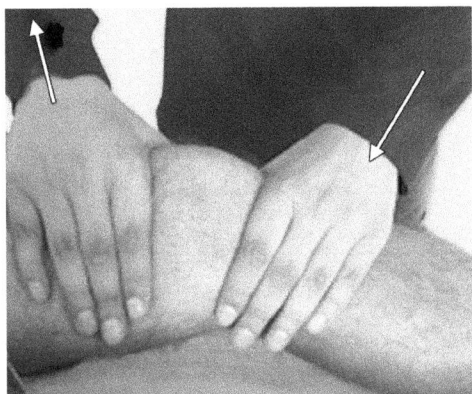

Fig. 81: Lachman's posterior test.

- **Palpation:**
  - Therapist palpate around the joint for areas of tenderness, warmth, swelling, etc.
  - Mild swelling, mild periarticular tenderness, minimal painful knee movements and normal gait in acute isolated PCL injury.

Special Tests
- **Posterior drawer test (Fig. 80):** Place the patient in supine position while keeping the knee in 90° of flexion. Therapist stabilizes the foot by siting on it and grasps proximal tibia with both hands by placing the thumb on anterior aspect of tibia. Then therapist pushes the tibia posteriorly. A positive test represents the feeling of soft end feel on the movement of tibia. Excessive posterior translation should also be noted.
- **Lachman's posterior test (Fig. 81):** Place the patient in supine position while keeping the knee in 15° of flexion. Therapist stabilizes the distal end of femur with one hand and pushes the proximal part of tibia posteriorly with other hand. A positive test represents feeling of soft end feel on the movement of tibia.
- **Posterior sag sign (Fig. 82):** Place the patient in supine position while keeping hip and knee in 90° of flexion. Therapist supports the heel in air. Positive test is

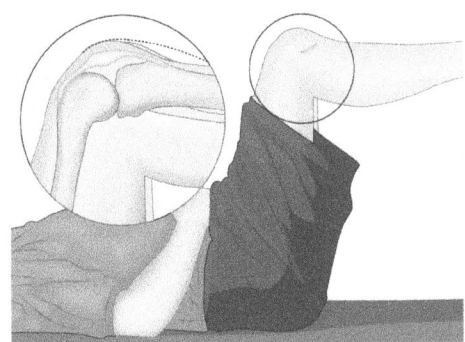

Fig. 82: Posterior sag sign.

indicated by inferior sagging of proximal tibia due to gravity.

Management
Conservative Treatment
Indications
- Acute isolated PCL injury
- Grade I and II PCL injuries.

Nonsurgical physiotherapy protocol

Precaution	Avoid more than 90° knee flexion for first 6 weeks post injury
	Posterior knee pain indicates that progression is too quick
Phase I	**Day 0–10**
ROM	0–60°
To reduce swelling	Ice, elevation, NSAIDs

Contd...

Contd...

Phase I	Day 0–10
WB/gait	Protected WB (50%) with crutches
Exercises	Isometric quadriceps as pain permits
Avoid	Avoid open chain hamstring strengthening exercises
Phase II	**Days 10–21**
ROM	Early ROM within limits of pain
	Active assisted and passive range of motion less than 60°
To reduce swelling	Ice, elevation, NSAIDs
WB/gait	WBAT with knee brace locked in extension
	Discontinue crutches when patient is able to and swelling is controlled
Exercises	Isometric quadriceps when pain permits
	Leg press: 0–60°
Avoid	Avoid open chain hamstring strengthening exercises
	Avoid posterior subluxation by placing a pillow under posterior aspect of lower leg when lying down
Phase III	**Weeks 3–5**
ROM	Progress as tolerated
To reduce swelling	Ice, elevation, NSAIDs, electrical stimulation
WB/gait	WBAT
	Discontinued the large hinged knee brace as tolerated
	Obtain a functional PCL brace
Exercise/ functional training	Increase strength and endurance of quadriceps
	Open chain knee extension exercises allowed only when no patellofemoral symptoms present
	Quadriceps sets and terminal knee extension
	Hip extension with knee extension

Contd...

Contd...

Phase III	Weeks 3–5
	No hamstring exercise with flexed knee
	Mini-squats: 0–60°
	Leg press: 0–60°
Phase IV	**Weeks 5–8**
ROM	Progress as tolerated
Gait/WB	WBAT
Exercise/ functional training	Closed chain exercises to improve functional strength, e.g. mini-squats, wall slides, steps-up, leg press
	Progressive resistance exercises of quadriceps
	Proprioceptive exercises: Slide board

Operative Treatment

Indications

- Grade III injury with marked knee instability
- Multiple ligamentous injuries
- Bony avulsion at insertion of PCL
- Symptomatic severe posterior knee instability
- There is almost no indication for reconstruction of an isolated intrasubstance rupture of PCL.

PCL reconstruction surgeries are done to repair the injured structures and to provide dynamic stability and maintaining full range of motion of knee. The grafts commonly used to replace the ACL include:

- **Autograft, i.e. of patient himself:** Hamstring tendon autograft.
- **Allograft (taken from another person):** Patellar tendon, Achilles tendon, semi-tendinosus, gracilis, or posterior tibialis tendon.

Postoperative physiotherapy protocol

Phase I	Immediate postoperative: Week 0–2
Goal	Control swelling and inflammation
	Obtain full passive extension

Contd...

Contd...

Phase I	Immediate postoperative: Week 0–2
	Gradually increases the flexion to 90°
	Patellar mobility
To reduce swelling	Ice and elevation
Brace	Wrap locked at 0° knee extension for ambulation and sleep only from 4th day onwards
WB	As tolerated with 2 crutches (50%)
ROM	PROM (0–90° of knee flexion) out of brace
Exercises	Patellar mobilization
	Stretching of hamstring and calf muscles
	Ankle pumps
	Quadriceps sets
	SLR for hip flexion, abduction and abduction
	Knee extension: 60–0°
EMS	To quadriceps during quadriceps sets
CPM	0–60° as tolerated
Phase II	Maximum protection: Weeks 2–6
Goals	Control extension forces to protect graft
	Restore motion
	Nourish articular cartilage
	Decrease swelling and fibrosis
	Prevents quadriceps atrophy
	Week 2
Brace	Wrap locked at 0° knee extension
WB	As tolerated with 1 crutch
ROM	PROM (0–90° of knee flexion) out of brace
Exercises	Multiangle isometrics 60, 40, 20°
	Quadriceps sets
	Knee extension 60–0°
	Leg press: 0–60°
EMS	To quadriceps during quadriceps sets
CPM	0–60° as tolerated

Contd...

Phase II	Maximum protection: Weeks 2–6
	Week 3
Brace	Wrap locked at 0° knee extension
WB	Full WB, no crutches
ROM	PROM (0–100° of knee flexion) out of brace
Exercises	Mini-squats: 0–45°
	Wall squats: 0–50°
	Knee extension: 60–0°
	Static cycling for ROM and endurance
Phase III	Controlled ambulation: Weeks 4–5
Goals	Restore full ROM
	Improve quadriceps strength
	Restore proprioception
	Discontinue knee immobilizer
	Quadriceps strength 70% of contralateral side
	Decrease joint effusion
ROM	PROM (0–120°)
Exercises	Knee extension: 60–0°
	Leg press: 0–75°
	Lateral step-ups
	Front and side lunges
	Heel toe raises
	Weeks 6–10
ROM	PROM (0–130°)
Phase IV	Light activity: Months 3–4
Goals	Develops strength, power and endurance
	Begin to prepare for return to functional activities
Exercises	Begin light running program
	Agility drills
	Initiate plyometrics

■ OSGOOD-SCHLATTER DISEASE (FIG. 83)

Osgood-Schlatter disease (OSD) is the inflammation of patellar tendon at its attachment

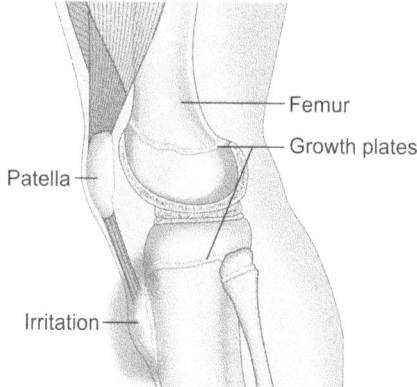

Fig. 83: Osgood-Schlatter disease.

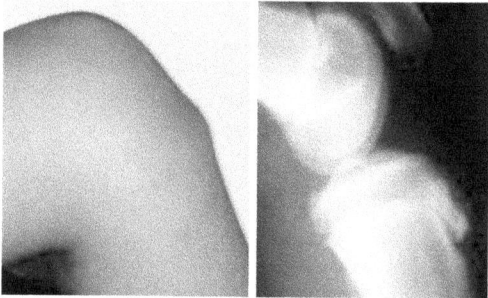

Fig. 84: X-ray findings for Osgood-Schlatter disease.

to the tibial tuberosity. It is also named as apophysitis of tibial tubercle.

Predisposing Factors
- Mostly occurs in adolescent athletes, i.e. 8–13 years girls and 10–15 years boys.
- Males are 3 times more affected than females.
- Repetitive stressful athletic activities, such as jumping, sprinting, etc.

Etiology
Cause is unknown. There are various theories for the cause of Osgood-Schlatter syndrome but the most accepted theory is repetitive contractions of quadriceps (during running, jumping, gym, and other sports) cause an extra-articular stress fracture or micro-avulsion of chondro-fibro-osseous tibial tubercle. It leads to the avulsion of patellar tendon from its attachment to bone that results in microfractures and an elevation of tibial tuberosity progressively during the reconstructive phase, the new bone deposits in avulsed space that results in a deviated and prominent tibial tuberosity.

It is a self-limiting condition that resolves after 1–2 years. It mostly occurs during growth spurts when the bone, muscles and growth plate area near tibial tubercle are weak and prone to get injured.

Clinical Presentation
- Localized pain on tibial tubercle.
- Swelling, tenderness or increased warmth below the patella and over the shinbone.
- Pain that gets worsen with exercise or high impact activities like jumping, running, squatting, ascending and descending stairs.
- Limping after physical activities.
- Enlarged area of calcification of tendon where it attaches to tibia.
- Symptoms are vague, gradual and intermittent in onset.

Diagnosis
Imaging Studies
- **X-ray findings (Fig. 84):** Enlargement or prominence of tibial tubercle.

Physical Examination
- **Observation:**
  - Erythema over proximal tibial.
  - Elevation of tibial tuberosity.
  - Silhouette appearance.
- **Palpation:**
  - Proximal tibial swelling.
  - Tenderness present over tibial tubercle (Fig. 85).
  - Pain with resisted knee extension.
  - Muscle tightness evaluation: Rectus femoris, hamstring
  - Quadriceps weakness and atrophy.
- **Examine gait pattern:** Antalgic gait is usually present because patient avoids

Soft Tissue Injuries

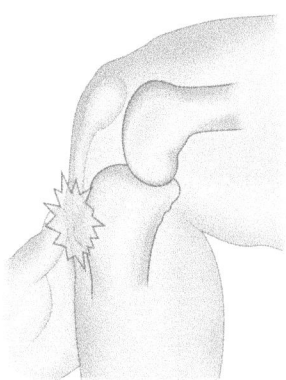

Fig. 85: Tenderness over tibial tubercle.

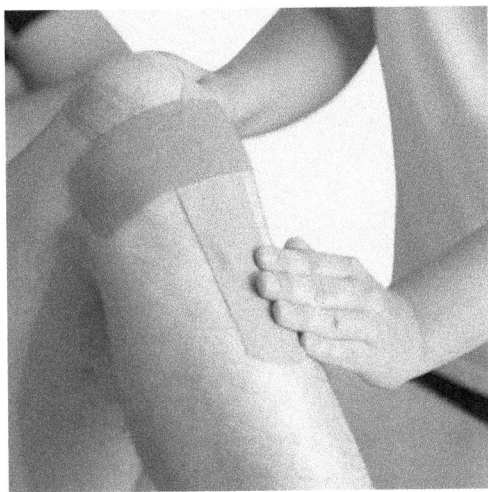

Fig. 87: Kinesiology taping.

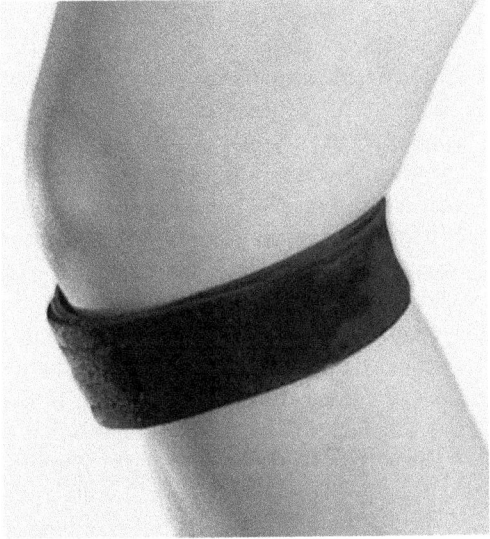

Fig. 86: Infrapatellar strap.

flexing the knee and prefers to ambulate with knee extension.

Management

Conservative Treatment
- **NSAIDs:** To decrease pain and inflammation.
- **Rest:** Avoidance of pain producing activities.
- **Infrapatellar strap, pads or braces (Fig. 86):** It provides support, reduces tension on affected area, absorbs stress and dissipates forces away from the site of OSD.

Physiotherapy Treatment
- **PRICE therapy:** Protection, rest, icing compression and elevation is used in acute phase to reduce pain and inflammation.
- **Taping (Fig. 87):** Taping helps to avoid or minimize undue stress on patellar tendon and support knee during activity.
- **Heat therapy** in chronic phase and pain relieving modalities like TENS/IFT are used to decrease pain.
- **Iontophoresis** using dexamethasone or lidocaine are used for 20 minutes duration and at intensity of 5 mA/min. It is helpful in reducing pain and inflammation.
- **Massage** over quadriceps, hamstring and calf muscles.
- **Stretching exercises:** Stretching of quadriceps, hamstring, hip flexors, calf muscles and iliotibial band is preferred because any tightness in muscle or tissue around knee can pull on patellar tendon and tibial tubercle.
- **Strengthening exercises:** Strengthening of quadriceps, hamstring, hip flexors, calf muscles and iliotibial band is done because the strength imbalance may also increase the stress on patellar tendon and tibial tubercle.

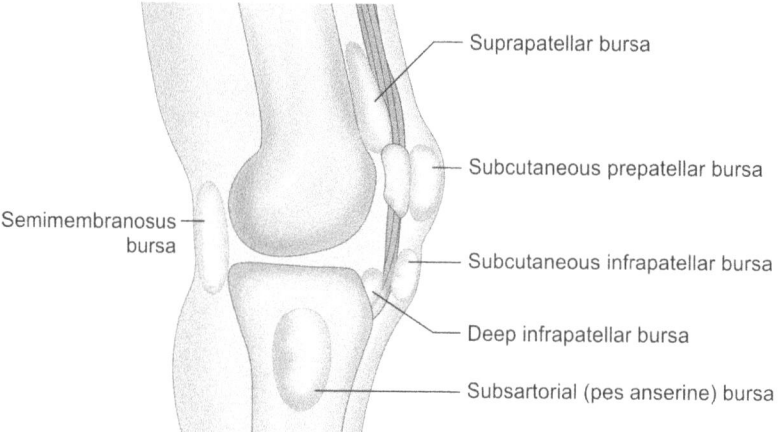

Fig. 88: Knee bursae.

- **Proprioception and balance exercises:** Exercises to improve balance and functional ability should be included in treatment protocol.

◼ KNEE BURSITIS

It is the inflammation of bursa around knee joint.

There are around 11 bursae that located around the knee. Frequently inflamed bursae are—prepatellar bursa, suprapatellar bursa, infrapatellar bursa, semimembranosus bursa and pes anserinus.

Following are most frequently occurring bursitis of knee (Fig. 88):

- **Prepatellar bursitis:** It is the inflammation of bursa present on anterior aspect of knee between skin and patella. It commonly occur due to prolonged kneeling, e.g. gardeners, plumber, roofers, housemaids, etc. It is also known as **housemaids knee.**
- **Pes anserine bursitis:** It is the inflammation of bursa present on medial side of knee between tibia and three adjoined medial knee tendons of semimembranosus, sartorius and gracilis. It commonly occurs due to repetitive activity of related muscles or direct hit in the region of Pes anserine. Overweight middle aged and athletes are commonly affected.
- **Semimembranosus bursitis:** It is the inflammation of bursa present in posteromedial aspect of knee beneath deep fascia of popliteal space between semimembranosus muscle and medial head of gastrocnemius muscle. It is commonly associated with OA knee and medial meniscal tear. It is also known as **popliteal or Baker's cyst.**
- **Infrapatellar bursitis:** It is the inflammation of one or both bursae present below patella. There are two infrapatellar bursa: Superficial and deep infrapatellar bursa.
  - Superficial bursa present between skin and patellar tendon, while deep bursa locates between patellar tendon and proximal tibia. It is also known as **Clergyman's knee.** It commonly occurs due to overuse of patellar tendon of knee with repetitive knee flexion, e.g. stair climbing, jumping or deep squats.
- **Suprapatellar bursitis:** It is the inflammation of bursa present above knee between quadriceps tendon and femur. It commonly occurs due to direct blow onto the knee or repetitive activities like running on uneven surface or occupation require prolonged kneeling.

Two most commonly occurring bursitis are prepatellar bursitis and semimembranosus bursitis.

Soft Tissue Injuries

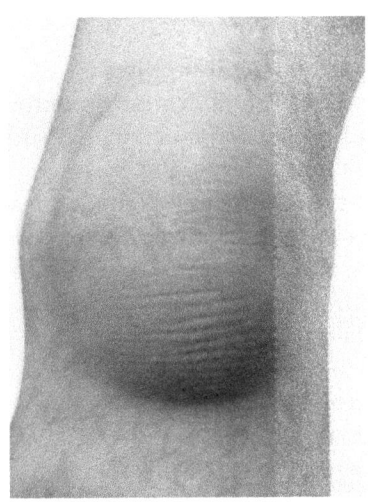

Fig. 89: Swelling.

Etiology

- Direct hit or blow to knee.
- Repeated or prolonged pressures on knee, such as activities require prolonged kneeling.
- Frequent falls on knee.
- Knee arthritis, e.g. gout, rheumatoid arthritis and osteoarthritis.
- Infection can be caused by cut, puncture or an insect bite.

Clinical Presentation

- Localized swelling or lump present over, above or below the patella (Fig. 89).
- Pain and tenderness: Particularly when the bursa gets squeezed during knee movement, i.e. extreme flexion or extension of knee.
- Warmth and redness: At the site of bursa.
- Chronic bursitis may lead to restricted end range of motion of knee joint.
- Pain aggravated by kneeling, squatting or repetitive knee bending.

Diagnosis

- **Imaging studies:**
  - **X-ray:** Radiography may be used to determine the cause of bursitis, such as a broken bone or a piece of bony growth (called a bone spur) or arthritis.
  - **Ultrasound:** Can be used to identify loose bodies or tophaceous gout as underlying causes of the bursitis.
  - **MRI scan:** Can be used for addition assessment in the presence of severe symptomatology and concern for osteomyelitis or abscess.
- **Laboratory test:**
  - **Blood test:** To check an infection, but this is not usually very helpful.
  - Sample of fluid from bursa using a needle is taken to lab for further testing. Presence of pus indicates that the bursa is infected.

Physical Examination

- **Patient history:** Detailed history about the onset of symptoms, pain pattern, history of injury or fall and occupation.
- **Observation:** Swelling and erythema on knee.
- **Palpation:**
  - Tenderness of affected area, i.e. on or near patella.
  - Fluctuant edema over the lower pole of patella.
  - Crepitus of knee.
  - Decreased knee flexion secondary to pain.

Preventive Measures

- Avoid kneeling for prolonged periods of time.
- Use knee pads or cushion during kneeling and other athletic activities to guard the knee joint.
- Avoid direct impact and persistent pressure at front of knee.

Management

Conservative Treatment

- **RICE therapy:**
  - **Rest:** Activities that may aggravate friction and pressure on affected bursa,

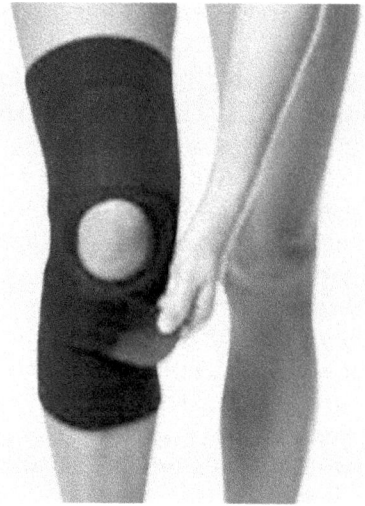

Fig. 90: Knee pad.

such as high impact sports and kneeling or crawling, should be avoided.
- **Cold therapy:** To decrease pain and inflammation for 15 minutes twice or thrice daily.
- **Elevation:** Affected limb should be elevated above the heart level to decrease the pooling of fluid.
- **Compression:** Application of elastic compression bandage over affected knee joint to reduce swelling.
- **Use of knee pads (Fig. 90):** Knee pads are used to decrease friction and pressure on affected bursa.
- **NSAIDs:** To decrease pain and inflammation.
- **Steroid injection:** To reduce pain and inflammation but because of its potential side effects it is commonly used for troublesome cases that are not managed with other possible conservative treatments.
- **Aspiration of fluid:** In this, the fluid is aspirated from inflamed bursa with help of syringe to decrease the pressure.
- **Antibiotics:** Orally or intravenously in septic or infected bursitis.

Physiotherapy Treatment
- **Reduce pain and swelling:**
  - **Activity modification:** Improve the technique and function, e.g. squatting, running, hoping, and walking
  - **Electrotherapeutic modalities (US, TENS, IFT, ES machines that use heat, light, or sound):** To reduce swelling and pain
  - Knee taping
  - Soft tissue massage.
- **Improve motion:** Initially passive and gradually progress to active ROM exercises to improve the ROM of lower limb.
- **Improve flexibility:** Stretching exercises for tight muscles surrounding the knee joint.
- **Improve strength:** Strengthening exercises for weak or injured leg muscles to restore strength and agility.
- **Improve proprioception, balance and agility:** Exercises to improve the balance skills.

Surgical Treatment

Indication: Chronic or septic knee bursitis that are not responding to conservative treatment.

Bursectomy: A surgery to remove the affected bursae called bursectomy.

ANKLE AND FOOT INJURIES

ANKLE SPRAIN

Ankle sprain is partial or complete tear of one or more ligaments of ankle. Lateral ankle sprain are most frequently occurring sprain that accounts for around 85% of all ankle sprains.

Mechanism of Injury (Table 2 and Figs. 91A to C)

It varies according to the different ligament injury.

Soft Tissue Injuries

Table 2: Mechanism of injury.

Aspect	Mechanism of injury	Ligaments
Lateral	Inversion and plantar flexion	• Anterior talofibular ligament • Calcaneofibular ligament • Posterior talofibular ligament
Medial	Eversion	• Posterior tibiotalar ligament • Tibiocalcaneal ligament • Tibionavicular ligament • Anterior tibiotalar ligament
High	External rotation and dorsiflexion	• Anterior-inferior tibiofibular ligament • Posterior-inferior tibiofibular ligament • Transverse tibiofibular ligament • Interosseous membrane • Interosseous ligament • Inferior transverse ligament

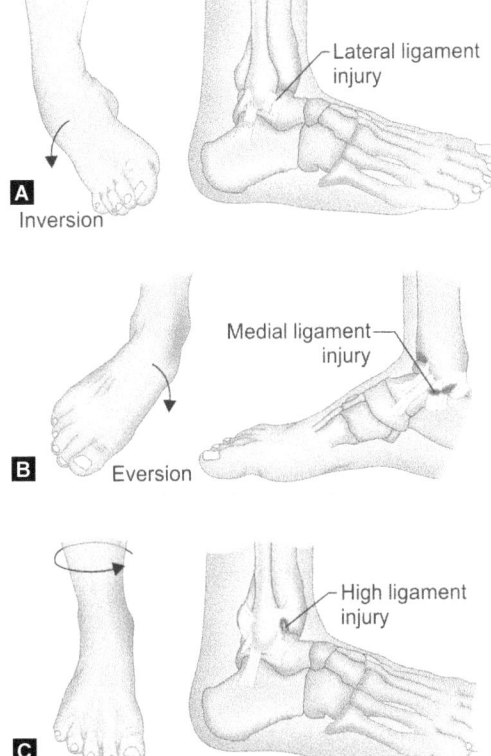

Figs. 91A to C: Mechanism of injury. A. Lateral ligament injury; B. Medial ligament injury; C. High ligament injury.

Clinical Presentation

- Complain of cold foot or paresthesia could be due to compromised neurovascular structure like peroneal nerve.
- Swelling and bruising around ankle joint.
- Inability to put weight on affected ankle.
- Stiffness of affected ankle joint.

Classification of Ankle Sprain on the Basis of Severity

- **Mild sprain/Grade I injury:** In this, affected ligament is stretched along with microscopic tear.
  - Symptoms: Mild swelling with no or mild joint instability.
  - Partial weight bearing.
  - Recovery time: 2–4 weeks.
- **Moderate sprain/Grade II injury:** In this, affected ligament is stretched with partial tear.
  - Symptoms: Mild to moderate swelling, bruising and joint instability.
  - Difficulty in weight bearing.
  - Recovery time: 4–8 weeks.
- **Severe sprain/Grade III injury:** Complete tear of ligament.
  - Symptoms: Acute and severe swelling, bruising and moderate to severe joint instability.
  - Weight bearing is not possible.
  - Recovery time: Up to 3 months.

Diagnosis

Imaging

- **X-ray:** Predominantly, ruling out the ankle fracture is essential particularly where weight bearing is affected.
- **MRI:** To find out the exact location, associated injuries and severity of sprain.

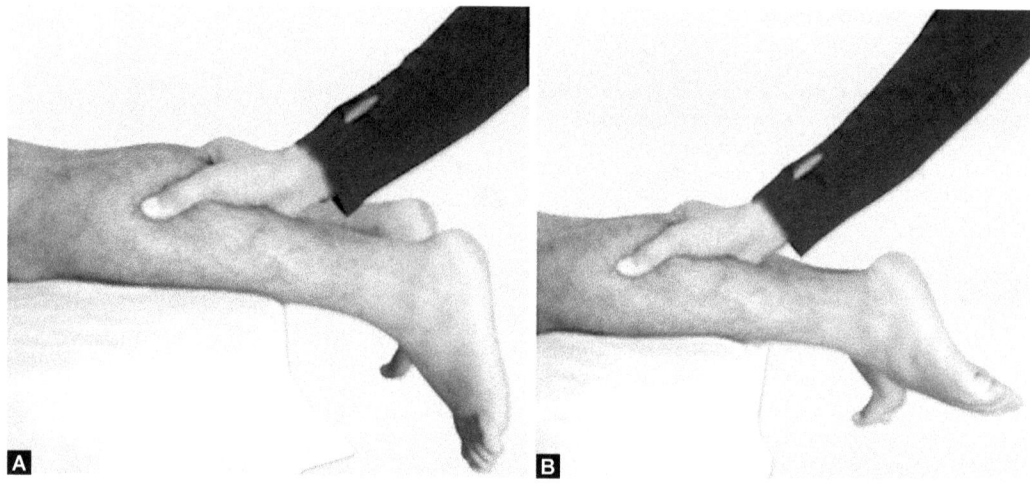

Figs. 92A and B: (A) Ruptured Achilles tendon; (B) Intact Achilles tendon.

Physical Examination

- **Inspection:**
  - Gait pattern
  - Any ankle deformity
  - Swelling, bruising or effusion around ankle or Achilles tendon
  - Any open wounds.
- **Palpation:** Palpate for tenderness around ankle joint, base of fifth metatarsal, calcaneus and whole length of fibula.
- **Examine for neurovascular injury:**
  - Sensation of affected foot.
  - Check the capillary refilling of toes.
  - Distal pulse, i.e. dorsalis pedis artery.
- **Range of Motion**
  - Both AROM and PROM of ankle should be assessed. PROM is usually pain-free as the muscles are not contracting but the end ROM may be painful due to the stretching of muscle.

Special Tests

- **Thompson's test (Figs. 92A and B):** It evaluates the integrity of Achilles tendon. Patient is in prone position with the foot hanging off the edge of the couch. Therapist compresses/squeezes the calf muscles. Absence of foot plantar flexion is interpreted as positive test and indicative of Achilles tendon rupture.
- **Anterior drawer test (Fig. 93):** To assess the ligamentous laxity or ankle instability. The therapist stabilizes the anterior aspect of distal leg with one hand and grasps the heel with the other hand and pulls the foot anteriorly. Excessive anterior translation of foot as compare to the contralateral leg is indicative of a positive test.

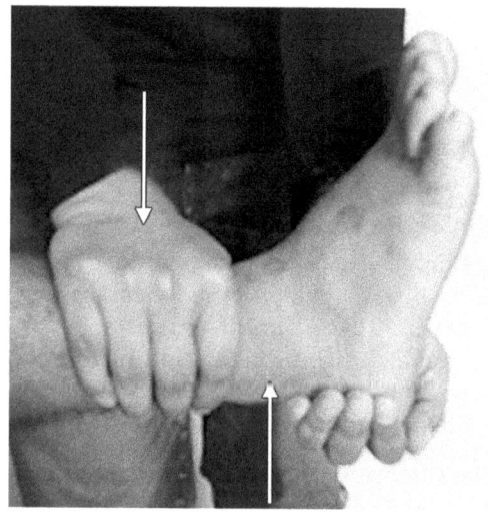

Fig. 93: Anterior drawer test.

Soft Tissue Injuries

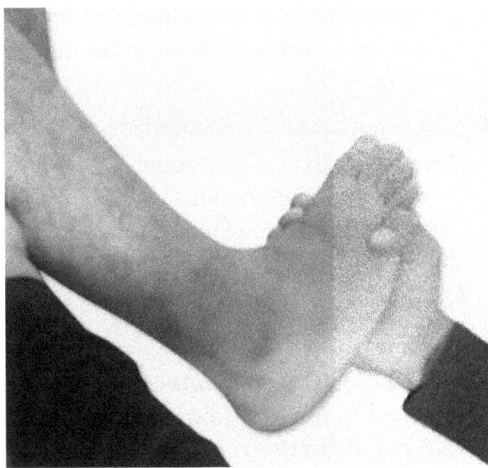

Fig. 94: Talar tilt test.

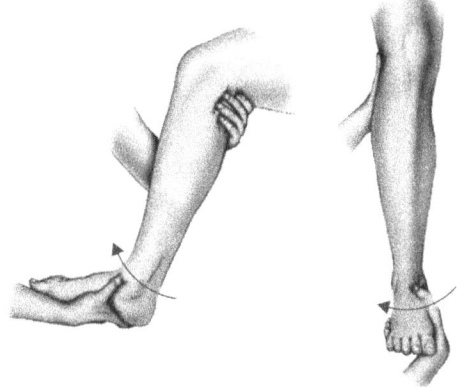

Fig. 96: Kleiger test.

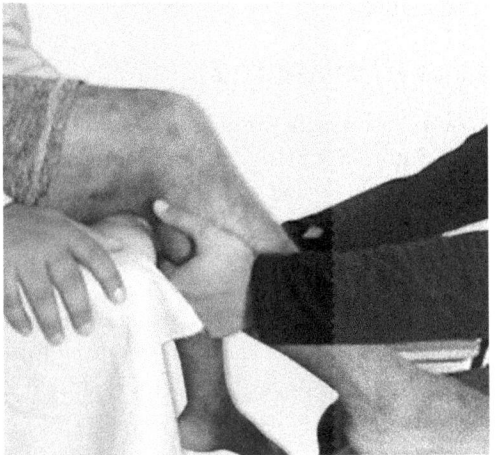

Fig. 95: Squeeze test.

- **Talar tilt test (Fig. 94):** It evaluates the integrity of lateral ligaments of ankle. Patient in high sitting position. Therapist stabilizes distal leg and inverts the ankle. He notices the range of inversion and compares it with contralateral side. Increased or painful inversion indicates the presence of lateral ankle ligament sprain. This test is also known as inversion stress test.
- **Tests for syndesmosis injury:**
  - **Squeeze test (Fig. 95):** Patient is in high sitting position, the therapist squeezes the proximal tibia against the fibula. Test is considered to be positive if it elicit pain in ankle joint or at the syndesmosis.
  - **Dorsiflexion external rotation stress test (Kleiger test) (Fig. 96):** Patient in high sitting position. Therapist stabilizes the proximal tibia with one hand and passively external rotate and then dorsiflex the ankle. A positive test is determined by the presence of pain at syndesmosis.

Management

Physiotherapy Treatment

1. *Acute Phase: From 0–3 Days-RICE Therapy*
- **Rest and activity modification:** Avoid activities that put direct pressure on the affected ankle joint. Crutch can be used to minimize stress over ankle joint.
- **Ice:** Cold pack application for 10–15 minutes, twice or thrice a day to decrease pain and inflammation.
- **Compression:** Application of elastic compression bandage over the ankle joint to reduce the swelling.
- **Elevation:** Keep the foot above the heart level to reduce the swelling.
- **Weight bearing as tolerated:** Higher the grade of sprain, longer the time required for nonweight bearing. Patient may need assistive device for pain-free gait.

2. Subacute Phase: From Day 3–2 Weeks

Goals: To decrease pain, increase pain free ROM, protecting from re-injury with brace or splint, prevent muscle weakness and to decrease swelling.

- **To reduce pain and swelling:** Ice, electrical stimulation (IFT, TENS, HVGS), ultrasound.
- **Joint mobilization:** Talocrural and subtalar joints mobilization to regain pain-free dorsiflexion and to improve stride.
- **ROM within pain-free range:**
  - Dorsiflexion and plantar flexion
  - Initiate inversion and eversion as pain and tenderness decreases
  - Toe curls
  - Ankle alphabets
  - Stationary bike.
- **Progress gait training:** Increase WB and gradually wean from assistive devices as tolerated.
- **Strengthening:** Initiate with isometric exercises
- **Stretching** of gastrocsoleus complex. Initially in nonWB than in WB position.
- **Protection:** Discontinue splint or brace.

3. Rehabilitation Phase: From 2–6 Weeks Post Injury

Goals: To regain ROM, strength and endurance

- Joint mobilization.
- **Stretching:** Achilles tendon, calf muscles.
- **Strengthening exercises:** Dorsiflexors, plantar flexors, evertors and invertors. Progress from active ROM to resisted exercises.
- **Close chain exercises:** For example, bilateral leg toe raise to single leg toe raise, bilateral squat to single squat, step-up and down.
- **Proprioceptive exercises:** Progress from sitting to standing on both legs than single leg, eyes open to eyes close, uneven surface, wobble board, foam pads, pillow, star excursion balance activities.
- **Gait training:** Wean from assistive device.
- **Endurance training:** Swimming, biking, walking.

4. Functional Phase: 6 Weeks Post Injury

- Return to activity and function.
- Progressive strengthening.
- Coordination and agility training: Lunges, hopping, step exercises, zigzag, jump rope, treadmill.

Treatment

- **For Grade III and syndesmotic sprain:** Immobilization in below knee cast is indicated over compression bandage.
- **Surgical treatment is indicated in Grade III injury** associated with fracture or joint instability.

PLANTAR FASCIITIS

Plantar fasciitis is chronic inflammation of the plantar fascia of foot characterized by heel pain. It is also named as Jogger's heel (Fig. 97).

Anatomy

Plantar fascia is a thick fibrous band of connective tissue that originates from anteromedial aspect of calcaneus, stretched underneath the sole of foot and inserted at the base of toes.

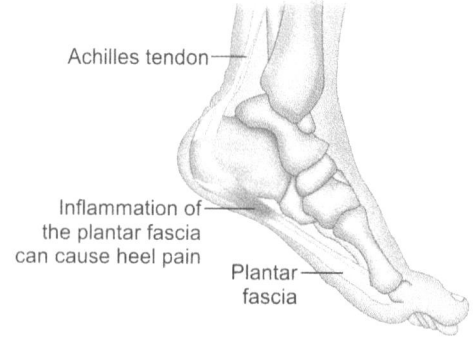

Fig. 97: Plantar fasciitis.

Etiology

Normally plantar fascia acts like a shock absorbing bowstring that also supports the arch of foot. Anatomical deformity of lower limb (like pes cavus, pes planus, excessive femoral anteversion), repetitive stress, tight Achilles tendon, overweight and many other factors that put extensive stress on plantar fascia, leads to collagen degeneration and microtrauma in the fascia progressively causes painful and inflamed plantar fascia.

Predisposing Factors

- Prolonged weight bearing like standing, walking, running, etc.
- Walking barefoot on hard surface
- Increase in physical activity, weight or age.

Commonly associated with:

- Flat feet (hyperpronation) that lead to increase tension of plantar fascia
- Obesity (leading to increase pressure on plantar fascia)
- Shoes with poor arch support
- Tight Achilles tendon
- Loss of fat pad of heel due to aging.

Clinical Presentation

- Stabbing pain on the medial side of heel.
- Most often the pain is worst with few steps after awakening or prolonged sitting. This can be due to the reason that at night or during prolonged rest, the front of foot hangs downward resulting in slight contraction of plantar fascia. In morning, sudden stretching of plantar fascia while walking soon after getting up can lead to heel pain.
- Pain increases on dorsiflexion of toes.
- Pain is severe after an activity than it is during an activity.
- Pain in heel increases gradually and becomes worse overtime.

Diagnosis

X-ray: X-ray finding helps to rule out the other associated condition that can cause heel pain like heel spur, etc (Fig. 98).

Ultrasound: Ultrasound is sometimes done to measure the plantar fascial thickness. A thickness of more than 0.4 cm is indicative of plantar fasciitis.

Physical Examination

- **Palpation:** Tenderness along medial plantar aspect of calcaneus (Fig. 99).
- Decreased dorsiflexion of foot is due to tight calf muscle.
- Dorsiflexion may elicit pain due to stretching of plantar flexors or plantar fascia.

Management

Plantar fasciitis is a self-limiting condition that resolves itself within 6 to 18 months.

Conservative Treatment

- **Medications:** Analgesic or NSAIDs to decrease pain and inflammation.
- **Injection of platelet rich plasma:** It is rich in growth factor that helps in healing process.

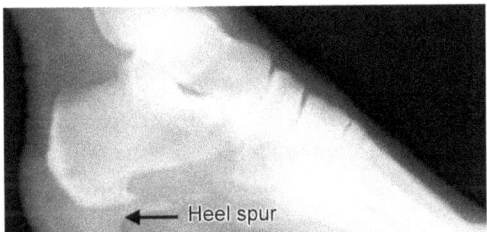

Fig. 98: X-ray findings of plantar fasciitis.

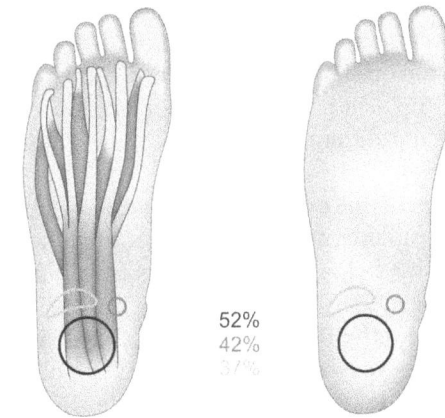

Fig. 99: Plantar fasciitis: Top 3 areas of pain.

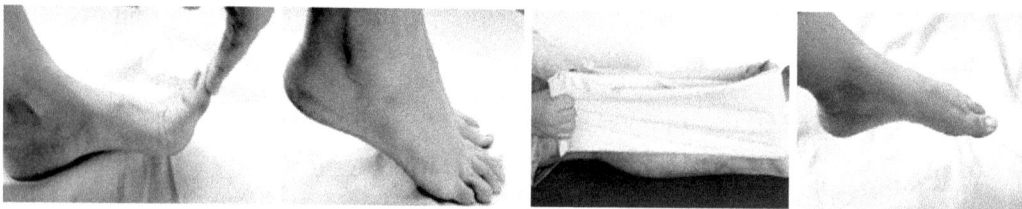

Fig. 100: Stretching exercises of plantar fascia and calf muscle.

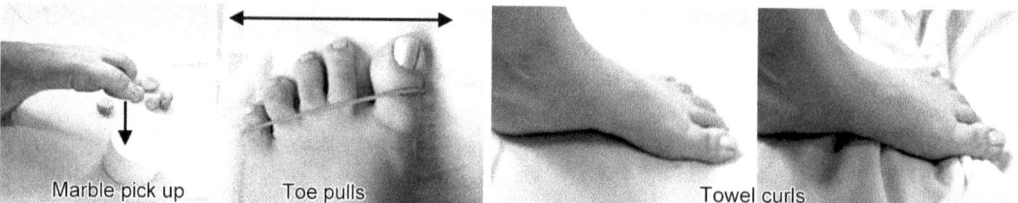

Fig. 101: Strengthening exercises of intrinsic foot muscles.

- **Corticosteroid injection:** In tender area it helps to improve pain and inflammation. It is given once or twice in 3 to 6 months.

Physiotherapy Treatment

- **General measures:**
  - Avoid walking bare foot.
  - Adequate rest to foot since plantar fasciitis often occurs due to overuse.
  - Avoid excessive physical activities to reduce stress on fascia.
- **Ice massage:** To reduce pain and inflammation.
  - Ice cube for 5-10 minutes.
  - Ice bath for 10-15 minutes.
  - Ice pack for 15-20 minutes
- **Pain relieving modalities:** Ultrasound, IFT, TENS, phonophoresis or iontophoresis using dexamethasone ions 2 to 3 times/week.
- **Stretching exercises (Fig. 100):** Stretching of calf muscle, Achilles tendon and plantar fascia helps to reduce stress over plantar fascia.
- **Strengthening exercises (Fig. 101):** Strengthening of intrinsic muscles of foot helps to restore stability of ankle joint and to support the arch of foot.

- **Marble pick up exercise:** Sit on the chair with both the feet in front. Scatter small pebbles or marbles and ask the patient to pick up with his toes, grip it and try to place it in the cup.
- **Toe pulls:** Wrap resistance band around the toes, ask the patient to spread toes outwards against the band's resistance.
- **Towel curls:** While sitting, place the foot on the towel spread on the floor, ask the patient to scrunch the towel with toes.
- **Footwear modifications:**
  - Shoes with thicker, well cushioned midsoles.
  - Firm heel counter to control hind foot.
  - Flat feet: Shoes with better longitudinal arch.
  - Heel cushion (12-15 heel raise).
- **Arch supports and orthotics:**
  - **Taping (Fig. 102):** Arch taping
    - Used to distribute force away from stressed and irritated fascia.
  - **Casting:** Short leg walking cast for 1 month with foot in neutral position.
  - **Orthotics (Fig. 103):** Patients with abnormal biomechanics, such as pes cavus or planus.
    - Semi-rigid, ¾ to full length orthotics with long arch support to limit

Soft Tissue Injuries

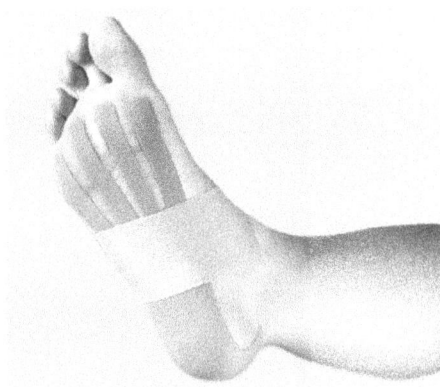

Fig. 102: Arch taping.

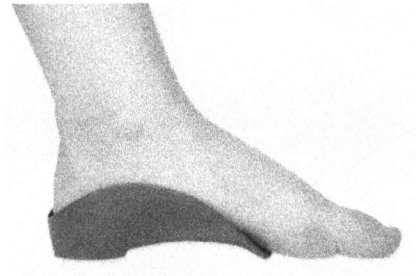

Fig. 104: Heel cups.

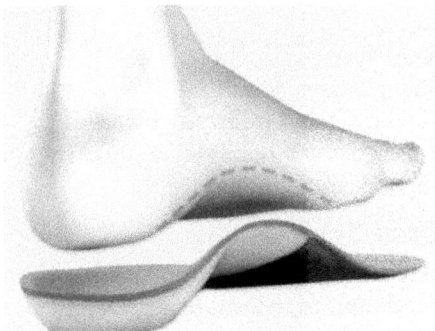

Fig. 103: Orthotics.

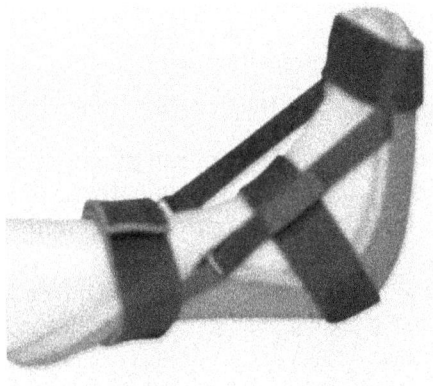

Fig. 105: Night splint.

overpronation of foot and movement of metatarsal heads especially first MT head.
- It reduce symptoms by diminishing and absorbing shock and correct postural deviation or muscular deficiencies that cause plantar fasciitis.
- **Heel cups (Fig. 104):** Heel cups are used to decrease the impact on calcaneus and decrease tension on plantar fascia by elevating the heel on a soft cushion.
- **Night splint (Fig. 105):** To maintain the ankle joint in neutral position or at 5° of dorsiflexion overnight. It helps to passively stretch the plantar flexors and calf muscles.

Surgical Treatment
Surgery for plantar fasciitis is done under rare conditions when the patient does not improve with conservative treatments over prolonged periods.

Plantar fasciotomy: It includes complete release of plantar fascia at its calcaneal attachment with/without the removal of calcaneal spur.

■ RETROCALCANEAL BURSITIS
It is the inflammation of bursa present between uppermost section of calcaneus and anterior to lower one-fourth of Achilles tendon.

It commonly associated with rheumatoid arthritis, gout, trauma and spondyloarthropathies (Fig. 106).

Anatomy
Retrocalcaneal bursa is a small, fluid filled cushioning sac that prevents friction between posterior aspect of calcaneus and Achilles tendon.

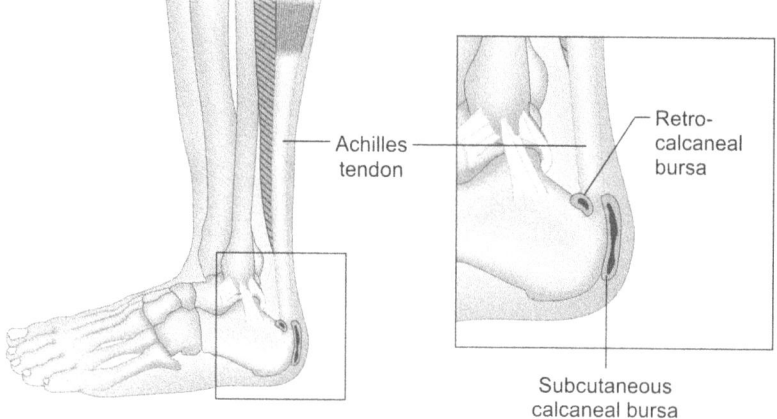

Fig. 106: Retrocalcaneal bursitis.

Etiology

Repetitive contraction of calf muscle, poorly fitted shoes, abnormal biomechanics of foot and many other factors causes continuous rubbing of Achilles tendon against retrocalcaneal bursa. These compressive forces and friction progressively leads to inflammation of bursa.

Predisposing Factors

- Wearing high heeled shoes for long term basis.
- Poor foot biomechanics (particularly flat feet).
- Repetitive athletic activities or overuse.
- Poorly fitted or tight shoes that cause extensive pressure at the posterior aspect of heel.
- Muscle weakness (calf, quadriceps and gluteals)
- Joint stiffness (ankle, subtalar joint or foot)
- Inadequate warm up.
- Being overweight.
- Poor proprioception and balance.
- Inadequate rehabilitation following previous Achilles injury.

Clinical Presentation

- Shooting pain at posterior aspect of heel.
- Swelling and redness of posterior heel (Fig. 107).
- Pain aggravates during activities that require strong and repetitive contractions of calf muscles, such as ascending and descending stairs, running, jumping, etc.
- Painful push off phase of gait.
- Pain worsens on toes standing or wearing high heels.
- In initial associated pain may 'warm up' with activity. But as condition progresses, pain increases during activity also.
- In chronic cases, limping and inability to bear weight on affected foot.

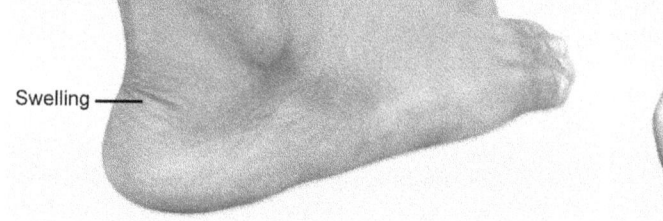
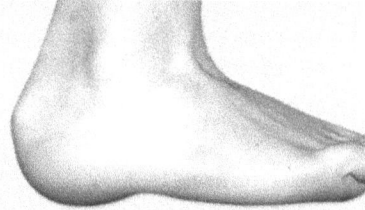

Fig. 107: Swelling and redness of heel.

Diagnosis

Imaging studies: Radiographs may be used to assess the presence of any anatomical deviation like increased prominence of posterosuperior aspect of calcaneus.

MRI shows bursal inflammation. Ultrasonography diagnosed the pathogenesis of Achilles tendon.

Physical Examination

Observation: Any bony prominence or local swelling should be observed.
Palpation: Warmth, tenderness and swelling may be present on posterior aspect of heel.

Preventive Measures

- Maintain good flexibility and strength around the ankle.
- Proper stretching of Achilles tendon.

Management

Conservative Treatment

- **NSAIDs:** To decrease pain and inflammation.
- **Steroid injection:** To reduce pain and inflammation.
- **Aspiration of fluid:** The fluid from the inflamed bursa is aspirated with help of syringe to decrease the pressure.
- **Antibiotics:** Orally or intravenously in case of septic or infected bursitis.
- **Orthotics:** Heel wedges used to:
  - To minimize stress in Achilles tendon.
  - To restore normal biomechanics of the foot.
  - To decrease friction over the bursa.
- **Footwear modification:**
  - Heel counter should be replaced with soft leather insert.
  - Shoes without laces should be avoided because these types of footwears are closely fitted to heel.
  - Heel cup inserts in shoes help to raise inflamed region slightly above heel counter of shoes.
  - Use of open backed shoes.

Physiotherapy Treatment

- **RICE therapy:**
  - **Rest:** Activities that may aggravate friction and pressure on affected bursa should be avoided.
  - **Cold therapy:** To decrease pain and inflammation for 15 minutes twice or thrice daily.
  - **Elevation of limb:** Affected limb should be elevated above the heart level to decrease the pooling of fluid.
  - **Compression:** Application of elastic compression bandage over the affected ankle joint to reduce swelling.
- **Contrast baths:** Contrast bath is used to decrease pain and inflammation by improving the circulation.
- **Ultrasound:** Helps to reduce pain, inflammation and facilitate the blood circulation and healing process.
- **Joint mobilization:** Ankle, subtalar, foot mobilization to accelerate blood circulation and fluid movement that may aid the healing process.
- **Stretching exercises:** Progressive stretching of Achilles tendon to relieve compression over the bursa.
- **ROM exercises:** To maintain mobility of joints, e.g. foot DF and PF, eversion/inversion, circles.

Surgical Treatment

Indications

- Presence of persistent or progressive symptoms
- Not responding to any conservative treatment.
- Causing functional disability

Types of Surgical Interventions

- **Bursectomy:** Surgical removal of inflamed bursa and resection of prominent bone if present.
- Repair of ruptured or avulsed Achilles tendon.

CHAPTER 2

Fractures and Dislocations

■ GENERAL INTRODUCTION OF FRACTURE

Definition

Break/crack in the bone or break in the continuity of bone is known as fracture. It occurs when the force applied against the bone is stronger than the actual mechanical strength of bone.

■ CLASSIFICATION OF FRACTURES

On the basis of integrity of skin and soft tissue:
- **Closed/simple fracture:** These are the broken bones that remain within the body and do not penetrate the skin.
- **Open/compound fractures:** These are the broken bones that penetrate through the skin and expose the bones and deep tissues to the external environment.

On the basis of location of fracture line (Fig. 1):
- **Epiphyseal fracture:** Fracture that involves the epiphysis of bone, (i.e. the rounded end part of bone).
- **Physeal fracture:** Fracture that involves the epiphyseal plate or growing plate (translucent, cartilaginous disc separating the epiphysis from the metaphysis and is responsible for the longitudinal growth of the bone). These fractures are also known as Salter-Harris fracture or growth plate fracture.
- **Metaphyseal fracture:** Fractures that involves the metaphysis (narrow portion of a long bone between epiphysis and diaphysis) of bone. These fractures are also known as corner fracture or bucket handle fractures.
- **Diaphyseal fracture:** Fractures that involve the diaphysis of bone (i.e. midsection or shaft of a long bone).

On the basis of extent of fracture line:
- **Incomplete fracture:** Also known as partial fracture. In these fractures, the bone does not break completely means it cracks without breaking all the way through.

  Types of Incomplete Fracture
  - **Greenstick fractures (Fig. 2):** These are incomplete fractures characterized

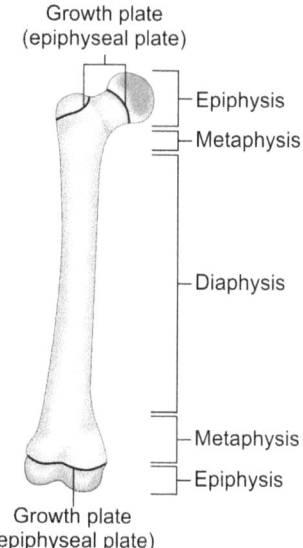

Fig. 1: Classification of fracture (on the basis of location of fracture line).

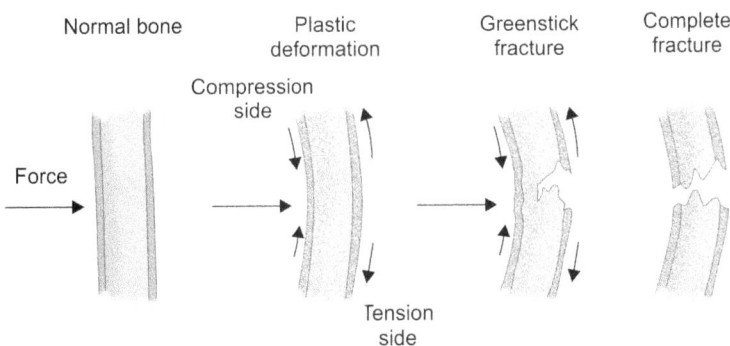

Fig. 2: Greenstick fracture.

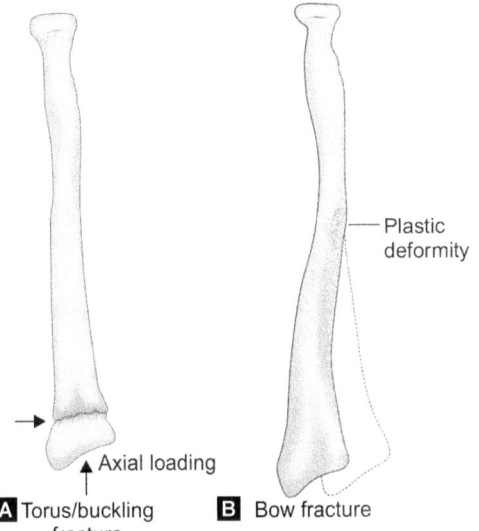

Figs. 3A and B: Buckle or bow fracture.

by the presence of breaks only on one side of the bone. It occurs by the application of perpendicular force along the longitudinal axis of the bone that eventually leads to fracture on the convex surface of the bent bone however the concave surface of the bone remains intact as the applied force is not strong enough to break the bone completely. They are commonly mid diaphyseal.
- **Buckle or torus fracture (Fig. 3A):** These are incomplete fractures of the shaft of long bone characterized by the bulging of cortex in which the bone is broken on one side and a bump or raised buckle develops on the other side. They result from trabecular compression from an axial loading force along the long axis of the bone. Commonly seen in children, frequently involving the distal radial metaphyseal.
- **Bowing fracture (Fig. 3B):** Angulated/curved bone along its longitudinal axis. It occurs when an angulated longitudinal force is applied to a bone. When the applied force is greater than the mechanical strength of the bone, the bone undergoes plastic deformation and remains in its bowed position even after the discontinuation of the force.
- **Hairline fracture:** A thin crack in the bone is known as hairline fracture.
- **Stress fracture:** Stress fractures are the small cracks in a bone caused by the repetitive stress or injury.
- **Complete fracture:** In a complete fracture, the bone breaks completely and snapped or crushed into two or more pieces. Types of complete fractures are (Fig. 4):
  - **Single fracture:** Fracture in which the bone is broken at one place or into two pieces.
  - **Segmental fracture:** Fracture in which the bone is broken at two places in a

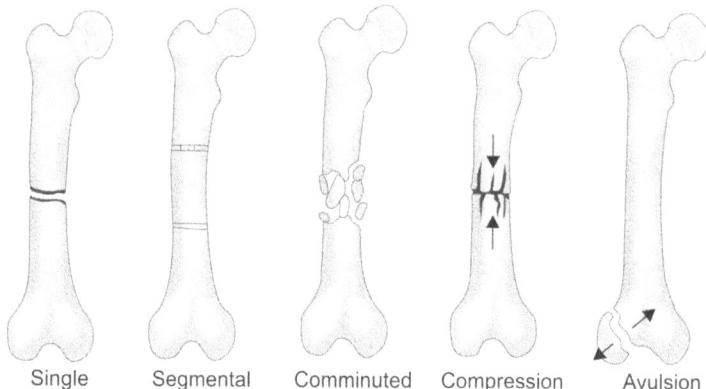

Fig. 4: Types of complete fracture.

way that leaves at least one segment floating and unattached.
- **Comminuted fracture:** Fractures in which the bone is broken into more than two fragments.
- **Compression fracture:** Fractures in which the bone is crushed and flattens under pressure.
- **Avulsion fracture:** Fracture in which a fragment of bone is pulled off often by a tendon or ligament.

On the basis of alignment of the fragments of fractured bone (Fig. 5):
- **Nondisplaced fracture:** When fracture fragments are in anatomical alignment.

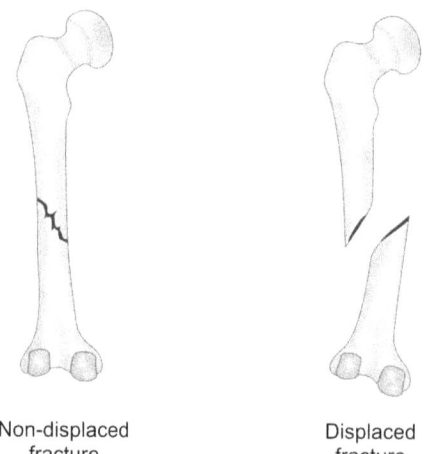

Fig. 5: Classification of fracture (on the basis of alignment of the fragments).

- **Displaced fracture:** When fracture fragments are not in their normal anatomical alignment.

Displacement can be of following types (Fig. 6):
- **Lateral displacement:** When the fragments of fractured bone are laterally displaced.
- **Angular displacement:** When the fragments of fractured bone forms an angle with each other, e.g. varus, valgus.
- **Overlapping/impacted fracture:** In buckled or impacted fracture the ends of the fractured fragments driven into each other.
- **Rotational displacement:** When the fragments of fractured bone rotates in relation to each other.
- **Distracted displacement:** When the fragments of fractured bone are pulled apart.

On the basis of the angle of the fractured line (Fig. 7): It depends on the direction of applied force to a bone.
- **Transverse fracture:** When the bone is fractured horizontally along its length. It occurs when the applied force is perpendicular to the long axis of a bone.
- **Oblique fractures:** These are the slanted fractures, i.e. the fracture line runs oblique to the long axis of the shaft of bone. It occurs when a force is applied at any angle other than a right angle to the bone.

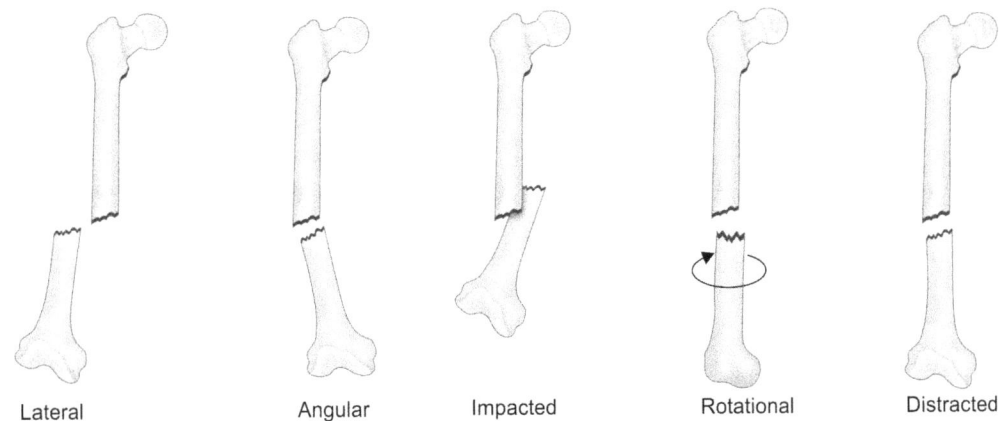

Fig. 6: Types of displacement.

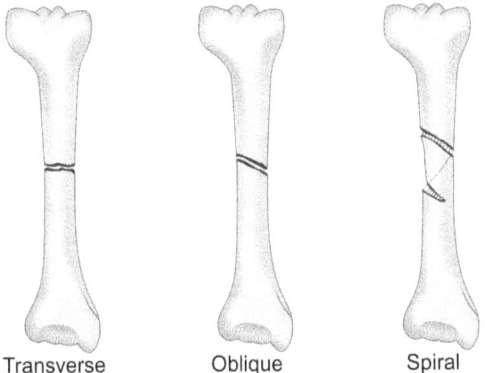

Fig. 7: Classification of fracture on the basis of angle of fracture line.

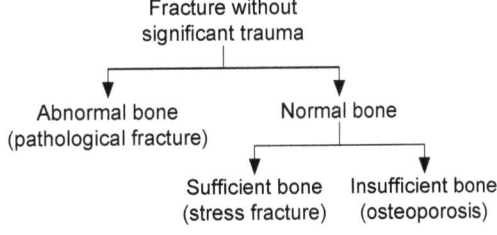

Fig. 8: Causes of fracture.

- **Spiral fractures:** It occurs when an extreme twisting force is exerted on a bone and the break is helical, i.e. fracture line spirals along the long axis.

Causes of Fracture (Fig. 8)
- **Direct injury:** Includes the traumatic incidents, such as direct high impact, fall or vehicle accidents.
- **Indirect injury:**
  - **Pathological fractures (Fig. 9):** Fractures caused by the medical conditions that weaken the bone and predispose them to fracture more easily, e.g. osteoporosis, infection, osteogenesis imperfect or some cancer conditions.

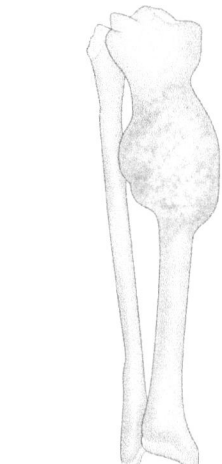

Fig. 9: Pathological fracture.

  - **Stress fracture:** Stress fractures are tiny cracks in a bone that develop over a period of time due to repetitive application of force. It is generally considered as overuse injury. They commonly occurs in athletes and military recruits.

Symptoms of Fracture

- **Intense pain:** In the area of fracture which get worsen with movement, weight bearing or applying pressure.
- **Swelling and tenderness:** Around the injured area
- **Bruising:** That is discoloration of the skin around the affected area.
- **Bleeding:** In case of open fracture.
- **Deformity:** Abnormal angulation of the affected area or limb.
- **Grating sensation** in the affected bone or joint.
- **Loss of function:** Inability to put weight or move the affected area.
- **Loss of mobility:** Inability to move the joint above or below an injury.

Diagnosis of Fracture

Diagnosis is made after carrying out physical examination and identifying the signs and symptoms.

X-ray is used to confirm the site, severity and the type of fractures.

CT scan and MRI scan helps to examine the associated soft tissue injuries along with bone condition.

■ COMPLICATIONS OF FRACTURE

Early Complications

Local Complications

- **Damage to blood vessels** that cause internal or external hemorrhage, e.g. damage to major branches of femoral artery in pelvic fracture.
- **Damage to viscera:** For example, fracture of skull, ribs, or pelvic bones may cause injury to brain, lungs or urinary bladder, respectively.
- **Damage to nerves:** For example, radial nerve injury in shaft of humerus fracture.
- **Damage to soft tissue:** Damage to surrounding soft tissue.
- **Hemarthrosis or articular bleeding:** It is the bleeding in the joint cavity. It is common associated with intra-articular fractures.
- **Compartment syndrome/Volkmann's ischemia:** It is a painful condition occurs due to increased interstitial pressure within the closed osseo-fasical compartment resulting in tissue ischemia in the affected area. It may leads to permanent disability in chronic stages.
- **Wound infection:** It is more common in open fractures.

Systemic Complications

- **Hypovolemic shock:** It is a condition results from rapid fluid loss leads to multiple organ failure due to inadequate organ perfusion and tissue oxygenation. It may occur due to excessive external or internal bleeding following fracture.
- **Thromboembolism:** It refers to the blockage of blood vessel by a thrombus (blood clot) that is detached from its original site of formation. It may cause disabling or even life-threatening complications. It includes both deep vein thrombosis (DVT) and Pulmonary embolism (PE).
- **Fat embolism:** It refers to the presence of fat globules in the circulation resulting in pulmonary and systemic symptoms like fever, respiratory distress, irregular heartbeats, petechial rashes, mental confusion, and may results in coma or death.

Late Complications

Local Complications

- **Delayed union:** It refers to the condition when the fracture takes longer than normal time to heal.
- **Nonunion:** When the fracture does not heal and there are no signs of healing even after 3 to 6 months.
- **Malunion:** When the fracture does not heal in normal alignment and heals in wrong position or alignment.
- **Joint stiffness:** It occurs due prolonged immobilization of joint in plaster of Paris (POP) cast.

- **Contracture:** It refers to the permanent shortening of muscles, tendons or other soft tissues leading to the deformity of joint. It commonly occurs due to prolonged immobilization.
- **Myositis ossificans:** It occurs when calcification and bony masses forms within the muscle near the fractured bone which restricts the movement of proximal joint, e.g. most common complication of supracondylar fracture of humerus.
- **Avascular necrosis/osteonecrosis:** It refers to the death of bone tissue that occurs due to the interruption of the blood supply to the affected bone.
- **Algodystrophy/Sudeck's atrophy:** It is a chronic and progressive neuroinflammatory condition that is characterized by continuous, intense pain with swelling, warmth, redness and trophic changes.
- **Osteomyelitis:** It refers to an infection and inflammation of bone that occurs when a bacteria or fungi enters the bone tissue from the bloodstream due to injury or surgery.
- **Growth disturbance or deformity:** Due to disruption of bone growth. It usually occurs in physeal fractures in children.

Systemic Complications
- **Gangrene:** Gangrene refers to the decay or death of tissue due to lack of blood supply. There are three major types of gangrene: dry, moist and gas gangrene. Gas gangrene is more prevalent in open fractures.
  Gas gangrene is an invasive anaerobic infection usually found in deep wound contaminated with anaerobic clostridia. It is characterized by massive, acute progressive muscle necrosis and severe intoxication of the organism.
- **Tetanus:** Tetanus is caused by infection with bacterium *Clostridium tetani*. It is characterised by stiffness of jaw and tetanic spasm of neck and back muscles. Open fractures are more prone as the bacteria enters through punctured wound.
- **Septicemia:** Septicemia is a life threatening complication that happens when infection enters the blood and spread throughout the body.
- **Pressure sore:** A pressure sore refers to the localized injury to the skin or underlying tissues as a result of constant pressure over a defined area, usually over the bony prominence. This constant pressure causes the disruption of the blood supply and results in the deprivation of the oxygen and nutrients to the area.

STAGES OF FRACTURE HEALING (FIG. 10)

Fracture healing is a natural process that persists for several months. It can be divided into three major phases:

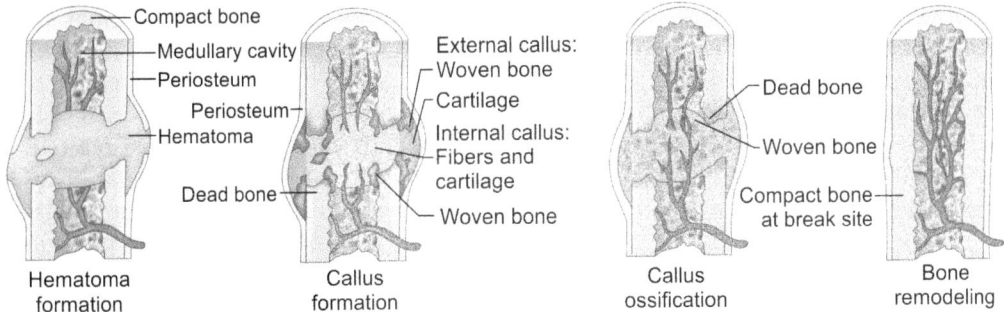

Fig. 10: Stages of fracture healing.

Stage 1: Inflammatory Phase

Duration: From 0 day to approx 2 weeks
The healing process starts immediately after the occurrence of fracture. Small blood clot known as hematoma, are formed around the fracture ends which attracts the white blood cells that causes inflammatory response, i.e. vasodilatation, hyperemia and proliferation of macrophages and polymorphonuclear neutrophils, etc. This in turn triggers the growth of new blood vessels and recruitment of some proteins and helps in bone building process. Gradually the hematoma becomes organized, infiltrated by fibrovascular tissue and replaced by the granulation tissue. Necrotic bones at fractured ends are removed by osteoclasts.

Stage 2: Reparative Phase

Duration: From 2nd week to 6–12 weeks
In this phase, gradual conversion of granulation tissue to fibrous tissue takes place due to intramembranous ossification. The ossified fibrous tissue with ingrowing vessels forms the soft callus or primary callus. Progressively this soft callus becomes organized and remodeled into hard callus over several weeks. The hard callus is the complete replacement of callus into calcified tissue due to intramembranous and endochondral ossification.

Stage 3: Remodelling Phase

Duration: From 6–12 weeks to several months or years
This phase is the longest phase that may continue for several years. It begins once the hard callus, (i.e. solidly united woven bone) has formed. In this phase, conversion of woven bone into lamellar bone occurs through surface erosion and osteonal remodeling. Now the bone is completely returned to its original anatomical morphology including the restoration of medullary canal.

Factors Affecting Fracture Healing

The rate and degree of fracture healing depends both on local and systemic factors:

Systemic Factors

- **Age:** Young patient heals rapidly with remarkable ability of remodeling and deformity correction. The rate of healing declines with increasing age.
- **Nutrition:** Good nutrition can influence the speed, comfort and completeness of bone renewal process. Vitamins (particularly B, C, D and K) and minerals (such as calcium, phosphorous, magnesium, silicon and zinc) have key role in bone healing.
- **Systemic diseases:** Diseases like diabetes, osteoporosis and other immune deficiency disease causes delay in healing process.
- **Hormones:** Growth hormone, thyroid hormone, calcitonin, insulin, etc. facilitates the healing process where as corticosteroids delays the healing.

Localized Factors

- **Degree of trauma:** The more extensive the bone and soft tissue injury, the poorer the outcome.
- **Type of bone:** Cancellous bones heal faster than cortical bones because cancellous bones are more stable, have greater surface area and better blood supply.
- **Blood supply to fracture site:** Associated vascular injuries impairs the blood supply that can significantly delays the fracture healing process.
  Talus, femoral head and scaphoid bones fracture have high incidence of delayed or malunion due to their vulnerable blood supply.
- **Alignment of bone ends:** Normal alignment of fractured fragments needed for optimal and faster union. Excessive traction, displacement and impaction of fracture ends could impede the migration of mesenchymal cells and vascular invasion that may result in malunion, delayed union, nonunion and other complications.
- **Type of fracture:**
  - Spiral or oblique fracture unites more rapidly than transverse fractures.

Transverse fracture approximately takes double time to heal as compared to spiral or oblique fracture because of their smaller surface area of contact and these fractures are often caused by high energy injuries.
- Closed fractures heal faster than open fractures. In open fractures extensive damage to soft tissues disrupt the blood supply to the fracture site and due to the exposure to external environment chances of infections are more that collectively delays the healing process.
- Segmental fractures have increase probability of delayed union or malunion because of disrupted intramedullary blood supply to the middle fragment.

- **Intra-articular fracture:** Healing of intra-articular fracture is comparatively slow because of dilution of fracture hematoma by synovial fluid. Excessive movement at the fracture site interferes with vascularisation of the fracture hematoma, causing high strain through the tissues and disturbs the bridging callus.

Treatment

The plan of the treatment depends on the site and type of fracture. The primary aim of the treatment is to determine the alignment of fractured bone. Proper alignment is compulsory for proper healing and restoration of original bone anatomy present before fracture with normal musculature, innervation and movements of joint.

Objective

The ideal objective of fracture treatment is to provide a completely rehabilitated patient as quickly as possible. Following steps are taken to fulfill the objective of treatment:

- **Reduction:** Reduction of bone ends of fractured bone is done to maintain the proper alignment of fractured bone and faster healing.
- **Immobilization:** Immobilization is done to maintain the ongoing healing process and to avoid unnecessary stress or load over the fracture site which can hinder the healing process, e.g. splints, plaster caster or inter/external applied metal fixators are used to immobilize the affected area.
- **Physiotherapy treatment:** Postoperatively or post-immobilization ROM exercises, strengthening exercises and mobilization of joints are given to prevent joint stiffness, fracture disease, and muscle atrophy.
- **Rehabilitation of the patient** with home exercise programs with regular follow-up is done to restore the functional abilities of patient's daily life.

Reduction and Immobilization

In case of displacement, the bone is re-positioned to maintain the proper alignment of fractured bone ends. This repositioning of bone is called "reduction." Reduction is followed by immobilization to stabilize the bone that allows the firm reunion of broken pieces. According to the severity, displacement and location of fracture there can be of two types of reduction which are as follows:

1. **Closed reduction:** Repositioning of bone without surgery is "closed reduction", i.e. the displaced bone ends are manually maneuvered back into its previous position. It is followed by a period of immobilization with casting or splinting for several weeks. It is indicated in non-displaced fracture or whenever a fracture can be reduced to the point at which the displacement is not more than one-half the width of the diaphysis of the broken bone.

2. **Open reduction:** Repositioning of bone using surgery is "open reduction." Internal or external rods and/or pins, screws or metal plates may be used to fix and immobilize the bone.
    - **Open reduction internal fixation (ORIF):** In this technique, the bone fragments are first repositioned or reduced in their normal alignment and

then held together by using screws, nails, wires, metal plates or by inserting rods down through the marrow space in the center of the bone. Even after the healing of fracture the metal hardware can be left within the body unless it is not causing any discomfort to the patient. It is most commonly indicated in displaced intra-articular fracture, inadequate closed reduction or irreducible fracture, pathological fracture, displaced epiphyseal fracture, fracture with compromised neurovascular structures and open fractures, etc.
- **External fixation:** In this technique, metal pins or screws are placed into the broken bone above and below the fracture site that are connected to a metal bar outside the skin. This forms a stabilizing frame that holds the bones in the proper position until the fracture is healed. Once it occurs, pins and frame are removed. This operative technique is indicated when there is extensive damage or loss of skin, surrounding soft tissues and bone.

Physiotherapy and Rehabilitation

Prolonged immobilization may results in restricted range of motion of proximal joints of fracture, muscle weakness and decreased functional ability. Physiotherapy during and after immobilization helps to:
- Restore complete joint ROM
- Strengthen the surrounding muscles
- Reduce pain and stiffness
- Improves the flexibility
- Improves balance and coordination
- Restore the functional ability.

UPPER LIMB FRACTURES

■ CLAVICLE FRACTURE

Clavicle fracture is a break in the collarbone. It is one of the most commonly fractured bones.

Mechanism of Injury
- Most often caused by direct fall on shoulder.
- Fall onto an outstretched arm (FOOSH).
- Direct blow or trauma to shoulder.
- In infant, clavicle fracture commonly occurs during passage through the birth canal.

Clinical Presentation
- Sagging of shoulder downward and forward.
- "A" deformity or bump over the break.
- Bruising, swelling and/or tenderness over collarbone.
- Inability to lift arm because of pain.
- Grinding sensation on raising the arm.

Classification of Fracture (Fig. 11 and Table 1)

Allman classification of clavicle fracture is based on the position of fracture line.

Fracture healing time: 6 to 12 weeks

Management

Nonsurgical Treatment
- **Closed reduction and immobilization:** Immobilization in a simple arm sling or eight brace/Gilchrist bandages for 3–4 weeks after closed reduction of fracture in an attempt to retain the normal position.
  Indications:
  - Closed undisplaced clavicle fracture.
  - Slightly displaced stable clavicle fracture.

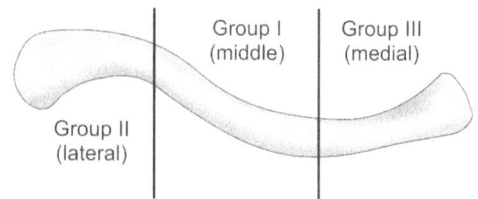

Fig. 11: Classification of clavicle fracture.

Table 1: Allman classification of clavicle fracture.

Group I	Middle third fractures (80% cases)
Group II	**Distal or lateral third fractures (15% cases)**
Type I	Minimally displaced/inter ligamentous
Type II	Displaced fractures. Fracture medial to the coracoclavicular ligaments
IIA	Both ligaments (conoid and trapezoid) attached to distal fragment
IIB	Conoid torn, trapezoid attached to distal fragment
Type III	Fracture involving articular surface
Type IV	Intact coracoclavicular ligaments attached to periosteal sleeve plus proximal fragment displaced
Type V	Comminuted
Group III	**Fracture of proximal or medial third (5% cases)**
Type I	Minimal displacement
Type II	Displaced
Type III	Intra-articular
Type IV	Epiphyseal separation
Type V	Comminuted

Surgical Treatment
- **Open reduction and internal fixation (ORIF):** The fragments are fixed with plate or pin fixation and limb is immobilized in sling for 3-4 weeks.
  Indications:
  - Open fractures
  - Associated neurovascular injury
  - Completely displaced fracture
  - Unstable clavicle fracture
  - Ipsilateral scapular neck fracture
  - Multiple injuries, such as ipsilateral injury to the sternum, ribs or contralateral clavicle.

Complications
- **Pneumothorax:** Clavicle fractures rarely causing (only around 1-3%) pneumothorax. It may develop secondary to perforation of the upper lobe of lung by sharp fractured fragment of clavicle.
- **Subclavin vessels injury:** Clavicle fractures are cited as the cause of around 50% of traumatic subclavin artery injuries usually causes life-threatening hemorrhages.
- **Brachial plexus paresis:** Middle cord of brachial plexus is commonly affected due to its close proximity to overlying clavicle. Brachial plexus compression commonly results from hypertrophic callus formation.
- **Nonunion:** Contributory factors to nonunion in clavicle fracture may include severe initial trauma, marked initial displacement and shortening, soft tissue interposition, inadequate initial immobilization, refracture, primary ORIF, and open fracture, etc.
- **Malunion or cosmetic deformity:** Shortening, angulation and displacement commonly occurs after closed management of fracture.
- **Increased chances for refracture:** As the clavicle is a flat bone, there are more chances of refracture. The chances of refracture increeaces further when the clavicle is healed in a bent position and treated nonoperatively.

Table 2: Postoperative physiotherapy protocol for clavicle fracture.

	Precaution	ROM exercises	Strengthening exercises
Week 0–2	Shoulder in adduction and IR and elbow in 90° flexion	• No ROM to shoulder when treated nonoperatively • Gentle pendulum exercise of shoulder in sling if treated with ORIF • AROM to wrist and hand	• No strengthening for shoulder. • Gentle isometric for elbow, wrist and hand
Weeks 2–4	Same as above	Gentle pendulum exercise for shoulder in sling	• Initiate gentle isometric exercise for shoulder muscle • Isotonic exercise of wrist and hand
Weeks 4–6	Limitation of shoulder abduction to 80°	Gentle AROM for shoulder	Pendular exercise with gravity elimination
Weeks 6–8	None	AAROM for shoulder	Resisted exercises for shoulder
Weeks 8–12	None	Complete PROM with gentle stretching to shoulder in all planes	PRE to shoulder

(ROM: range of motion; AROM: active range of motion; ORIF: open reduction and internal fixation; PRE: Progressive resistance exercises)

Postoperative physiotherapy treatment: Table 2 shows the postoperative physiotherapy protocol for clavicle fracture.

■ SCAPULAR FRACTURE

Scapular fractures are quiet uncommon injuries and accounts for only 3% of all shoulder fractures and approximately 1% of all skeletal injuries.

Mechanism of Injury

- **Direct injuries:** High energy trauma, e.g. motor vehicle accidents (MVA) or falling from significant height.
- **Indirect injury:** FOOSH when the load is transmitted axillary through arm on the outstretched arm.
- **Traction injuries:** Due to pull of muscles or ligaments that may results in avulsion fractures.

Clinical Presentation

- Sudden pain and swelling on the posterior aspect for shoulder at the time of injury.
- Pain during shoulder and upper back movement.
- Tenderness over shoulder blade.
- Inability to perform overhead activity.

Classification

Classification Based on the Location of Fracture

Type I: Scapular body fractures (54%)
Type II: Coracoid, spine and acromion fractures (17%)
Type III: Glenoid (rim and fossa) and neck (surgical and anatomic necks) fractures (29%).

Coracoid fracture classification (Fig. 12)

Type I	Fractures proximal to coracoclavicular ligament
Type II	Fractures distal to coracoclavicular ligament

Acromial fracture classification

Type I	Nondisplaced or minimally displaced
Type II	Displaced but does not compromise subacromial space
Type III	Displaced and compromises subacromial space

Fractures and Dislocations

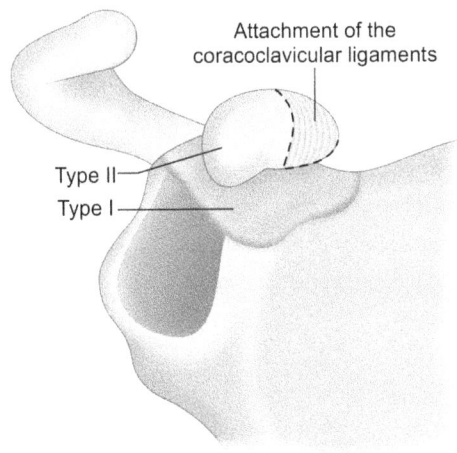

Fig. 12: Coracoid fracture classification.

Figure 13 and Table 3 shows the classification of glenoid and neck fracture of scapula.

Complications
- **Nonunion or malunion:** Commonly associated with nonoperative treatment.
- **Early post-traumatic arthritis:** Postoperative arthritis commonly occurs due to articular incongruity after nonoperative treatment.
- **Glenohumeral instability:** Recurrent shoulder subluxation or dislocation may occur due to the failure of anatomic reduction of large glenoid rim fractures.
- **Subacromion impingement syndrome:** It may occur due to malunion of a displaced acromion fracture.
- **Neurovascular injury:** Suprascapular nerve injury and subclavin vessels are commonly associated with scapular fracture.
- **Compartment syndrome of supraspinatus and infraspinatus fossa:** Fracture of scapula increase the pressure in ossseofasical compartment in supraspinatus or infraspinatus fossa that may lead to compartment syndrome.
- **Associated injuries:** About 80–90% cases of scapular fractures are associated with injuries of adjacent or distant osseous and soft tissue structures.
  - Fracture of rib, spine, and ipsilateral clavicle fracture.
  - Anterior or posterior shoulder dislocation
  - Brachial plexus injury
  - Pulmonary injury
  - Head injury
  - Vascular injury, e.g. axillary artery injury.

Fracture healing time: 6–12 weeks

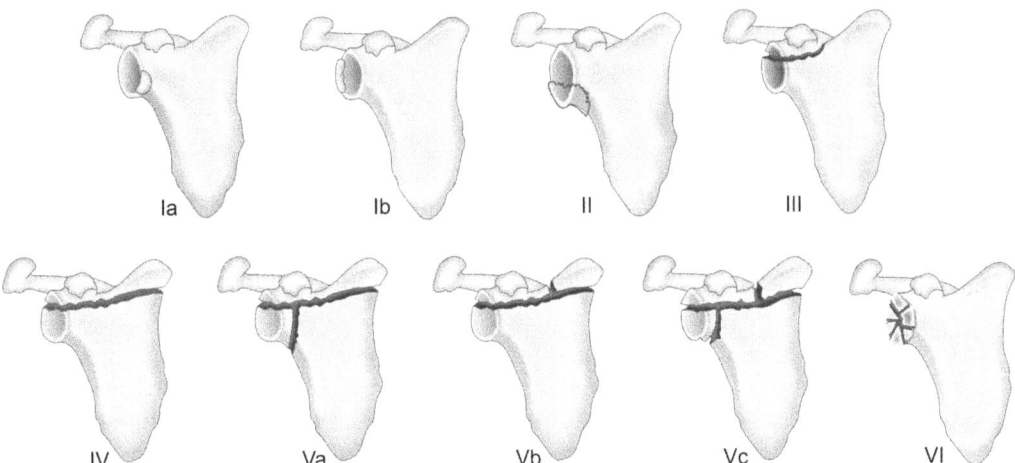

Fig. 13: Intra-articular glenoid and neck fracture of scapula.

Table 3: Classification of glenoid and neck fracture of scapula.

1.	Intra-articular glenoid fracture
Type I	Fractures of glenoid rim fracture
Type IA	Anterior glenoid rim fracture
Type IB	Posterior glenoid rim fracture
Type II	Fracture line through the glenoid fossa exiting at lateral border of scapula
Type III	Fracture line through the glenoid fossa exiting at superior border of scapula
Type IV	Fracture line through the glenoid fossa exiting at medial border of scapula
Type V	Fracture in combination with other fracture patterns
Type VA	Combination of types II and IV
Type VB	Combination of types III and IV
Type VC	Combination of types II, III and IV
Type VI	Comminuted fracture
2.	**Extra-articular glenoid fracture** These might be associated with acromioclavicular separation or clavicular fracture
Type I	Glenoid neck fracture without clavicular fracture
Type II	Glenoid neck fracture with clavicular fracture and acromioclavicular dislocation

Management

Nonsurgical Treatment

Vast majority of scapular fractures are managed nonoperatively.

- **Sling immobilization and early movement:** The shoulder is immobilized using sling for 2–3 weeks followed by early shoulder movement, i.e. pendular exercises and protected ROM within 1 week after injury to reduce the risk of shoulder and elbow stiffness.
  Indications:
  - Nondisplaced or minimally displaced scapular fractures
  - Scapular body fracture.

Surgical Treatment

- **Open reduction and internal fixation:**
  Indications:
  - Open fractures
  - Intra-articular glenoid fractures with subluxation and instability of humeral head.
  - Glenoid rim fractures displaced >10 mm and involve >25% of joint surface that are more likely to be associated with instability.
  - Glenoid fossa fractures that are displaced >5 mm.
  - Scapular neck fracture with >10 mm medial displacement, >40° angulation, with associated clavicle fracture or articular step off greater than 2 mm.
  - Depressed acromion fractures that encroach on subacromial space and interfere with rotator cuff function.
  - Fractures associated with neurovascular injuries and scapulothoracic dislocation.

Physiotherapy treatment: Table 4 shows the nonoperative physiotheraphy protocol for scapular fracture.

■ PROXIMAL HUMERAL FRACTURE

Proximal humerus fractures are among the most common broken bones in the shoulder. In elderly people, proximal humeral fractures are the third most frequently occurring fractures after hip and wrist fractures.

Table 4: Nonoperative physiotherapy protocol for scapular fracture.

	Precaution	ROM exercises	Strengthening exercises
Week 0–3	• No shoulder movement • Shoulder immobilized in sling	• No ROM at shoulder • Flexion, extension at elbow with forearm pronation and supination • Gentle shoulder pendular exercises after 6-7 days after injury	• No strengthening exercises to shoulder • Postural awareness, i.e. brings the shoulder back and squeezes the scapular blades together
Weeks 3–6	No weight lifting	• Gentle pendular exercises • Active assisted shoulder flexion and ER with arm at side of trunk	• Isometric exercises for elbow flexors and wrist musculature
Weeks 6–9	None	• AROM of shoulder flexion abduction, ER	• Isometric exercises for shoulder muscles
Weeks 9–12	None	• Full AROM of shoulder flexion extension, ER-IR, abduction-adduction	• Resisted exercises to shoulder muscle

(ROM: range of motion; AROM: active range of motion; ER: external rotation; IR: internal rotation)

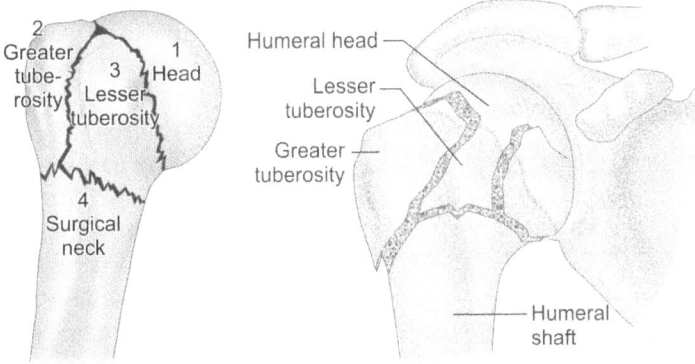

Fig. 14: Parts of proximal humerus.

Mechanism of Injury

- **Low impact injuries:** Usually in older people due to a fall from standing height on the outstretched arm.
- **High impact injuries:** Falling directly on shoulder or due to direct blow to shoulder.

Clinical Presentation

- Pain, swelling and bruising over shoulder.
- Inability to move the shoulder.
- Grinding sensation on shoulder movement.
- An unusual appearance of upper arm.

Classification

Most commonly used classification: Neer classification divides the proximal humerus in four major parts (Fig. 14).
1. Humeral head (with articular surface)
2. Greater tuberosity
3. Lesser tuberosity
4. Humeral shaft (diaphysis).

Neer Classification of Proximal Humeral Fractures (Fig. 15 and Table 5)

Two main components of classification:
1. **Number of fracture parts:** Undisplaced (1 part), 2 part, 3 part and 4 part fractures.

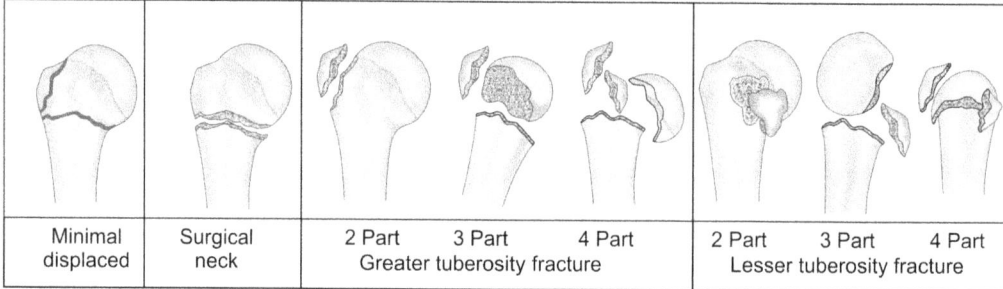

Fig. 15: Neer classification of proximal humeral fracture.

Table 5: Neer classification of proximal humeral fracture.

Type		Subtype
I	Minimal displacement	1 part
II	Anatomical neck	2 part
III	Surgical neck	2 part
IV	Greater tuberosity	2, 3 or 4 part
V	Lesser tuberosity	2, 3 or 4 part
VI	Fracture dislocation	Anterior 2, 3, 4 part or articular surface involvement Posterior 2, 3, 4 part or articular surface involvement

2. **Displacement:** A fracture fragment is considered displaced when it is displaced by at least 1 cm or angulated by 45° or more.

Complications

- **Nonunion:** It occurs in about 1.1–10% following closed treatment commonly associated with 2 part surgical neck fractures. Disruptions of blood supply, severe osteopenia, heavy smoking, nutritional deficiencies and/or metabolic bone diseases are the common factors that cause nonunion.
- **Malunion:** It occurs in about 4–20% cases of nonoperative treatment. Greater tuberosity malunion commonly occurs because of pull of rotator cuff muscles. According to Beredjiklian there are main three types of malunion: Malposition of tuberosities, incongruity of articular surface and malalignment of tuberosities and humeral head relative to shaft malunion.
- **Post-traumatic arthrofibrosis/post-traumatic stiffness or frozen shoulder:** It occurs due to prolonged immobilization. Therefore early gentle movement of shoulder after 3 weeks of injury is necessary.
- **Neurologic and brachial plexus injuries:** It occurs in about 50% cases. The risk of nerve injuries escalates in elderly patients, surgical neck fracture, shoulder dislocation, trauma associated with hematoma and in unsuccessful ORIF.
- **Vascular injuries:** Axillary artery injury may occur in displaced proximal humerus fracture. Therefore it is necessary to examine radial pulse and sign of vascular compromise like pallor, paresthesia, pulselessness, hypotension, etc.
- **Avascular necrosis:** It commonly occurs in 3 or 4 part fractures treated with closed reduction.

Fracture healing time: 6–8 weeks

Management

Nonsurgical Treatment
- **Sling immobilization:** The shoulder is immobilized for 2–3 weeks using sling or shoulder immobilizer.

Indications: Nondisplaced, impacted or minimally displaced fractures.

Surgical Treatment

- **Closed reduction and percutaneous fixation:** Threaded pins or cannulated screws are used for fixation after closed reduction of fragments.
  Indications: 2 part fractures in younger patients without any significant rotator cuff tear. It is commonly done for displaced surgical neck fracture.
- **Open reduction and Internal fixation:** Locking plates, screws, pins or tension bands are used for fixation of fractured fragments.
  Indications: 2, 3 and 4 part fractures in younger patients that may also require the rotator cuff repair.
- **Prosthetic arthroplasty:**
  Indications:
  - Anatomic neck fractures in elderly (initial varus malalignment >20°) or in severely comminuted fracture.
  - 4 part fractures and fracture dislocations (3 part when stable internal fixation is unachievable).
  - Head splitting fractures with incongruity of humeral head.
- Disrupted of articular blood supply (3 and 4 part fractures).
- Humeral head impression defect of more than 40% of articular surface.

Postoperative physiotherapy treatment: Table 6 shows the postoperative physiotherapy protocol for proximal humeral fracture.

■ HUMERAL SHAFT FRACTURE

Humeral shaft fractures accounts for around 3–5% of all fractures. It commonly occurs in young males in third decade and elderly or osteoporotic females in the seventh decade. The most common site of humeral shaft fracture is in middle third of humerus.

Mechanism of Injury

- **Low impact injuries:** Usually in older people due to a fall from standing height on the outstretched arm.
- **High impact injuries:** Falling directly on shoulder or due to direct blow to shoulder.

Clinical Presentation

- Pain in the upper arm.
- Significant swelling commonly occurs from shoulder to hand.

Table 6: Postoperative physiotherapy protocol for proximal humeral fracture.

	Precaution	ROM exercises	Strengthening exercises
Week 0–2	No shoulder movement	• No ROM at shoulder and elbow • Gentle pendular exercises for nondisplaced fractures and arthroplasty	No strengthening exercises to shoulder or elbow
Weeks 2–4	Avoid IR/ER of shoulder	• Gentle pendular exercises • Passive assistive exercises to shoulder	• No strengthening exercises for extensors of elbow • Isometric exercises for elbow flexors and wrist musculature
Weeks 4–6	None	AROM to AAROM for elbow including flexion, extension	Isometric exercises for elbow and wrist in flexion and extension
Weeks 6–10	None	Full AROM and PROM exercise for elbow and wrist in all planes	Progressive resisted exercises for elbow and wrist muscles

(AROM: active range of motion; AAROM: active-assisted range of motion; ROM: range of motion; PROM: passive range of motion)

- Inability to raise the arm.
- Tendency of arm to flop and bend.

Classification of Fracture

Although no standard classification system is present for humeral shaft fractures.

Fractures are classified on following basis:
- **On the location of fracture:**
  - **Proximal fractures:** Fractures above the insertion of pectoralis major muscle.
  - **Middle fractures:** Fractures below pectoralis major insertion and above deltoid muscle.
  - **Distal fractures:** Fractures below the insertion of deltoid muscle.
- Other criterias are used to describe fractures are fracture patterns (transverse, oblique, spiral, comminuted, segmental), open or closed, amount and direction of angulation and displacement.

Complications

- **Nerve injury:** Radial nerve more commonly affected than ulnar or medial nerve. It is usually affected in midshaft humeral fracture due to its proximity to posterior aspect of bone.
- **Brachial artery injury:** Although uncommon but injury to brachial artery may occur. It has greater risk of injury in proximal and distal 1/3rd of humerus.
- **Malunion:** Varus angulation usually occurs in humeral shaft fracture but it rarely has any functional or cosmetic sequel.
- **Postfracture joint stiffness:** Adhesive capsulitis of shoulder and elbow stiffness resulting in a decreased range of motion due to prolonged immobilization during healing process.
- **Nonunion or delayed union:** Because of biological and mechanical factors, such as significant bone gap, soft tissue interposition, bone loss, uncontrolled fracture motions, disrupted blood supply, vitamin D deficiency, osteoporosis and is more commonly occurs in transverse fracture and segmental fracture pattern.

Fracture healing time: 8–12 weeks

Management

Nonsurgical Treatment

Majority of humeral shaft fractures can be managed nonoperatively.
- **Coaptation splint followed by functional brace:** Coaptation splint is applied until the swelling is reduced followed by application of functional brace for at least 8 weeks to prevent refracture.
  Indications: When the fracture is non-displaced or minimally displaced, i.e. <20° anterior angulation, <30° varus/valgus angulation or < 3 cm shortening.

Surgical Treatment

- **Intramedullary nailing:** Intramedullary rod is commonly interlocked with screws on either ends.
  Indication:
  - Pathological fractures
  - Segmental fractures
  - Severe osteoporotic bone
  - Multiple trauma.
- **Open reduction and internal fixation with plates:**
  Indications:
  - Open fractures.
  - Vascular injury that require repair
  - Brachial plexus injury
  - Ipsilateral forearm fracture
  - Compartment syndrome.

Postoperative physiotherapy treatment: Table 7 shows postoperative physiotherapy protocol for humeral shaft fracture.

■ DISTAL HUMERAL FRACTURE

Fracture of distal humerus in adults comprises 2% of all the skeletal injuries and around 30% of all humeral fractures. It occurs most commonly in young males and older females.

Table 7: Postoperative physiotherapy protocol for humeral shaft fracture.

	Precaution	ROM exercises	Strengthening exercises
Week 0–2	No weight lifting with affected limb	• Gentle AROM and AAROM of elbow and shoulder when treated with ORIF • ROM exercises not recommended for shoulder and elbow when treatment with brace or splint	• No strengthening exercises for elbow and shoulder
Weeks 2–4	Same as above	• Same as above for ORIF treatment • No abduction to shoulder beyond 60° when treatment with brace or splint	• Gentle pendulum exercises for the shoulder • No strengthening exercises for elbow and shoulder
Weeks 4–6	Same as above	AROM to AAROM to shoulder and elbow	Isometric and isotonic exercises for forearm muscles
Weeks 6–10	No contact sports	AROM, AAROM and PROM exercise for shoulder and elbow	Progressive resistance exercises for shoulder and elbow muscles

(AAROM: active-assisted range of motion; ROM: range of motion; AROM: active range of motion; ORIF: open reduction and internal fixation)

Mechanism of Injury

- **Low impact injuries:** In older people having osteoporotic bone, fracture may occur even after a minor fall.
- **High impact injuries:** Falling directly on the elbow, falling on outstretched arm with the elbow held tightly to brace against the fall or receiving direct blow to the elbow.

Clinical Presentation

- Severe pain, swelling, bruising and tenderness around the elbow joint.
- Inability to move the elbow joint.
- Feeling of instability in joint or feeling of "popping out" of elbow.

Classification of Fracture

Fractures of distal humerus is classified on the basis of the surgical anatomy of distal humerus. Figure 16 and Table 8 shows the ASIF classification of distal humeral fracture.

Complications

- **Heterotopic ossification:** It occurs in around 50% of cases after the acute treatment. Heterotopic ossification (HO) commonly occurs on the posterolateral aspect of elbow from lateral humeral condyle to posterolateral olecranon. The risk of the development of HO formation increases with forced manipulation and massage.
- **Postfracture stiffness:** Commonly occurs due to prolonged immobilization and often results in painful shoulder stiffness and reduced ROM.
- **Volkmann's ischemia:** It occurs due to abnormal pressure build up within the muscles of the elbow that leads to the inhibition of nourishment and oxygen to the soft tissues due to compromised blood circulation of the area.
- **Injury to neurovascular structures:** They occur in around 7–15% cases. Radial nerve is commonly affected in posteromedial displaced fractures, whereas median nerve injuries mostly occur with posterolateral angulated fractures. An ulnar neuropathy particularly anterior interosseous nerve injury is frequently associated with ORIF of distal humeral fractures or with closed pediatric supracondylar fractures.
- **Malunion:** It commonly occurs after lateral condylar fracture. Fusion of bony

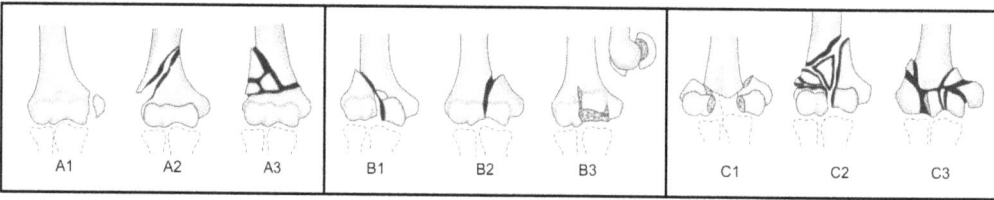

Fig. 16: ASIF classification of distal humeral fracture.

Table 8: ASIF classification of distal humeral fracture.

Type	Description		Type	Description
A	Extra-articular	Supracondylar	A1	Epicondylar avulsion fracture
			A2	Simple metaphyseal fracture
			A3	Comminuted metaphyseal fracture
B	Intra-articular	Unicondylar	B1	Sagittal plane: Lateral condylar including capitellum
			B2	Sagittal plane: Medial condylar including trochlea
			B3	Frontal plane i Capitellum
				ii Medial condylar capitellum
C	Intra-articular	Transcondylar: Bicondylar or intercondylar	C1	Simple articular, simple metaphyseal
			C2	Simple articular, comminuted metaphyseal
			C3	Comminuted articular

fragments in malaligned position leads to deformity of the elbow known as cubitus varus deformity/angulation.

Fracture healing time: 12–16 weeks

Management

Nonsurgical Treatment

- **Cast/posterior splinting and immobilization:** The limb is immobilized in a long arm cast or posterior long arm splint with elbow in 90° flexion and forearm in neutral position. In nondisplaced fracture, the limb is immobilized for 2–3 weeks, whereas immobilization following closed reduction is done for 4–6 weeks.
  - Medial condyle fractures are immobilized with forearm in pronation and wrist in 30° flexion to relax the common flexor pronator muscles.
  - Lateral condyle fractures are immobilized with forearm in supination and wrist in slightly extended position to relax the extensor muscles.

Indications: Undisplaced fractures especially extra-articular.

Surgical Treatment

- **Closed reduction and percutaneous pinning:** In this the pins are left in place with the arm in a splint or cast with elbow 90° flexion and forearm in neutral position for 4–6 weeks
  Indications: Extra-articular undisplaced fractures commonly used in children.
- **Open reduction and internal fixation:** Fixation with medial and lateral plates or with screws is performed to fix the fracture.
  Indications: Intra-articular and displaced fractures commonly supracondylar and intercondylar fractures.
- **Total joint replacement:**
  Indication: Distal bicolumnar fractures in elderly patients.

Postoperative physiotherapy treatment: Table 9 shows postoperative physiotherapy protocol for distal humeral fractures.

Table 9: Postoperative physiotherapy protocol for distal humeral fractures.

	Precaution	ROM exercises	Strengthening exercises
Week 0–2	No IR/ER of shoulder and no PROM of elbow joint	• Gentle AROM for elbow flexion and extension when treated with ORIF • ROM exercises not recommended in other methods of fixation	No strengthening exercises
Weeks 2–4	Same as above	• Same as above for ORIF treatment • Gentle AAROM elbow flexion and extension for non-displaced stable fracture	Same as above
Weeks 4–6	Same as above	AROM to AAROM for elbow including flexion, extension	Same as above
Weeks 6–10	No heavy lifting and pushing activities	Full AROM and PROM exercise for elbow	Progressive resisted exercises for elbow muscles

(IR: internal rotation; ER: external rotation; PROM: passive range of motion; AROM: active range of motion; AAROM: active-assisted range of motion; ROM: range of motion; ORIF: open reduction and internal fixation)

■ ULNAR OLECRANON FRACTURE

Olecranon fractures are common because of its exposed anatomical position on the point of elbow directly under the skin without much of muscular and soft tissue protection.

Mechanism of Fracture
- Falling directly on the elbow.
- Direct blow to elbow against something hard.
- Fall on outstretched hand with elbow flexed and hand strikes the ground that can cause the forceful contraction of triceps muscle that pull a piece of bone off the ulna. It is more common in elderly patient.
- Fall on semi-flexed supinated forearm may lead to avulsion fracture.
- Repeated hyperextension of elbow can cause stress fracture of olecranon due to recurrent impaction of olecranon against the olecranon fossa. It is relatively common in children and adults.

Clinical Presentation
- Sudden, intense pain and tenderness that prevent the movement of elbow.
- Swelling at the tip of elbow.
- Bruising around the elbow that may spread up the arm or down the forearm.
- Numbness of one or more fingers.
- Feeling of instability of joint.
- Pain with elbow movement.

Classification of Olecranon Fracture

Fracture of olecranon process is classified on the basis of stability, displacement and comminution of the fragments.

Figure 17 and Table 10 shows Mayo classification.

Complications
- **Ulnar nerve injury:** The proximity of the ulnar nerve to the olecranon makes it more prone to get injured (2–5%) when olecranon fractures occur.
- **Postfracture joint stiffness:** Limitation or restriction of elbow movement including flexion contracture and extensor lag of elbow joint particularly when associated with intra-articular fracture or dislocation of elbow.

Fracture healing time: 8–12 weeks.

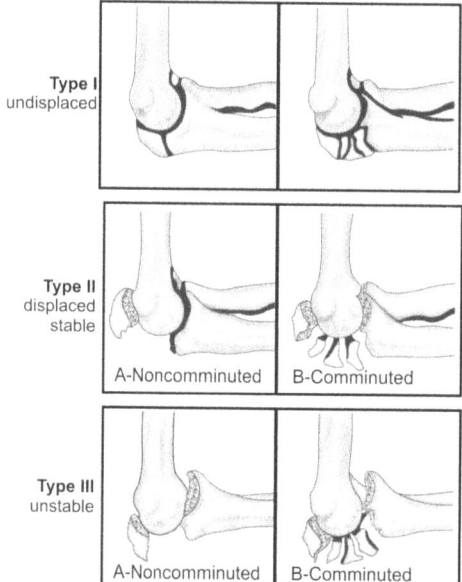

Fig. 17: Classification of olecranon fracture.

Table 10: Mayo classification.

Type	Description	
I	Undisplaced	Noncomminuted
		Comminuted
II	Displaced >3 mm, stable	Noncomminuted
		Comminuted
III	Displaced >3 mm, unstable	Noncomminuted
		Comminuted

Management

Nonsurgical Treatment

- **Cast/splinting and immobilization:** The arm is immobilized in long arm cast with elbow in 90° flexion for 3–4 weeks.
  Indications: Nondisplaced stable fracture.

Surgical Treatment

- **Open reduction and internal fixation:**
  Indications: Displaced and comminuted fractures.
  The choice of implant depends on the fracture pattern:
  - Transverse fractures are well treated by tension band wiring.
  - Oblique fractures are treated preferably by intramedullary screw with or without tension band wiring over the screw.
  - Plate fixation with a lag screw provides excellent stability for oblique fractures. It is also recommended in severely comminuted fractures.
  - Excision and triceps advancement may be indicated for severely comminuted fractures or in osteoporotic patients.

Postoperative physiotherapy treatment: Table 11 shows postoperative physiotherapy protocol for ulnar olecranon fracture.

■ RADIAL HEAD FRACTURE

Radial head fractures account for around 1.5–4% of all skeletal injuries. It is among the most common elbow fractures, i.e. around 33%. It is more frequent in females than males and likely to happen between 30–40 years.

Mechanism of Injury

Commonly caused by fall on to an outstretched arm with elbow in extension and forearm in pronation that leads to the transmission of force from wrist to radial head that strikes against the capitellum.

Clinical Presentation

- Pain on lateral aspect of elbow.
- Swelling in elbow joint.
- Pain on elbow movement.
- Inability in turning the forearm (pronation and supination).

Classification of Radial Head Fracture

Figure 18 and Table 12 shows the Mason classification modified by Hotchkiss and Broberg-Morrey.

Complications

- **Forearm compartment syndrome:** It occurs due to swelling associated with soft tissue injuries which results in increased pressure inside muscle compartment.

Fractures and Dislocations

Table 11: Postoperative physiotherapy protocol for ulnar olecranon fracture.

	Precaution	ROM exercises	Strengthening exercises
Week 0–2	No elbow movement	• Gentle active elbow flexion when treated with ORIF • ROM exercises for elbow and wrist are not recommended in other nonsurgical methods of fixation	• No strengthening exercises for elbow • Gentle isometric exercise to wrist
Weeks 2–4	Cast or splint: No extension for elbow less than 90°	Same as above	• No strengthening exercises to extensors of elbow • Isometric exercises for elbow flexors and wrist musculature
Weeks 4–6	None	AROM to AAROM to elbow including flexion, extension	Isometric exercises for elbow and wrist in flexion and extension
Weeks 6–10	None	Full AROM and PROM exercise for elbow and wrist in all planes	Progressive resisted exercises for elbow and wrist muscles

(AROM: active range of motion; ROM: range of motion; AAROM: active-assisted range of motion; ORIF: open reduction and internal fixation; PROM: passive range of motion)

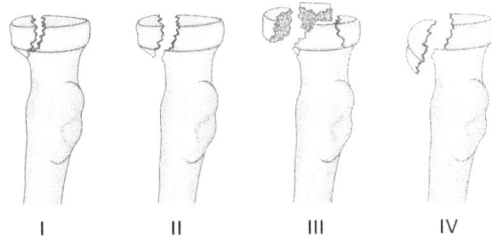

Fig. 18: Classification of radial head fracture.

- **Neurovascular injuries:** The posterior interosseous nerve is commonly injured due to its proximity to radial head.
- **Nonunion/malunion:** It may occur due to improper reduction of displaced fracture or due to continuous movement of the fractured bone after injury.
- **Postfracture stiffness of elbow joint:** Loss of elbow extension is common in radial head fracture.

Fracture healing time: 6–8 weeks

Management

Nonsurgical Treatment

- **Sling or splint:** Type I fracture is usually treated with immobilization in a simple arm sling or splint for 5–7 days. If associated with elbow dislocation, the splinting should be continued for a greater period and days usually 3 weeks.

Table 12: Mason classification modified by Hotchkiss and Broberg-Morrey.

Type I	Nondisplaced or minimally displaced (<2 mm). No mechanical block to rotation.
Type II	Displaced >2 mm or angulated. Possible mechanical block to forearm rotation
Type III	Comminuted and displaced. Mechanical block to motion.
Type IV	Radial head fracture with associated elbow dislocation.

Indications: Fractures with minimum displacement and angulation.

Surgical Treatment

- **Open reduction and internal fixation**
  Indications:
  - Masson type II with mechanical block
  - Masson type III where ORIF is feasible
  - Presence of other complex ipsilateral elbow injuries.
- **Excision of fracture fragments or entire radial head:** Recent studies recommend the repair of articular surface to maintain the stability rather than opting for the excision of the fragment. Prosthetic spacers are used to provide stability in case of observable instability secondary to the bone loss and ligament damage.

88 Simplified Approach to Orthopedic Physiotherapy

Table 13: Postoperative physiotherapy protocol for radial head fracture.

	Precaution	ROM exercises	Strengthening exercises
Week 0–2	No PROM for the forearm	AROM for elbow in flexion and pronation	Gentle isometric exercise for deltoid, biceps and triceps
Weeks 2–4	Same as above	AROM for elbow	Isometric exercise for deltoid, biceps and triceps
Weeks 4–6	Avoid valgus stress to elbow	AROM to AAROM for elbow and wrist including flexion, extension, supination and pronation	Gentle isometric exercise for forearm muscles
Weeks 6–10	No heavy lifting and pushing activities	Full AROM and PROM exercise for elbow and wrist. Including supination and pronation for forearm	Progressive resisted exercises for forearm muscles, i.e. flexors, extensors, supinators and pronators

(PROM: passive range of motion; ROM: range of motion; AROM: active range of motion; AAROM: active-assisted range of motion)

Indications: Comminuted fractures that are amenable to repair, i.e. when the fragments have <25% of surface area of radial head or 25-33% of capitellar surface area.

Postoperative physiotherapy treatment: Table 13 shows postoperative physiotherapy protocol for radial head fracture.

▪ FOREARM FRACTURES

It refers to fracture of ulna or radius or both of the bones of forearm.

Mechanism of Injury
- Direct blow on the forearm
- Fall on an outstretched arm
- Motor vehicle accidents.

Clinical Presentation
- Sudden severe pain, tenderness and swelling on forearm
- Inability to rotate the forearm, i.e. supination and pronation
- Abnormal appearance, i.e. bent and shorten forearm
- Patient need to support the injured arm with other hand.

Classifications

A. Classification on the Basis of the Location of Fracture
- Upper part or proximal third of bone
- Lower part or distal third of bone
- Mid shaft/diaphysis or middle third of bone

B. Classification of Forearm Fractures used for Adults
On the basis of closed versus open fractures, pattern of fractures (transverse, oblique, spiral and segmental), and displaced or non-displaced fractures.

C. Classification of Forearm Fractures used for Children
- **Growth plate fracture (Fig. 19):** It occurs in children. It refers to the fracture which

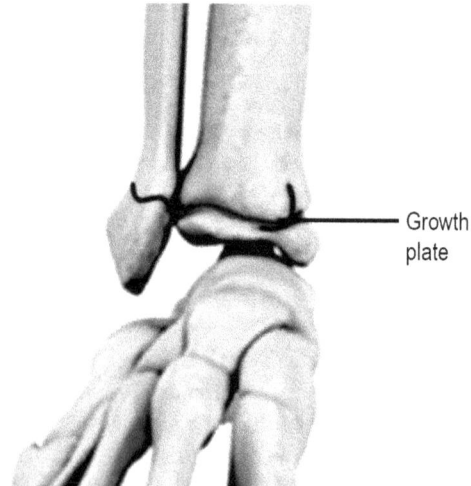

Fig. 19: Growth plate fracture.

Fractures and Dislocations

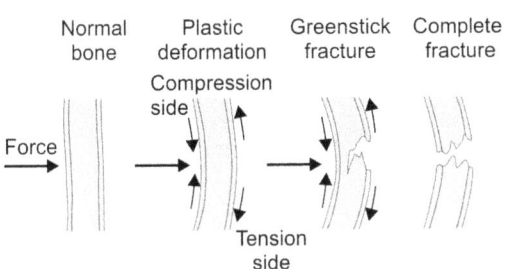

Fig. 20: Greenstick fracture.

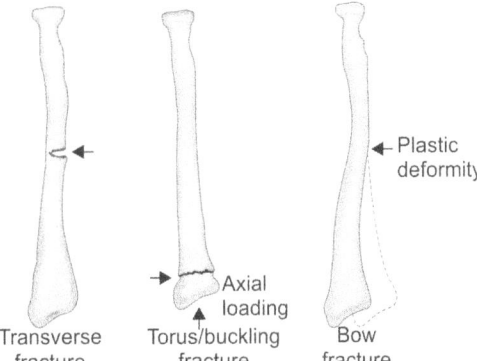

Fig. 21: Different forms of greenstick fracture.

include epiphysis (epiphyseal plate or growth plate are the area at either end of the bone where cartilage grows and becomes ossified bone).

- **Greenstick fracture (Fig. 20):** It occurs in infants and young children of less than 10 years when the bones are soft. These are incomplete fractures characterized by the presence of breaks only on one side of the bone. It occurs by the application of perpendicular force along the longitudinal axis of the bone that eventually leads to fracture on the convex surface of the bent bone however the concave surface of the bone remains intact as the applied force is not strong enough to break the bone completely. They are commonly mid diaphyseal.

Following are the three basic forms of greenstick fracture (Fig. 21):

1. **Transverse fracture:** It refers to the fracture that occurs around the cortex that extends to the middle of bone caused by a force perpendicular to the long axis of bone.
2. **Buckle or torus fracture:** These are incomplete fractures of the shaft of long bone characterized by the bulging of cortex in which the bone is broken on one side and a bump or raised buckle develops on the other side. They result from trabecular compression from an axial loading force along the long axis of the bone. Commonly seen in children, frequently involving the distal radial metaphyseal.
3. **Bowing fracture:** Angulated/curved bone along its longitudinal axis. It occurs when an angulated longitudinal force is applied to a bone. When the applied force is greater than the mechanical strength of the bone, the bone undergoes plastic deformation and remains in its bowed position even after the discontinuation of the force.
- **Metaphyseal fracture:** It is a fracture of upper or lower part of bone shaft, outside the growth plate.
- **Diaphyseal fractures:** Orthopedic Trauma Association (OTA) gives the classification of shaft of ulna and radius. (Table 14)

Some common forearm fractures are:
- **Monteggia fracture/dislocation (Fig. 22):** Fracture of proximal third of ulna with dislocation of proximal head of radius.
- **Galeazzi fracture/dislocation (Fig. 23):** Fracture of distal third of radius with dislocation of distal radioulnar joint.

Table 14: OTA classification of radial and ulnar shaft fractures.

Type	Description
A	Simple fracture of ulna (A1), radius (A2) or both (A3)
B	Wedge fracture of ulna (B1), radius (B2) or both (B3)
C	Complex fractures

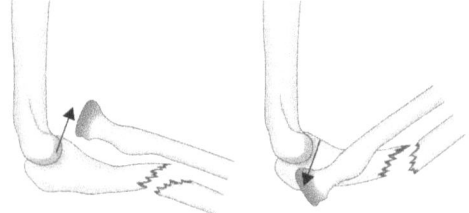

Fig. 22: Monteggia fracture/dislocation.

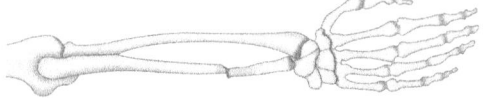

Fig. 24: Nightstick fractures.

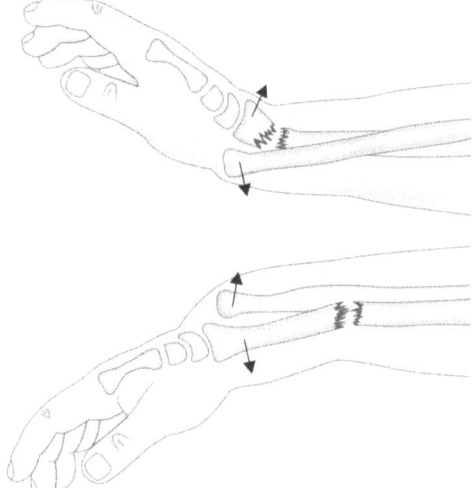

Fig. 23: Galeazzi fracture/dislocation.

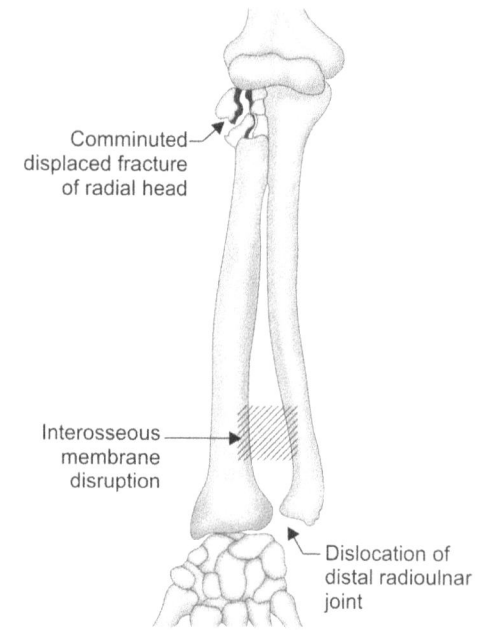

Fig. 25: Essex-Lopresti fracture.

- **Nightstick fractures (Fig. 24):** Isolated fractures of ulna in the midshaft. It usually results from direct blow on forearm.
- **Essex-Lopresti fracture (Fig. 25):** Fracture of radial head with dislocation of distal radioulnar joint due to the disruption of interosseous membrane.

Complications
- **Post-traumatic radioulnar synostosis:** It is a condition which is characterized by osseous union of the radius and ulna.
- **Posterior interosseous nerve (PIN) injury:** It occurs in around 3.1 to 31.4% cases of forearm fractures, more commonly associated with monteggia fracture/dislocation. Mostly neuropraxia, that recovers spontaneously with conservative treatment.
- **Compartment syndrome:** It refers to the elevated swelling and pressure in the forearm muscular compartments.
- **Ulnar/radial artery injury:** Incidence of radial and ulnar arterial injuries is present in the forearm fractures.
- **Malunion or nonunion:** It may occur due to inadequate reduction or continuous movement of fracture fragments after injury.

Fracture healing time: 8–12 weeks

Management
Nonsurgical Treatment
- **Closed reduction and cast immobilization:** The forearm is immobilized in the long arm cast with elbow in 90° flexion for 4 weeks followed by short arm cast or functional brace for 2 weeks.

- Middle third fractures are immobilized in neutral rotation.
- Proximal third radius fractures are immobilized in supination.
- Distal third radius fractures are immobilized in pronation.

Indications: Isolated nondisplaced or distal 2/3 ulnar shaft fracture (nightstick fracture) with <50% displacement and <10° of angulation.

Surgical Treatment
- **Open reduction and internal fixation:**
  Indications:
  - Isolated radial fractures
  - Both forearm bones fractures
  - Fractures associated with radial head dislocation or distal radioulnar joint dislocation.

Postoperative physiotherapy treatment: Table 15 shows postoperative physiotherapy protocol for forearm fracture.

■ WRIST FRACTURE/DISTAL RADIUS FRACTURES

Fracture of distal radius commonly occurs due to fall on outstretched hand (FOOSH) when the subject extends his arm and hands to stabilize him against an impact. The extension of arm puts the whole impaction stress on the wrist. It commonly occurs in adolescents (5–14 years) and elderly people.

Clinical Presentation
- Immediate pain, tenderness, bruising and swelling in and around the wrist joint.
- Wrist may be deformed, i.e. wrist hangs in an odd or bent way.

■ COLLES' FRACTURE (FIG. 26)

It is an extra-articular fracture of distal radius usually at its corticocancellous junction (about 2–3 cm from distal articular surface) associated with dorsal displacement and dorsal angulation of distal fragments of radius. This deformity is known as dinner fork deformity.

Mechanism of Injury
Fall on outstretched hand with wrist in 40–90° extension.

■ SMITH'S FRACTURE (FIG. 27)

It is also known as reverse Colles' fracture. It is an extra-articular fracture of distal radius associated with volar displacement and volar

Table 15: Postoperative physiotherapy protocol for forearm fracture.

	Precaution	ROM exercises	Strengthening exercises
Week 0–2	No PROM for the forearm	Gentle AROM exercises for elbow and wrist including supination and pronation in case of adequate fixation and if forearm is not in cast	• Gentle isometric exercise for deltoid, biceps and triceps if treated with ORIF • No strengthening exercises for forearm if treated nonsurgically
Weeks 2–4	Same as above	Gentle AROM exercise for elbow and wrist in the case of adequate fixation and if forearm is not in cast	Same as above
Weeks 4–6	Same as above	AROM to AAROM for elbow and wrist including flexion, extension, supination and pronation if forearm is out of cast	Gentle isometric and isotonic exercise for forearm muscles
Weeks 6–10	No heavy lifting and sports activities	Full AROM and PROM exercises for elbow and wrist including supination and pronation of forearm	Progressive resisted exercises for forearm muscles

(PROM: passive range of motion; ROM: range of motion; AROM: active range of motion; AAROM: active-assisted range of motion; ORIF: open reduction and internal fixation)

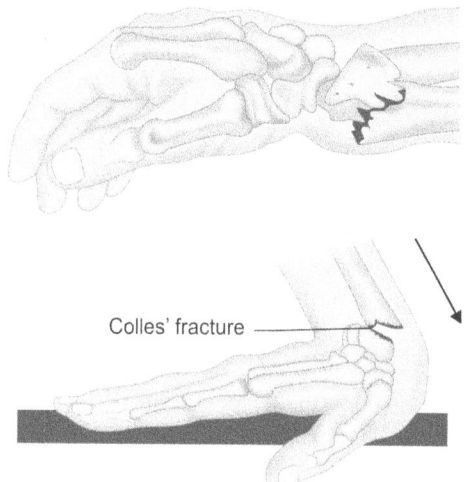

Fig. 26: Colles' fracture.

angulation (apex dorsal) of distal fragment of radius. This deformity is known as garden spade deformity.

Mechanism of Injury
- Direct blow on dorsal forearm
- Fall on the dorsal aspect of flexed wrist
- Fall on outstretched hand with forearm in supination followed by pronation around a fixed extended wrist.

■ BARTON'S FRACTURE (FIG. 28)

It is an intra-articular fracture of distal radius with dislocation of radiocarpal joint. There are two types of Barton fracture:
1. **Dorsal Barton fracture:** It is a fracture dislocation of dorsal rim of radius.
2. **Volar Barton fracture:** It is a fracture dislocation of volar rim of radius.

Mechanism of Injury

Fall on an extended and pronated wrist that increases the carpal compression force on the dorsal rim.

■ CHAUFFEUR FRACTURE (FIG. 29)

It is also known as Hutchinson fracture or Backfire fracture. It is an intra-articular fracture of radial styloid process.

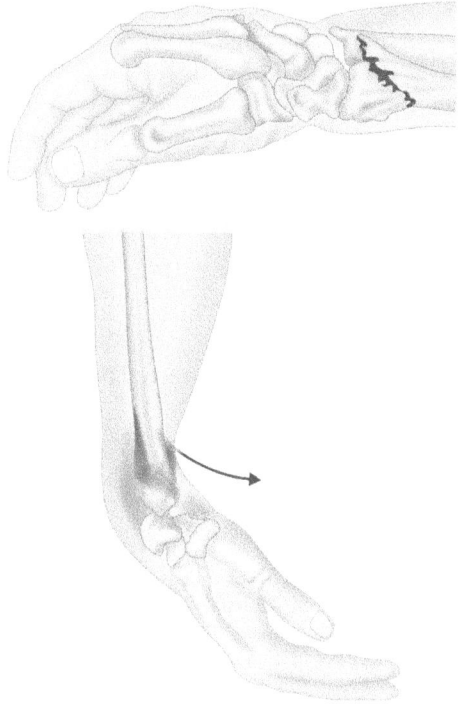

Fig. 27: Smith's fracture.

Mechanism of Injury
- Direct blow on dorsum of wrist
- Forced dorsiflexion and abduction.

■ DIE PUNCH FRACTURE (FIG. 30)

It is an intra-articular depression fracture of lunate fossa of distal radius. It is the result of compressive load of lunate through lunate on distal radius.

Mechanism of Injury

Wrist hyperextension.

Complications
- **Disruption of triangular fibrocartilage complex (TFCC):** TFCC is a disc interposed between proximal row of carpals and distal ulna. It enhances the joint stability of distal radioulnar joint and also absorbs the compressive force through wrist or hand. It is commonly injured in FOOSH injury

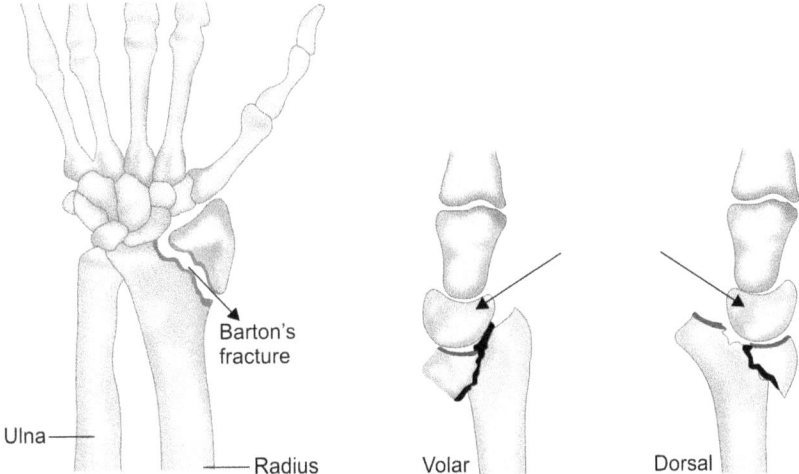

Fig. 28: Barton's fracture and its types.

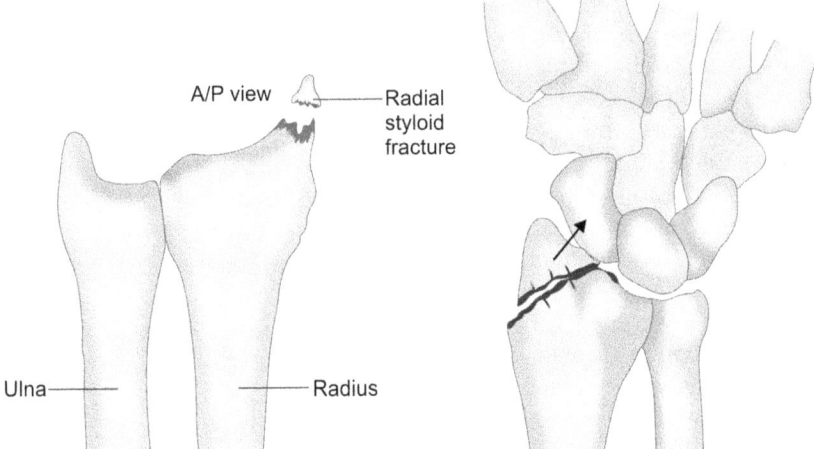

Fig. 29: Chauffeur fracture.

with forearm in pronated position. Patient complains of pain just distal to ulnar styloid process that worsens with ulnar deviation and hand/wrist movements.
- **Carpal tunnel syndrome:** It refers to the contusion or compression of median nerve that occurs due to direct trauma from the fragments of fracture, edema, and forced hyperextension of wrist.
- **Nerve injury:** Median nerve is the most commonly affected nerve because of its close proximity to the area and its confinement within the carpal tunnel.
- **Post-traumatic radiocarpal osteoarthritis:** Wrist fracture may damage the cartilage and leads to altered joint mechanics and making it wear out more quickly.
- **Heterotrophic ossification:** It is condition in which the injured bodily tissues are replaced by heterotopic bone causing pain and eventually leading to the immobilization and fusion of radioulnar

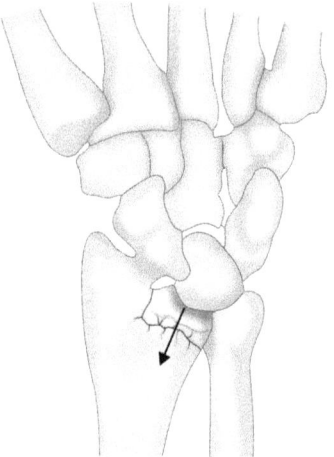

Fig. 30: Die punch fracture.

and radiocarpal joints due to abnormal growths of bone.
- **Reflex sympathetic syndrome:** It presents with excessive pain, swelling, stiffness and vasomotor changes in the affected limb.
- **Tendon rupture:** Most commonly tendon of extensor pollicis longus is injured because of compromised blood supply caused by edema within the compact edges of the extensor retinaculum.
- **Malunion:** It is due to displacement or angulation of distal fragment of radius. Dinner fork and garden spade deformity are the most commonly occurring deformities due to the malunion of distal radius fracture.
- **Postfracture stiffness of wrist joint:** Prolonged immobilization of joint may lead to residual limitation of wrist mobility as well as of grip strength.

Fracture healing time: 6–8 weeks

Management

Nonsurgical Treatment
- **Closed reduction and cast immobilization:** After closed reduction long arm cast is applied for 4–6 weeks followed by the removal or shortening of cast on the basis of fracture union. Postreduction X-rays are obtained at 7th, 14th and 21st day.

Indications: Non-displaced or minimally displaced fractures without much comminution.

Surgical Treatment
- **Open reduction and internal fixation:** Postoperative cast is applied for 2–6 weeks depending on the stability of fixation.
  Indications:
  - Comminuted displaced intra-articular fractures
  - Associated carpal fractures
  - Associated neurovascular or tendon injury.

Post-operative physiotherapy treatment: Table 16 shows postoperative physiotherapy protocol for wrist/distal radius fracture.

■ CARPAL FRACTURE

Carpal fractures worldwide account for 8–19% among all hand injuries.

Relative Incidence of Carpal Bones Fracture:
- Scaphoid: 68.2%
- Triquentrum: 18.3%
- Trapezium: 4.3%
- Lunate: 3.9%
- Capitate: 1.9%
- Hamate: 1.7%
- Pisiform: 1.3%
- Trapezoid: 0.4%.

Clinical Presentation
- Sharp pain at wrist
- Presence of Tenderness
- Pain increases with movement of wrist
- Presence of swelling.
- Decreased grip strength.
- Restricted wrist movements.
- Instability of wrist.

■ SCAPHOID FRACTURE

Scaphoid is the most frequently fractured carpal bone accounting for approx 60–80% of all bone fractures. The classical sign of

Fractures and Dislocations

Table 16: Postoperative physiotherapy protocol for wrist/distal radius fracture.

	Precaution	ROM exercises	Strengthening exercises
Week 0–2	• Avoid supination and pronation • Avoid ROM for wrist	• Full AROM at MCP joint • Full opposition of thumb	Gentle isometric exercises for intrinsic muscles of hand
Weeks 2–4	• Avoid supination and pronation • Avoid PROM	• Full AROM at MCP and IP joints • Gentle AROM of wrist when treated with ORIF	Gentle isometric exercises for intrinsic muscles of hand, and flexors and extensors of wrist
Weeks 4–6	Avoid PROM	• Full AROM at MCP, IP and wrist joints • Begin UD, RD, supination and pronation	• Gentle resisted exercises for the fingers to improve the power grip • Gentle resisted exercises for the wrist when treated with ORIF
Weeks 6–10	No heavy lifting and sports activities	Full AROM and PROM exercises for hand and wrist including supination and pronation of forearm	Progressive resisted exercises for hand and wrist muscles

(ROM: range of motion; PROM: passive range of motion; AROM: active range of motion; MCP: metacarpophalangeal; IP: interphalangeal; ORIF: open reduction and internal fixation; UD: ulnar deviation; RD: radial deviation)

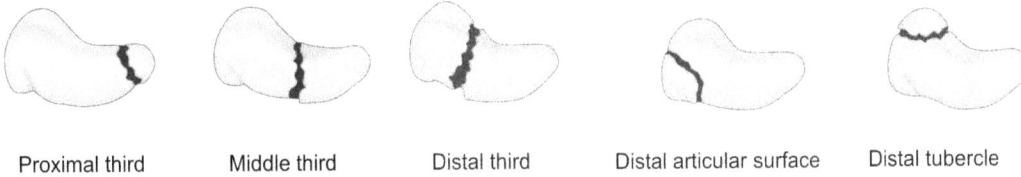

Proximal third Middle third Distal third Distal articular surface Distal tubercle

Fig. 31: Mayo classification of scaphoid fracture.

scaphoid fracture is tenderness in anatomical snuffbox.

Mayo Classification of Scaphoid Fracture (Fig. 31)
- Proximal third fracture: 20%.
- Middle third fracture (waist of scaphoid): 70–80%.
- Distal third fracture: 10%.
- Distal articular surface fracture.
- Distal tubercle fracture (most commonly occurs in children).

Mechanism of Injury (Fig. 32)
Fall on outstretched hand with wrist in extension and radial deviation.

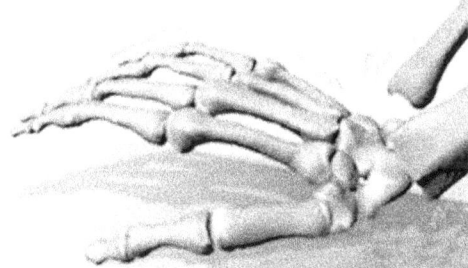

Fig. 32: Mechanism of injury of scaphoid

Complications
- **Avascular necrosis:** It most commonly occurs in proximal portion of scaphoid because arterial supply of scaphoid enters distal to proximal. Fracture of waist of scaphoid bone leads to the interruption

of blood flow in proximal pole of scaphoid that progressively results in the necrosis of the bone.
- **Nonunion:** It occurs due to poor blood supply.

Fracture healing time: 4–12 weeks
Depending on the fracture location.

Management

Nonsurgical Treatment

Most scaphoid fractures are treated non-operatively.
- **Thumb spica cast immobilization:** Duration of the immobilization depends on the site of fracture i.e.
  - Distal waist fracture are immobilized for 3 months
  - Mid-waist fractures are immobilized for 4 months
  - Proximal third fractures are immobilized for 5 months

Early immobilization is suggested as the chances of nonunion increases with delayed immobilization i.e.> 4 weeks after trauma.

Indications: Stable non-displaced fractures.

Surgical Treatment
- ORIF and percutaneous screw fixation
  Indication:
  - Unstable fractures
    - proximal pole fracture
    - displacement more than 1mm
    - 15 degree humpback scaphoid deformity
  - Comminuted fractures
  - Non-displaced waist fracture.

■ TRIQUENTRUM FRACTURE (FIG. 33)

Triquentral is the second most commonly fractured carpal bone after scaphoid. It represents around 18–20% of all carpal bone injuries. It can either be dorsal chip fracture or through the body of triquentrum.

Mechanism of Injury
- Fall on outstretched hand with wrist in extension and ulnar deviation that could lead to the impingement of hamate or ulnar styloid on dorsal triquentrum.
- A direct impact from a hard object on the dorsum of the wrist that can lead to fracture of body of triquentrum.

Management

Nonsurgical Treatment
- **Immobilization for 4-6 weeks**
  Indications:
  - Non-displaced body fracture
  - Stable palmar or dorsal cortical fractures

Surgical Treatment
Indication
- Displaced body fracture
- Unstable palmar or dorsal cortical fractures.

■ TREPEZIUM FRACTURE

Fracture of trapezium is the third most common fracture of carpal bone, accounting for approximately 4 to 5% of all carpal bone fractures.

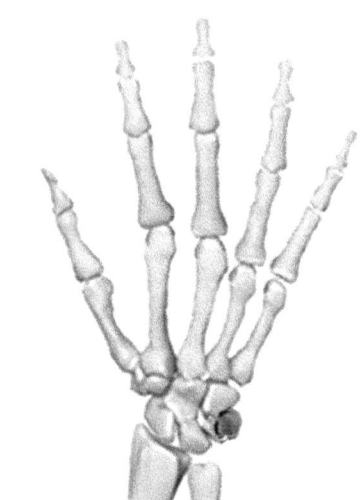

Fig. 33: Triquentrum fracture.

Fractures and Dislocations

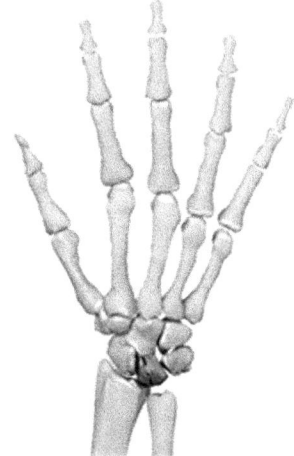

Fig. 34: Lunate fracture.

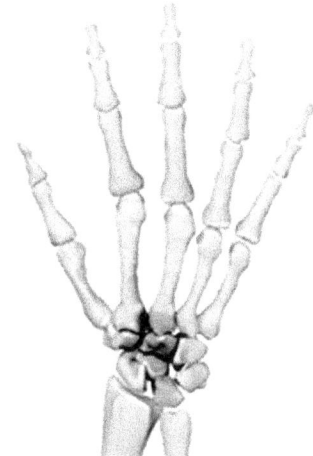

Fig. 35: Capitate fracture.

Mechanism of Injury
- Fall on outstretched hand with wrist in radial deviation
- Direct blow on the dorsum of hand.

■ LUNATE FRACTURE (FIG. 34)

Lunate is the fourth most fractured carpal bone following scaphoid, triquentrum and trapezium. It accounts for approximately 3–4% of all carpal bone fracture.

Mechanism of Injury
- Direct blow to wrist
- Fall on outstretched hand with hyperextended wrist.
- Push forcefully with extended wrist.

■ CAPITATE FRACTURE (FIG. 35)

Capitate is the largest carpal bone and rarely fractured in isolation. It commonly occurs in complex injury to wrist and accounts for only around 1–1.5% of all carpal bone fractures. The combination of capitate fracture along with scaphoid waist fracture is known as "scaphocapitate syndrome".

Mechanism of Injury
- Direct blow to wrist
- Fall on outstretched hand with extended wrist.

■ HAMATE FRACTURE

Hamate fracture comprises of about 1.5–2% of all carpal fractures.

Milch Classification of Hamate Fracture (Fig. 36 and Table 17)

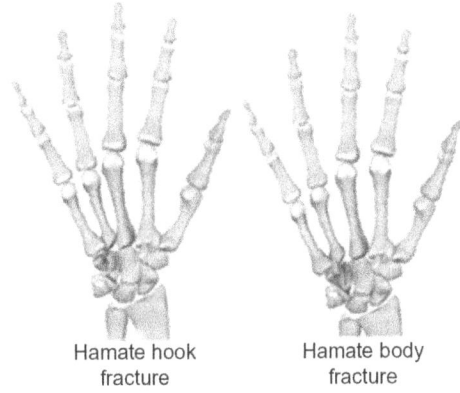

Hamate hook fracture   Hamate body fracture

Fig. 36: Milch classification of hamate fracture.

Table 17: Milch classification of hamate fracture.

Type	Description
Type I	Hook of hamate fracture
Type II	Body of hamate fracture. It is commonly associated with dislocation of 4th and 5th metacarpals

Mechanism of Injury

Frequently seen in golfers, baseball and racket sport players.
- Direct blow to wrist
- Fall on outstretched hand with extended or while holding an object.
- Type II fractures are more associated with the mechanism of a clenched fist striking a wall.

Management

Nonsurgical Treatment
- **Application of cast for 6 weeks**
  Indication:
  - Stable Non-displaced fracture
  - Acute hook of hamate fracture
  - Extra-articular non-displaced fracture of body of hamate

Surgical Treatment
- **Open reduction internal fixation**
  Indication:
  - Intra-articular displaced fracture of body of hamate
- **Excision of hamate fractured fragment**
  Indication:
  - Chronic hook of hamate fracture with non union

Postoperative physiotherapy treatment: Table 18 shows postoperative physiotherapy protocol for carpal fracture.

■ METACARPAL FRACTURE

Fracture of metacarpals accounts for around 10% of all the fractures and around 18–44% of all hand injuries. Fractures of metacarpals are classified as head, neck and shaft fracture. Metacarpal neck is the most common site of fracture.

Mechanism of Injury

It is often caused by a traumatic axial impact on metacarpal. Compression along the metacarpal bone is often caused when a person punches against a hard object.

Clinical Presentation

- Severe pain, tenderness, swelling and bruising over hand
- Inability to move the finger
- Shortening of involved finger
- Stiffness of the fingers and pain when trying to form a fist.
- Injured finger crosses over its neighbor finger when trying to make a partial fist.

Some common metacarpal fractures are:
- **Bennett fracture dislocation (Fig. 37):** This is an intra-articular two part fracture dislocation of the base of first metacarpal bone.
- **Rolando fracture (Fig. 38):** This is three parts or comminuted intra-articular fracture dislocation of the base of first metacarpal

Table 18: Postoperative physiotherapy protocol for carpal fracture.

	Precaution	ROM exercises	Strengthening exercises
Week 0–2	Avoid PROM	AROM for shoulder and digits	Gentle isometric exercise to intrinsic muscle of hand
Weeks 2–4	Same as above	Gentle AROM exercise for elbow and wris	Isometric exercise for deltoid, biceps and triceps
Weeks 4–6	Same as above	AROM to AAROM for elbow and wrist including flexion, extension, supination and pronation	Gentle for isometric exercise for forearm muscles
Weeks 6–10	No heavy lifting and sports activities	Full AROM and PROM exercises for elbow and wrist including supination and pronation for forearm	Progressive resisted exercises for forearm muscles

(ROM: range of motion; PROM: passive range of motion; AROM: active range of motion; AAROM: active-assisted range of motion)

Fractures and Dislocations

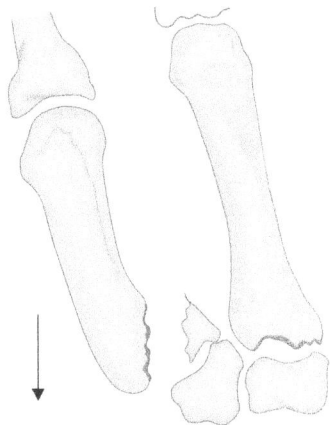

Fig. 37: Bennett fracture dislocation.

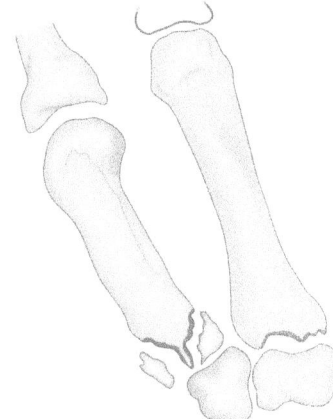

Fig. 38: Rolando fracture.

bone. It is also termed as comminuted Bennett fracture as the mechanism of injury is as of Bennett fracture.
- **Reverse Rolando fracture:** This is a three part intra-articular fracture of the base of first metacarpal.
- **Boxer's fracture (Fig. 39):** This is the fracture of the neck of fifth metacarpal bone.

Complications
- **Postfracture stiffness:** It commonly occurs due to prolonged immobilization.
- **Malunion:** Dorsal apex angulation and rotational deformity.

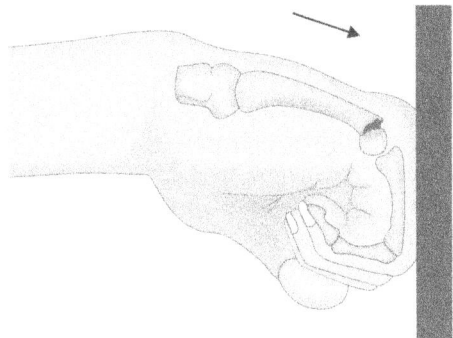

Fig. 39: Boxer's fracture.

Fracture healing time: 4–6 weeks

Management

Nonsurgical Treatment
- **Cast and immobilization:** Short cast is applied for 4 weeks with wrist in 30° extension, MCP joint in between 60–90° flexion and DIP and PIP joint in 5–10° of flexion to maintain the collateral ligaments in elongated position. Along with this the affected finger is buddy taped with the adjacent finger to maintain the alignment.

Indications:
- Stable fracture of neck and shaft of metacarpal
- No rotational deformity.
- Acceptable neck angulation (i.e. 10–15° of index and long finger, 30–40° of ring finger and 50–60° of little finger).
- Acceptable shaft angulation (i.e. 10–20° of index and long finger, 20° of ring finger and 30° of little finger).
- Acceptable shaft shortening (i.e. 2–5 mm).

Surgical Treatment
Closed reduction and percutaneous pinning: Variety of methods including intramedullary pin fixation, crossed Kirschner wires (K-wires) and transfixation to other metacarpals are used. Applications of pins are followed by immobilization of hand in cast or splint for proper fixation. Pins and cast are removed after 3–4 weeks.

Indications:
- Unstable metacarpal neck and shaft fracture.
- Intra-articular basal fractures of first and fifth metacarpal bone.

■ **Open reduction and internal fixation:** Fractured fragments are fixed with multiple small screws in collateral recess, headless screws or K-wires. Postoperatively the hand is immobilized in cast or splint for 3–4 weeks.

Indications:
- Intra-articular fracture
- Rotational malalignment of digit
- Significantly displaced fractures
- Multiple metacarpal shaft fractures
- Loss inherent stability from border digit during healing process.

Postoperative physiotherapy treatment: Table 19 shows the postoperative physiotherapy protocol for metacarpal fracture.

LOWER LIMB FRACTURES

■ PELVIC FRACTURE

Pelvic fractures are uncommon and accounts for only about 3% of all adult fractures. The pelvis is a butterfly shaped group of bones at the base of the spine. It consists of three bones: pubis, ilium and ischium.

Mechanism of Injury

- **High energy trauma:** Most commonly occurs in motor vehicle crashes. It may also occur due to fall from height.
- **Low energy trauma:** Commonly occurs in adolescents and elderly. In elderly, sacrum and anterior pelvic ring fracture frequently results from falls while ambulating. In adolescents, avulsion fractures of superior or inferior iliac spines, iliac apophyses or ischial tuberosity occurs due to athletic activity injury.

Clinical Presentation

- Severe pain, swelling and bruising occurs in groin, hip or low back region.
- Pain is aggravated by weight bearing or moving the legs.
- Abdominal pain may present.
- Numbness, tingling sensation in groin or legs.
- Patient tries to keep his hip or knee flexed in a specific position to avoid pain.

Classification

Pelvic fractures are commonly described by one of the two classification system.

1. **Modified Tile classification (Fig. 40 and Table 20):** It is based on the integrity of the posterior sacroiliac complex.

Table 19: Postoperative physiotherapy protocol for metacarpal fracture.

	Precaution	ROM exercises	Strengthening exercises
Week 0–2	No PROM for the affected fingers	AROM for nonsplinted fingers	Isometric exercise for nonsplinted fingers within the cast
Weeks 2–4	Same as above	• AROM for affected fingers. • AROM, AAROM and PROM for nonsplinted fingers	Same as above
Weeks 4–6	Same as above	Full ROM for fingers and wrist (including pronation, supination, UD and RD)	• Grip strengthening exercises • Progressive resistance exercises for fingers adduction and abduction
Weeks 6–10	None	Same as above	Progressive resisted exercises for all fingers and wrist muscles

(PROM: passive range of motion; ROM: range of motion; AROM: active range of motion; AAROM: active-assisted range of motion; UD: ulnar deviation; RD: radial deviation)

Fractures and Dislocations

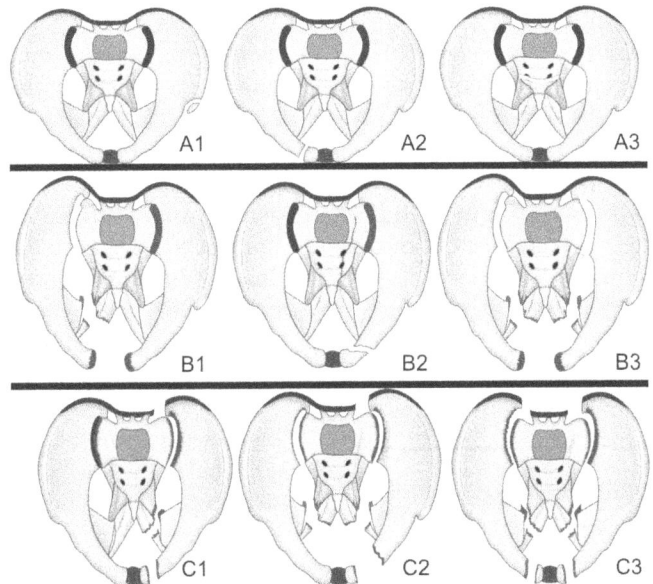

Fig. 40: Modified Tile classification of pelvic fracture.

Table 20: Modified Tile classification for pelvic fracture.

Type	Description
Type A	**Stable (posterior arch intact)**
A1	Avulsion of the innominate bone
A2	Iliac wing or anterior arch fracture caused by a direct blow
A3	Transverse sacrococcygeal fracture
Type B	**Partial stable (incomplete disruption of posterior arch):** Rotational unstable and vertical stable
B1	Open book injury (external rotation)
B2	Lateral compression injury (internal rotation)
B2.1	Ipsilateral anterior and posterior injuries
B2.2	Contralateral anterior and posterior (bucket handle) injuries
B3	Bilateral
Type C	**Complete unstable (complete disruption of posterior arch):** Rotational and vertical unstable
C1	Unilateral
C1.1	Iliac fracture

Contd...

Contd...

Type	Description
C1.2	Sacroiliac fracture dislocation
C1.3	Sacral fracture
C2	Bilateral with one side type B and one side type C
C3	Bilateral with both side type C

2. **Young-Burgess classification (Fig. 41 and Table 21):** It is based on the mechanism of injury, i.e. predominant direction of force vector at the time of injury.

Complications

Complications of pelvic fractures are often frequent and severe. In acute phase, patients are susceptible to the development of adult respiratory distress syndrome, thromboembolic disease, pneumonia and multiple organ failure.

- **Infection:** Approximately 6% of pelvic fractures suffer from infection. Incidence of infection increases when associated with open bowel injury, obesity, diabetes and delay in treatment.

- **Nerve palsy:** Injuries to L5 or S1 nerve roots usually occurs in pelvic fractures. Particularly peroneal component of sciatic nerve is involved. L4 nerve may also be involved in severe injuries.
- **Thromboembolic problems:** Significant pelvic hemorrhage may occur in up to 75% of pelvic fractures. It increases the risk of developing DVT or pulmonary embolism.
- **Nonunion/malunion:** These may occur due to inadequate initial treatment of displaced pelvic fractures.
- **Genitourinary complications:** Around 37% of patients with pelvic fractures have genitourinary complication due to disruptions of bladder, ureter and kidney.
- **Sexual dysfunction:** Around 29% of patients with pelvic ring injuries suffered from dyspareunia and erectile dysfunction.
- **Associated injuries:** The most significant complications of pelvic fractures are those that results from accompanying injuries to adjacent or distant osseous and soft tissues structures. Most common associated injuries are:
  - Morel-Lavalle lesion: It is a significant soft tissue injury associated with pelvic trauma. In this, subcutaneous tissues are torn away from the underlying fascia, creating a hematoma and liquefied fat filled cavity. A soft fluctuant area may be present over greater trochanter or in dorsolumbar region.

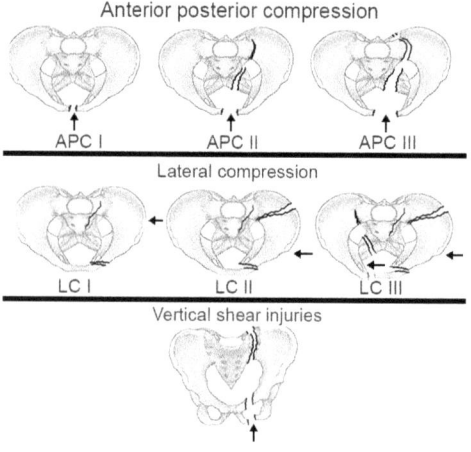

Fig. 41: Young Burgess classification of pelvic fractures.

Table 21: Young Burgess classification for pelvic fracture.

Type	Description
Type 1	**Anteroposterior compression (APC):** Common feature is diastasis of pubic symphysis or vertical fracture of pubic rami
APC I	Pubic symphysis diastasis, <2.5 cm, no significant posterior ring injury (stable)
APC II	Pubic symphysis diastasis, >2.5 cm, tearing of anterior sacral ligaments (rotational unstable, vertically stable)
APC III	Hemipelvis separation with complete disruption of pubic symphysis and posterior ligament complexes (completely unstable)
Type 2	**Lateral compression (LC):** Common feature is a transverse fracture of pubic rami
LC I	Posterior compression of sacroiliac (SI) joint without ligament disruption (stable)
LC II	Posterior SI ligament rupture, sacral crush injury or iliac wing fracture (rotationally unstable, vertically stable)
LC III	LC II with open book (APC) injury to contralateral pelvis (completely unstable)
Type 3	**Vertical shear injuries (VS):** Common feature is a vertical fracture of pubic rami Displaced fractures of anterior rami and posterior columns including SI dislocation (completely unstable)
Type 4	**Combined mechanism (CM) fractures:** Massive pelvic injuries that do not fit the other categories (completely unstable)

- **Soft tissue injuries:** It can vary from superficial abrasion and lacerations to closed internal degloving injuries to open wounds. Perineal, rectal and vaginal lacerations are indicative of severe injuries.
- **Urogenital injuries:** Around 12% of pelvic injuries are associated with urogenital injuries characterized by hematuria, presence of blood at external urethral meatus, swelling in perineal and genital region and high riding prostate gland in male.
- **Skeletal injuries:** Axial and appendicular skeletal injuries are frequently associated with pelvic ring fractures.

Bone healing time: 8–12 weeks

Management

Nonsurgical Treatment

- **Weight bearing as tolerated using assistive device:** Crutches or walker for up to 3 months or until the bones are fully healed. Wheelchair for sometime may be needed to avoid weight bearing.
  Indications: Nondisplaced or minimally displaced fractures.

Surgical Treatment

- **Open reduction and internal fixation:** The displaced fragments of bone are first repositioned or reduced to their normal alignment and then held together with screws or metal plates.
  Indications:
  - Symphysis diastasis >2.5 cm
  - Sacroiliac (SI) joint displacement >1 cm
  - Sacral fracture with displacement >1 cm
  - Displacement or rotation of hemipelvis
  - Chronic pain and diastasis in parturition induced diastasis.
- **External fixation:** In this metal pins or screws are inserted into the bones through small incisions into the skin and muscles and then projected out of the skin on both the sides of pelvis to attach them to the carbon fire bars outside the skin.

Indications:
- Complex pelvic ring fracture
- Severe open fractures
- Crushing injuries
- Pelvic ring injuries with an external rotation component (APC, VS, CM)
- Unstable ring injury with ongoing bleeding.

Postoperative physiotherapy treatment: Table 22 shows the postoperative physiotherapy treatment protocol for pelvic stable fractures.

■ PROXIMAL FEMORAL FRACTURE

Proximal part of femur includes head of femur, neck of femur and trochanteric region of femur.

Classification of Proximal Femur Fracture

On the basis of their location with regard to the joint capsule, i.e. intracapsular and extracapsular fractures (Fig. 42).

Intracapsular Fractures

These fractures include the sites within the lining of hip joint capsule and associated with injury to blood supply to head of femur. A compromised blood supply may result in avascular necrosis of femoral head.

- **Femoral head fractures:** Usually occurs secondary to femoral head dislocation.
- **Femoral neck fractures:** Depending on fracture location the femoral neck fractures are classified as:
  - **Subcapital fracture:** Fractures just below the head of femur.
  - **Transcervical fracture:** Fractures through midneck of femur.
  - **Basicervical fracture:** Fractures through base of neck of femur.

Extracapsular Fractures

These fractures are present outside the capsule and do not cause the same degree of vascular damage as intracapsular fractures and therefore can be treated differently.

Simplified Approach to Orthopedic Physiotherapy

Table 22: Postoperative physiotherapy treatment protocol for pelvic stable fractures.

	Precaution	ROM exercises	Strengthening exercises	Weight bearing
Week 0–2	Do not roll or lie towards the operated side	• Ankle toe movement • AROM of hip adduction, abduction • AROM of knee flexion, extension, i.e. heel slide	Isometric exercise for glutei, quadriceps, hamstring	NWB
Weeks 3–6	High impact activities	AROM, AAROM and gentle PROM for hip and knee	• Same as above • PRE of surrounding muscles of pelvic area and trunk muscles	PWB and gait re-education in parallel bars
Weeks 7–8	High impact activities	Complete AROM and PROM for hip and knee	• Same as above • Upper body strengthening exercises	FWBAT with assistive device
Weeks 8–12	High impact activities	Complete AROM and PROM exercise for hip and knee	• Same as above • Cardiovascular exercises	FWB

(ROM: range of motion; AROM: active range of motion; AAROM: active-assisted range of motion; PROM: passive range of motion; PRE: progressive resistance exercises; NWB: noweight bearing; PWB: partial weight bearing; FWBAT: full weight bearing as tolerated; FWB: Full weight bearing)

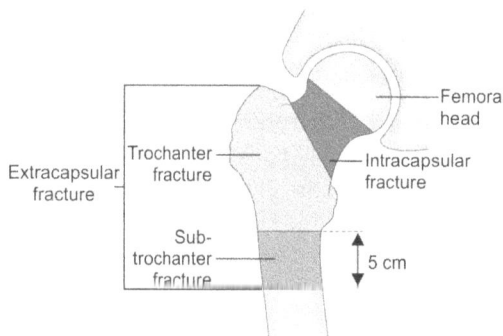

Fig. 42: Classification of proximal femur fractures on the basis of their location with regard to joint capsule.

The trochanteric fractures are extracapsular injuries:
- Intertrochanteric fractures
- Subtrochanteric fractures

Fracture of Head of Femur

It is a rare fracture which is commonly associated with dislocation of hip.

Mechanism of Injury
- Falling from height.
- Motor vehicle accident in which the knees strikes against the dashboard of vehicle.

Classification of Femoral Head Fracture
Figure 43 and Table 23 shows the Pipkin classification of fracture of head of femur.
Complications: Avascular necrosis.

Fracture of Neck of Femur

It is most frequently occurs in elderly osteoporotic patients. Elderly females are more affected than males.

Neck of femur fracture is considered as an intracapsular fracture. According to anatomical location femoral neck fractures are further classified in the following types (Fig. 44):
- **Subcapital fracture:** Head and neck junction of femur.
- **Transcervical fracture:** Mid portion of neck of femur.
- **Basicervical fracture:** Base of neck of femur.

Classification of Femoral Neck Fracture
Garden classification: Based on the degree of valgus displacement on anterior posterior (AP) radiograph (Fig. 45 and Table 24).

Pauwels classification: Based on vertical orientation of fracture line (Fig. 46 and Table 25).

Fractures and Dislocations

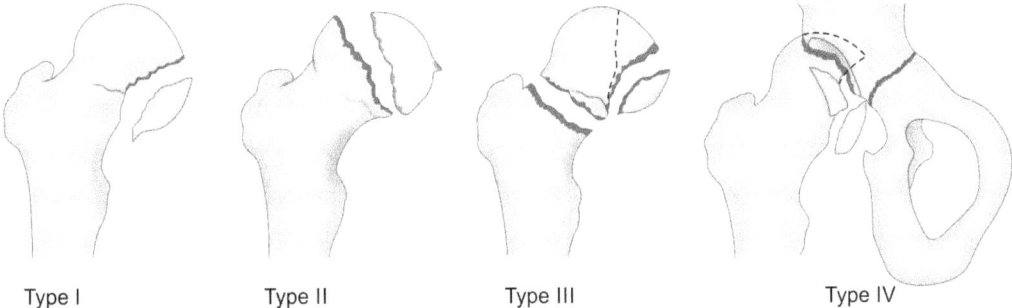

Type I Type II Type III Type IV

Fig. 43: Pipkin classifiaction of femoral head fracture.

Table 23: Pipkin classification of femoral head fracture.

Type	Description
I	Fracture inferior to fovea capitis. Small fracture that does not involve the weight bearing surface of femoral head
II	Fracture superior to fovea capitis. Large fracture that involves the weight bearing surface of femoral head
III	Type I or II associated with femoral neck fracture. Increase risk of avascular necrosis
IV	Type I or II associated with actabular fracture usually posterior wall

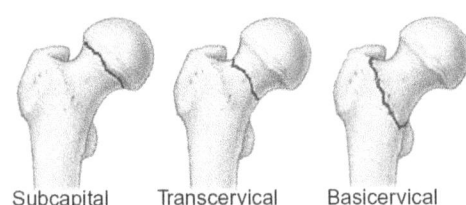

Subcapital Transcervical Basicervical

Fig. 44: Types of femoral neck fracture.

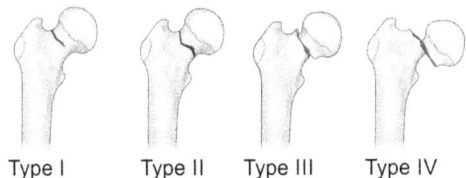

Type I Type II Type III Type IV

Fig. 45: Garden classification.

OTA Classification

Table 26 shows the orthopedic trauma association (OTA) classification.

Table 24: Garden classification of femoral neck fracture.

Type	Description
I	Incomplete/valgus impacted
II	Complete and nondisplaced
III	Complete with partial displacement
IV	Completely displaced

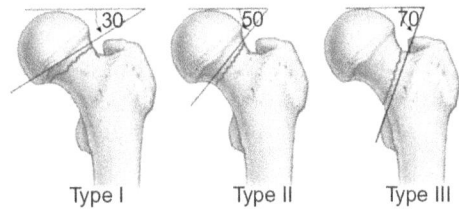

Type I Type II Type III

Fig. 46: Pauwels classification.

Table 25: Pauwels classification of femoral neck fracture.

Type	Description
I	Less than 30° from horizontal
II	30–50° from horizontal
III	More than 50° from horizontal. Most unstable with greater risk of avascular necrosis and nonunion

Mechanism of Injury
- Motor vehicle accident that causes axial loading during high force trauma with an abducted hip in young patients.
- Fall directly onto the hip in elderly patients.

Table 26: Orthopedic trauma association (OTA) classification of femoral neck fracture.

B1 Group fracture	Nondisplaced to minimally displaced subcapital fractures
B2 Group fracture	Transcervical fracture (through middle to base of neck)
B3 Group fracture	All displaced nonimpacted subcapital fractures

Complication
- **Avascular necrosis:** Higher incidence of avascular necrosis (AVN) of femoral head in femoral neck fracture is due to the extensive interruption of blood supply to femoral head.

Trochanteric Fracture

It is the fracture that involves greater and/or lesser trochanter of femur.

Classification on the Basis of Anatomical Location (Fig. 47)
- Intertrochanteric region
- Subtrochanteric region: It lies between the lesser trochanter and 5 cm distal.
- Greater trochanteric avulsion fracture
- Lesser trochanteric avulsion fracture.

Complication
Malunion: Malunion results in coxa vara deformity, rotational deformity or shortening of limb.

Intertrochanteric Fracture of Femur

It is an extracapsular fracture of proximal femur that lies between the greater and lesser trochanter. It is also more prevalent among elderly patients. Females are more affected than males.

Mechanism of Injury
Same as for femoral neck fracture.
- High energy trauma in young individuals.
- Low energy trauma like trivial fall in elderly people.

Evans Classification of Intertrochanteric Fracture
Based on the stability of fracture fragments (Fig. 48 and Table 27).

Subtrochanteric Fracture

Subtrochanteric fracture is between the lesser trochanter and the adjoining proximal third, i.e. isthmus of femoral shaft.

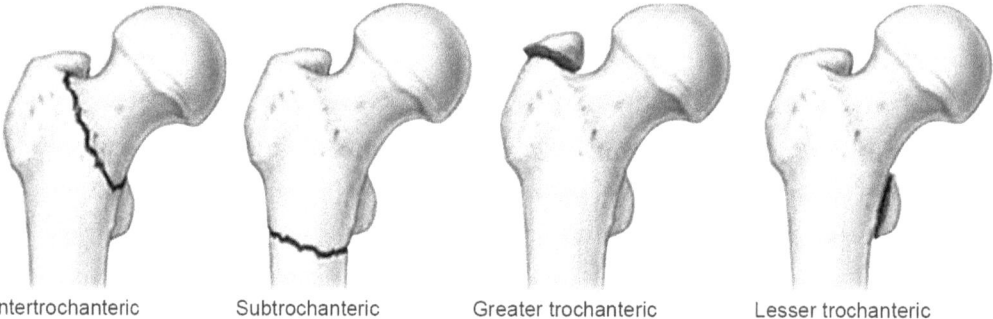

Fig. 47: Classification of trochanteric fracture.

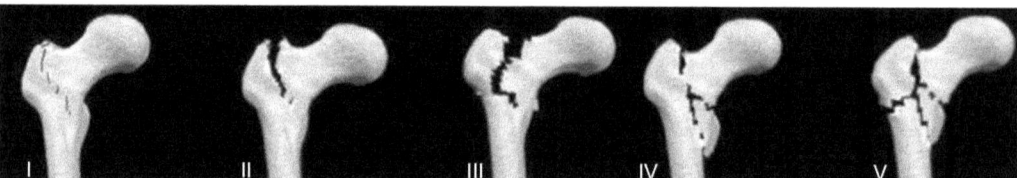

Fig. 48: Evans classification of stable intertrochanteric fracture.

Table 27: Evans classification.

Type	Description
I	**Stable fracture** Fracture line extends upwards and outwards from lesser trochanter
A	2 fragment undisplaced fracture
B	2 fragment displaced fracture
C	3 fragment fracture without posterolateral support. Displaced greater trochanter fragment
D	3 fragment fracture without medial support. Displaced lesser trochanter fragment
E	4 fragment fracture without posterolateral and medial support
II	**Unstable fracture** Fracture line extends downwards and outwards from lesser trochanter

Mechanism of Injury
Same as for neck of femur fracture and intertrochanteric fracture.
- Motor vehicle accident that causes axial loading during high force trauma with an abducted hip in young patients.
- Fall directly onto the hip in elderly people.

Complications
- **Nonunion:** Inability to resume full weight bearing (WB) within 3-6 months indicates nonunion.
- **Malunion:** Malunion of subtrochanteric fracture causes limp, leg length discrepancy or rotational deformity.

Bone healing time: 12–16 weeks

Management
Patients with hip fracture should be admitted to the hospital by keeping the hip in slight flexion and external rotated and supported by keeping the pillows under the knees.

Surgical Options
- **Closed or open reduction and internal fixation:**

Indications: Younger patient of less than 65 years having impacted, nondisplaced or adequately reduced fractures.
- **Prosthetic replacement of femoral head: Indications:** Patients of more than 65 years having unstable fractures or when satisfactory reduction cannot be obtained.

Postoperative physiotherapy treatment: Table 28 shows the postoperative physiotherapy treatment for proximal femur fracture.

■ FEMORAL SHAFT FRACTURE
It is diaphyseal fracture of femur. Femur is longest and strongest bone of our body. Therefore high energy force is required to break it. It usually occurs in individuals of less than 25 years and more than 65 years.

Mechanism of Injury
- High energy trauma such as direct trauma to thigh associated with motor vehicle accidents, high impact sport, falling from height or direct blow, gunshot wound or any other violence.
- Low energy trauma such as minor fall from standing position in elderly patients.

Clinical Presentation
- Pain with weight bearing.
- Tenderness, swelling and bruising over thigh.
- The leg may appear shorter and crooked.

Classification
On the basis of the angle of fracture line:
- **Transverse fracture:** When the shaft is fractured horizontally along its length.
- **Spiral fracture:** It results from twisting force and the break is helical, i.e. fracture line spirals along the long axis.
- **Oblique fracture:** When the fracture line runs oblique to the long axis of shaft.
- **Segmental fracture:** When the shaft is broken at two places in a way that leaves at least one segment floating and unattached.
- **Comminuted:** When the shaft is broken in three or more fragments.

Table 28: Postoperative physiotherapy treatment for proximal femur fracture.

	Precaution	ROM exercises	Strengthening exercises	Weight bearing
Week 0–2	• Avoid hip adduction and abduction • Avoid isometrics of quads and hams	AROM for hip and knee flexion, extension	Isometric exercise for glutei	• TTWB in unstable fracture treated with ORIF • WBAT in stable fracture treated with IM nail
Weeks 2–4	Avoid end range adduction and abduction	AROM, AAROM and gentle PROM for hip in flexion and extension	Isometric exercise for glutei, quadriceps and hamstrings	Same as above
Weeks 4–8	Avoid torsional force at fracture site	• Same as above. • AROM for hip adduction and abduction	Same as above	Same as above
Weeks 8–12	None	Complete AROM and PROM exercises for hip and knee	Progressive resisted exercises for hip and knee muscles	Progress from TTWB to PWB to FWB

(ROM: range of motion; AROM: active range of motion; AAROM: active-assisted range of motion; PROM: passive range of motion; TTWB: toe touch weight bearing; ORIF: open reduction and internal fixation; WBAT: weight bearing as tolerated; IM: intramedullary; PWB: partial weight bearing; FWB: full weight bearing)

On the basis of the level of fracture on shaft of femur:
- Proximal third
- Middle third
- Distal third.

On the basis of the Degree of Fracture Comminution: Winquist's Classification

Figure 49 and Table 29 shows the Winquist's classification of femoral shaft fracture.

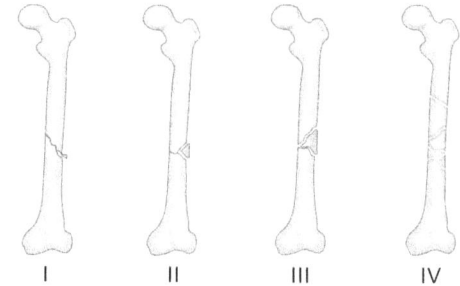

Fig. 49: Winquist's classification.

Complications
- **Shock (hypovolemic shock):** The most immediate complication is blood loss. As the femur is very vascular bone, the fracture of femur may result in massive blood loss (e.g. in adults up to 1500 ml may readily be lost) that eventually cause hypovolemic shock.
- **Compartment syndrome of thigh:** Femoral shaft fracture often leads to compartment syndrome of thigh that needs an early surgical intervention.

Table 29: Winquist's classification of femoral shaft fracture.

Type	Description
1	A tiny cortical fragment
2	Butterfly fragment is larger but still at least 50% cortical contact between the main fragments
3	Butterfly fragment involves more than 50% of bone width
4	Comminuted fracture

- **Neurovascular injuries:** Femoral shaft fracture may be associated with sciatic nerve, pudendal nerve, femoral nerve and arterial injury.
- **Fat embolism:** There is a high incidence of fat embolism with this injury. This usually occurs within 48-72 hours of the injury.
- **Malunion and rotational malalignment:** Angular deformity and rotational deformity occurs due to malalignment and muscular action on the fractured fragments.
- **Limb length discrepancy:** The incidence of limb length discrepancy is high in children. Both overgrowth and shortening may be noted by following femoral shaft fracture in the child. Children of 2-10 years are at greater risk for overgrowth by following shaft fracture.

Fracture healing time: 6 to 8 weeks

Management

Nonsurgical Treatment

Most femoral shaft fractures require surgery. Very rarely it is treated nonoperatively.

- **Closed reduction and cast immobilization:** Very young children are sometimes treated with cast. Children between 7 months to 5 years are treated with application of spica cast for the proper alignment of the fragments till the bone is fused.
  Indications: Nondisplaced femoral shaft fractures

Surgical Treatment

- **Intramedullary nailing:** Intramedullary nail is dynamically or statically interlocked with screws. Interlocking offers stability and rotational control. Antegrade and retrograde intramedullary nailing techniques are used. It is the gold standard treatment of diaphyseal femur fractures.
- **Open reduction and internal fixation:** It is preferred for femur shaft fracture with periarticular or intra-articular extension that precludes placement of an intramedullary nail.

  Indications:
  - Ipsilateral neck fracture requiring screw fixation.
  - Fracture at distal metaphyseal-diaphyseal junction.
  - Inability to access medullary canal.
- **External fixation:** It is often a temporary measure and conversion to intramedullary nail is done within 2-3 weeks.
  Indications:
  - Type 3 open fractures (wound larger than 10 cm with extensive soft tissue and bone loss).
  - Severely comminuted and displaced fractures.

Postoperative physiotherapy treatment: Table 30 shows postoperative physiotherapy treatment for femoral shaft fracture.

DISTAL FEMORAL FRACTURE

■ SUPRACONDYLAR FRACTURE

It is a metaphyseal fracture of femur that includes distal 8 to 15 cm of the femur. It accounts for approximately 4-7% of all femoral fracture.

Mechanism of Injury

- High energy trauma in young patients.
- Low energy fall in elderly patients.

Clinical Presentation

- Pain with weight bearing.
- Swelling and bruising around knee or thigh.
- Tenderness to touch around the knee or may be also in thigh region.
- Knee may look out of place and the leg may appear shorter and crooked.

Classification

Figure 50 and Table 31 shows the Muller's classification of distal femoral fracture.

Complications

- **Knee osteoarthritis:** Most likely to occur when fracture line involves the articular surface due to the disruption of smooth cartilaginous layer.

Table 30: Postoperative physiotherapy treatment for femoral shaft fracture.

	Precaution	ROM exercises	Strengthening exercises	Weight bearing
Week 0–4	• Avoid PROM for hip or knee • Avoid rotatory movement with foot on ground	AROM for hip and knee	Isometric exercises for quadriceps and glutei	• FWBAT in stable fractures • TTWB or NWB in unstable fractures
Weeks 4–8	Avoid rotatory movement with foot on ground.	AROM, AAROM and Gentle PROM for hip and knee	• Same as above. • SLR	• FWBAT in stable fractures. • TTWB or PWB in unstable fractures
Weeks 8–12	Avoid rotatory movement with foot on ground	AROM, AAROM and PROM for hip and knee	Progressive resistance exercises for quads, hams and glutei	• FWBAT in stable fractures. • PWB in unstable fractures
Weeks 12–16	None	Complete AROM and PROM for hip and knee	Same as above	Progress from PWB to FWB

(PROM: passive range of motion; ROM: range of motion; AROM: active range of motion; AAROM: active-assisted range of motion; SLR: straight leg raising; FWBAT: full weight bearing as tolerated; TTWB: toe touch weight bearing; PWB: partial weight bearing; NWB: no weight bearing; FWB: full weight bearing)

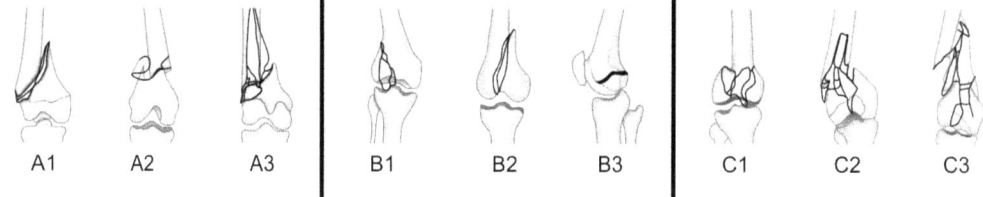

Fig. 50: Muller's clasification.

Table 31: Muller's classification of distal femoral fracture.

A   Extra-articular fracture
- A1   Simple metaphyseal component
- A2   Wedge fracture in metaphyseal region
- A3   Complex metaphyseal involvement

B   Partial articular fracture
- B1   Sagittal lateral condyle fracture
- B2   Sagittal medial condyle fracture
- B3   Coronal/Hoffa fracture:
  - B3.1   Anterior and lateral flake fracture
  - B3.2   Unicondylar posterior fracture
  - B3.3   Bicondylar posterior fracture

Contd...

C   Complete articular fracture
- C1   Supracondylar/intercondylar femur fracture with simple metaphyseal and articular fracture
- C2   Supracondylar/intercondylar femur fracture with complex metaphyseal and simple articular fracture
- C3   Supracondylar/intercondylar femur fracture with complex articular fracture

- **Knee stiffness:** It usually occurs due to prolonged immobilization of limb.
- **Infection:** It is more common in case of open fracture. It can be minimized or prevented by using proper antibiotics.

- **Surgical complications:** It could be due to the failure of the implant used for the fixation of bony fragments which can cause persistent pain and irritation.
- **Compartment syndrome:** Associated trauma can lead to inflammation and bleeding which can further lead to the compression of vessel, nerves and muscle in the thigh compartment.
- **Nonunion:** Most commonly occurs that is in comminuted fractures.
- **Malunion:** Commonly valgus occurs that is often associated with plating.

Fracture healing time: 12–16 weeks

Management

Nonsurgical Treatment

- **Casting and traction:** This treatment is associated with severe potential risks of prolonged bed rest and malunion (valgus, varus or rotational deformities).
  Indications: Severe life threatening or other medical condition in which the risks of anesthesia are high.

Surgical Treatment

- **Open reduction and internal fixation:** Almost all the distal femur fracture is treated with operative interventions because of greater risks of prolonged immobilization.
  Indications:
  - Unicondylar fracture
  - Fracture in coronal plane (Hoffa fracture)
  - Open intra-articular fracture
  - Ipsilateral fracture of tibial plateau or patellar fracture
  - Ipsilateral fracture of tibia (floating knee)
  - Associated neurovascular injuries
  - Multiple injuries
  - Pathological fractures.

Postoperative physiotherapy treatment: Table 32 shows postoperative physiotherapy treatment protocol for distal femoral fracture.

■ PATELLAR FRACTURE

It is the break in kneecap or patella. Patellar fracture comprises only 1% of all skeletal injuries.

Mechanism of Injury

- **Direct injury:** Direct fall or blow onto the knee or due to the hitting of patella against the dashboard in motor vehicle accidents (MVA).

Table 32: Postoperative physiotherapy treatment for distal femoral fracture.

	Precaution	ROM exercises	Strengthening exercises	Weight bearing
Week 0–4	Avoid PROM	• AROM • Full knee extension • 60–90° knee flexion	Isometric exercises for quadriceps and hamstrings	None
Weeks 4–8	Same as above	• >90° knee extension • AROM, AAROM in flexion and extension	Isometric exercises for quadriceps and hamstrings	None
Weeks 8–12	Avoid aggressive PROM	AROM, AAROM and Gentle PROM exercise	Isometric and isotonic exercises for quadriceps and hamstring	None
Weeks 12–16	Avoid aggressive PROM	Complete AROM and PROM exercises of knee	Isometric, isotonic and progressive resisted exercises to quads and hams	Progress from TTWB to PWB to FWB

(PROM: passive range of motion; ROM: range of motion; AROM: active range of motion; AAROM: active-assisted range of motion; TTWB: toe touch weight bearing; PWB: partial weight bearing; FWB: full weight bearing)

Simplified Approach to Orthopedic Physiotherapy

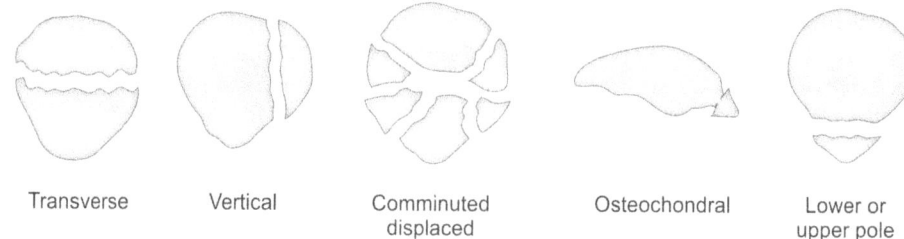

Fig. 51: Classification of patellar fracture on the basis of pattern of fracture.

- **Indirect injury:** Excessive tension through the extensor mechanism results from forceful contraction of quadriceps muscles with knee in flexed position.

Clinical Presentation
- Severe pain in and around the kneecap.
- Bruising and swelling in the front of the knee.
- Inability to walk and extend the knee.
- Deformed appearance of knee.
- Tenderness when pressing on the kneecap.

Classification
On the basis of displacement of fragments:
- **Displaced fracture:** More than 3 mm of fragment separation or more than 2 mm of articular incongruity.
- **Undisplaced fracture:** Less than 3 mm of fragment separation or less than 2 mm of articular congruity.

On the basis of the pattern of fracture (Fig. 51):
- **Transverse fracture:** when the patella splitted occurs through the midline dividing the patella into upper and lower part. It usually requires surgical interventions to put the patellar fragments back together.
- **Longitudinal/vertical fracture:** When the patella is splitted vertically and divides the patella in two parts right and left.
- **Comminuted (stellate) fracture:** When the patella shatters into more than two fragments. It can be further classified into:
  - Undisplaced comminuted fracture
  - Displaced comminuted fracture
- **Osteochondral fracture:** It refers to an injury to the cartilage and the underlying bone of patella. It is usually associated with acute patellar dislocation.
- **Pole:** Fracture of upper or lower pole.

Complications
- **Postfracture knee stiffness:** It occurs due to prolonged immobilization in healing phase.
- **Extensor mechanism insufficiency:** Weakness of the quadriceps muscle along with some loss of extension and flexion in the knee is also common.
- **Post-traumatic arthritis:** Severe arthritis is less prevalent whereas mild to moderate arthritis known as chondromalacia patella is more common. It occurs due to the disruption of articular cartilage.
- **Chronic pain:** It may be related to post-traumatic arthritis, stiffness, and muscle weakness.
- **Loss of reduction:** May occur in osteoporotic bone.
- **Osteonecrosis of proximal fragment:** It may occur due to excessive initial fracture displacement.

Fracture healing time: 8–12 weeks

Management
Nonsurgical Treatment
- **Knee immobilized in extension (brace or cylinder cast):** The limb is immobilized in cylinder cast for 4–6 weeks. Progression in flexion done after 2–3 weeks.

Indications:
- Intact extensor mechanism
- Extra articular fracture
- Nondisplaced or minimally displaced fractures
- Vertical fracture patterns.

Surgical Treatment
- **Open reduction and internal fixation:**
  Indications:
  - Extensor mechanism failure
  - Open fractures
  - Comminuted fracture
  - Fracture articular displacement > 2 mm
  - Displaced patella fracture > 3 mm
  - Patella sleeve fractures in children.
- **Partial/Total patellectomy:** It refers to partial or complete excision of patella. After excision, the limb is immobilized in full extension for approximately 4 weeks.
  Indications: Severely comminuted fracture that cannot be repaired and ONLY when open reduction interal fixaton (ORIF) is also not possible.

Postoperative physiotherapy treatment: Table 33 shows postoperative physiotherapy treatment for patellar fracture.

PROXIMAL TIBIAL FRACTURE

It is also termed as tibial plateau fracture that involves the proximal metaphysis of tibia. Lateral plateau is more commonly fractured than medial plateau because large amount of force is required to injure medial plateau.

Mechanism of Injury
- High energy trauma in young people, such as MVA, fall from height or any strenuous sports activity.
- Low energy trauma in elderly people; trivial fall from standing.
- Due to metastatic disease or infection of bone.
- Valgus or varus loading with/without axial loading.

Clinical Presentation
- Severe pain, tenderness, swelling and/or bruising over the fracture site.
- Inability to bear weight on affected limb.
- Appearance of deformed leg.
- Numbness and coldness below the foot or lower leg due to vascular damage.

Table 33: Postoperative physiotherapy treatment for patellar fracture.

	Precaution	ROM exercises	Strengthening exercises	Weight bearing
Week 0–4	• Avoid PROM	• Not possible if in cast. • AROM for knee in sitting position when treated with ORIF	No strengthening for knee muscles	FWB with assistive device
Weeks 4–8	• Same as above	• AROM for knee flexion and extension	Isometric exercise for quadriceps and hamstrings	FWB
Weeks 6–8	• Avoid aggressive PROM	• AROM, AAROM and Gentle PROM exercise	• Same as above • Isotonic exercise for quads with active knee extension initially from 45° flexion to 0° extension and then gradually from 90° flexion to 0° extension	FWB
Weeks 8–12	• None	• Complete AROM and PROM exercises of knee	• Progressive resisted exercises to quads and hams • Closed chain exercises	FWB

(PROM: passive range of motion; ROM: range of motion; AROM: active range of motion; ORIF: open reduction and internal fixation; AAROM: active-assisted range of motion; FWB: full weight bearing)

Table 34: Schatzker classification of tibial plateau fracture.

Type	Description
I	Wedge shaped or split fracture of lateral tibial plateau
II	Splitting and depression of lateral tibial plateau
III	Pure depression of lateral tibial plateau
IV	Medial tibial plateau fracture with split or depressed component
V	Bicondylar fracture involving both plateaus and also as Inverted Y fracture
VI	Fracture of proximal tibial diaphyseal-metaphyseal junction, along with any type of tibial plateau fracture (metaphyseal-diaphyseal discontinuity)

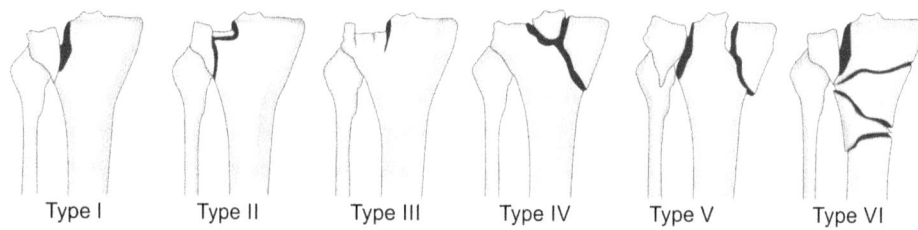

Fig. 52: Schatzker classification.

Classification

Table 34 and Figure 52 shows the Schatzkar classification of tibial plateau fracture.

Complications

- **Compartment syndrome of leg:** Increased pressure in leg compartment due to soft tissue swelling that may compromise the blood circulation of muscles and nerves of affected leg.
- **Secondary knee osteoarthritis:** Post-traumatic arthritis occurs because of the involvement of articular surface and associated knee ligament injuries.
- **Associated neurovascular, ligaments and meniscal injuries:** Fracture of proximal tibia is commonly associated with anterior cruciate ligament (ACL), collateral ligaments (commonly MCL) and meniscal injuries.
- **Malunion:** Malunion commonly causes genu valgus and procurvatum deformities.
- **Post fracture stiffness:** Prolonged immobilization in long arm casts often leads to the knee or ankle stiffness.
- **Fat embolism syndrome (FES):** Incidence of FES is about 16.3% but sometimes it is as high as 50-62%. Most cases have certain predisposing factors like fatty patient, longer injury-surgery interval, reamed nailing, etc.

Fracture healing time: 10-12 weeks

Management

Nonsurgical Treatment

- **Closed reduction and cast immobilization:** Long leg cast is applied with knee in 10-20° of flexion for 4 weeks. The cast is followed by functional brace for 4 weeks.

Indications:
- Undisplaced fractures
- Closed low energy fractures with acceptable alignment
- <5° varus or valgus angulation
- <10° anterior/posterior angulation
- 50% cortical apposition
- <1 cm shortening
- <10° rotational alignment.

Surgical Treatment

- **Intramedullary nailing:** This is the preferable treatment for unstable and segmental tibial fractures. In this the intramedullary nail is interlocked dynamically or statically by screws.
  Indications: When there is enough proximal bone to accept two locking screws.
- **Fixation with percutaneous locking plates:** This is the most preferred technique that enables the surgeon to do percutaneous plating without extensively opening the fracture and with minimum soft tissue dissection. The plate may be used on lateral side or medial side. The lateral plate is preferred because of better available soft tissue cover.
  Indications:
  - Inadequate proximal fixation for intramedullary (IM) nailing.
  - Best suited for transverse or oblique fractures.
- **External fixator:** This is used as a temporary measure to maintain limb length till the soft tissue heals well enough for performing surgery or the patient can become stable enough to be operated.
  Indications:
  - Fractures with extensive soft tissue compromise and bone loss.
  - Multiple trauma.

Postoperative physiotherapy treatment: Table 35 shows postoperative physiotherapy treatment for proximal tibial fracture.

■ TIBIAL SHAFT FRACTURE

It refers to diaphyseal fracture of tibia. Tibial shaft fracture is the most frequently fractured bone of the body.

Mechanism of Injury

- **Low energy fracture:** In this oblique or spiral fracture occurs due to indirect trauma from torsional injury. Often occurs in sports injuries like fall while skiing,

Table 35: Postoperative physiotherapy treatment for proximal tibial fracture.

	Precaution	ROM exercises	Strengthening exercises	Weight bearing
Week 0–4	Avoid rotatory movement with foot on the ground	• Elevated ankle pumps and toe curling • AROM of hip extension, flexion, abduction adduction • Wall slides • AROM for knee and ankle if not in cast	Isometric exercise for quadriceps, tibialis anterior and gastrosoleus	• WBAT with assistive device for stable fracture • NWB to TTWB for unstable fracture
Weeks 4–8	Same as above	Same as above	Isometric and isotonic exercises for knee and ankle	Same as above
Weeks 8–12	None	AROM, AAROM and gentle PROM exercises	Progressive resisted ROM exercises for quads, DF and PF	WB as tolerated
Weeks 12–16	Avoid aggressive PROM	• Complete AROM and PROM exercises for knee • Proprioceptive exercises	Isometric, isotonic and progressive resisted exercises for quads and hams	Progress from TTWB to PWB to FWB

(PROM: passive range of motion; ROM: range of motion; AROM: active range of motion; AAROM: active-assisted range of motion; DF: dorsiflexion; PF: plantar flexion; WBAT: weight bearing as tolerated; NWB: no weight bearing; TTWB: toe touch weight bearing; WB: weight bearing; PWB: partial weight bearing; FWB: full weight bearing)

skating or collapse with other player in soccer or football.
- **High energy fracture:** Transverse or comminuted fracture commonly occurs due to direct impact or force. It is often occurs in motor vehicle accidents.

Clinical Presentation
- Immediate severe pain, swelling and bruising on the leg
- Inability to bear weight on the fractured limb.
- Appearance of deformed leg.
- Numbness or tingling in the foot.
- Bone "tenting" the skin or protruding through a break in the skin.

Classification
On the basis of anatomical location of fracture:
- Proximal one-third.
- Middle one-third.
- Distal one-third.

On the basis of fracture pattern:
- Transverse fracture
- Oblique fracture
- Spiral fracture
- Segmental fracture
- Comminuted fracture.

Table 36 and Figure 53 shows OTA classification of tibial shaft fracture.

Complications
- **Compartment syndrome:** The leg is susceptible to compartment syndrome (4.7% in closed fractures, 3.3% in open fractures) especially anterior and posterior compartment of leg. It is characterized by five P's, i.e. increased pressure, pulselessness, paresthesia, pain and pallor to the distal affected extremity.
- **Nonunion:** When no visible signs of healing present for the past 3 months. It may occur due to variety of causes like infection, malnutrition, unstable fracture fixation or incomplete fracture reduction.
- **Neurovascular injury:** Common peroneal nerve and popliteal artery are more susceptible to injure in tibial shaft fracture.
- **Posttraumatic subtalar and ankle joint stiffness:** It may occur due to prolonged immobilization.
- **Malunion:** High incidence of valgus and procurvatum (apex anterior) malalignment in proximal third fractures. Malalignment, rotation or angulation of the

Table 36: OTA classification for tibial shaft fracture.

Type	Description
A	**Simple fractures**
A1	Simple spiral fractures
A2	Simple oblique fractures ≥ 30°
A3	Simple transverse fractures <30°
B	**Wedge fractures**
B1	Spiral wedge fractures
B2	Bending wedge fractures
B3	Fragmented wedge fractures
C	**Complex fractures**
C1	Spiral fractures
C2	Segmental fractures
C3	Irregular fractures

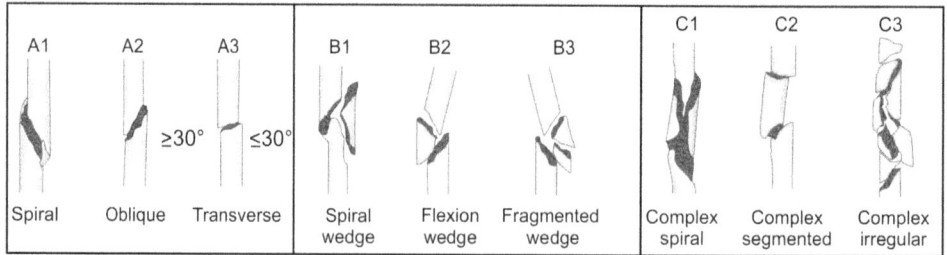

Fig. 53: OTA classification of tibial shaft fracture.

shaft of tibia may occur that may result in an increased risk of ankle osteoarthritis due to uneven weight loading.
- **Osteomyelitis:** Deep bony infection is more prone to occur in open fracture.

Fracture healing time: 10–12 weeks

Management

Nonsurgical Treatment

- **Closed reduction and cast immobilization:** Limb is immobilized in long leg cast followed by functional (patellar tendon bearing) brace upto 4 weeks. When the fracture is displaced then closed reduction is performed under general anesthesia.
  Indications:
  - Closed low energy fractures with acceptable alignment
    - <5° of varus-valgus angulation.
    - <10° of anterior/posterior angulation
    - >50% cortical apposition
    - <1 cm shortening
    - <10° of rotational malalignment
    - Nonambulatory (i.e. paralyzed) patients or those who are unfit for surgery.

Surgical Treatment

- **Intramedullary nailing:**
  Indications:
  - Unacceptable alignment with closed reduction and casting
  - Segmental fractures
  - Comminuted fractures
  - Ipsilateral injury
  - Multiple trauma
  - Bilateral tibial fracture.
- **External fixation:**
  Indications: Often used in open fractures with significant bone and soft tissue loss.
- **Open reduction and internal fixation with plates:**
  Indications:
  - Proximal tibial fractures with inadequate proximal fixation from IM nailing
  - Distal tibial fractures with inadequate distal fixation from IM nailing.

Postoperative physiotherapy treatment: Table 37 shows postoperative physiotherapy treatment for tibial shaft fracture.

■ DISTAL TIBIAL FRACTURE/TIBIAL PLAFOND FRACTURE

It is the metaphyseal fracture of tibia which involves the tibial plafond, i.e. horizontal weight bearing surface of distal tibia. It is also known as **pilon fracture**.

Mechanism of Injury

High impact energy trauma:
- Often caused by high energy rotational force or axial loading
- Fall from height or MVA

Low impact energy trauma:
- Low energy rotational force and some axial compression
- Following activities, such as skiing.

Clinical Presentation

- Immediate severe pain, swelling, tenderness and/or bruising around the ankle and lower leg.
- Inability to bear weight on affected limb
- Deformed ankle (ankle may look angled or crooked).

Classification

Figure 54 and Table 38 shows OTA classification of tibial plafond fracture.

Complications

- **Shortening of limb:** Shortening of involved limb occurs due to proximal impaction of distal tibia particularly associated with fibular fracture in approximately 75% of plafond fractures.
- **Neurovascular injury:** Posterior tibial artery, dorsal pedis artery and tibial nerve are at potential risk to get injured in distal tibial fracture.
- **Tendon injury:** Higher risk of rupture or incarceration of proximate tendons

Table 37: Postoperative physiotherapy treatment for tibial shaft fracture.

	Precaution	ROM exercises	Strengthening exercises	Weight bearing
Week 0–4	Avoid rotatory movement with foot on the ground	AROM for ankle and knee if not immobilized in cast	Isometric exercise to quadriceps, tibialis anterior and gastrosoleus	• WBAT with assistive device for stable fracture • NWB to TTWB for unstable fracture
Weeks 4–8	Same as above	Same as above	Isometric and isotonic exercises for knee and ankle	Same as above.
Weeks 8–12	None	AROM, AAROM and gentle PROM of knee and ankle	Progressive resisted ROM exercises for quads, DF and PF	WBAT
Weeks 12–16	Avoid aggressive PROM	• Complete AROM and PROM exercise for knee • Proprioceptive exercises	Isometric, isotonic and progressive resisted exercises to quads and hams	Progress from TTWB to PWB to FWB

(PROM: passive range of motion; ROM: range of motion; AROM: active range of motion; AAROM: active-assisted range of motion; DF: dorsiflexion; PF: plantar flexion; WBAT: weight bearing as tolerated; NWB: normal weight bearing; TTWB: toe touch weight bearing; PWB: partial weight bearing; FWB: full weight bearing)

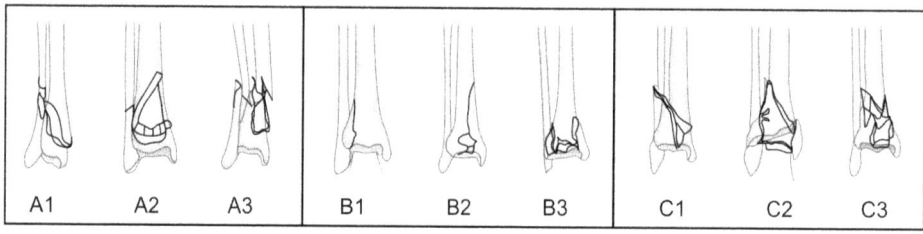

Fig. 54: OTA classification of tibial Plafond fracture.

Table 38: OTA classification of tibial plafond fracture.

Type	Description
A	**Extra-articular fracture**
A1	Simple fracture
A2	Wedge fracture
A3	Multifragmentary fracture
B	**Partial articular fracture**
B1	Split fracture
B2	Split depression fracture
B3	Depression fracture
C	**Complete articular fracture**
C1	Simple articular, simple metaphyseal fracture

Contd...

Type	Description
C2	Simple articular, multifragmentary metaphyseal fracture
C3	Multifragmentary articular and metaphyseal fracture

frequently in the flexor halluces longus or posterior tibial tendons.
- **Foot compartment syndrome:** Irreversible ischemic injury to muscle and/or nerve occurs due to increased pressure in ossseofascial compartment of foot.
- **Nonunion or delayed union:** Great chances of non or delayed union occur

due to poor blood supply of distal one third of tibia.
- **Malunion:** Varus or valgus malalignment of distal part of tibia may occur following displaced fracture.
- **Avascular necrosis:** Post-traumatic AVN of distal tibia occurs due to relatively tenuous blood supply of lateral tibial plafond.
- **Post-traumatic arthritis of ankle joint:** Axial load injuries often lead to cartilage damage that eventually results in degenerative arthritis.

Fracture healing time: 6 to 8 weeks

Management

Nonsurgical Treatment
Most closed tibial fractures are treated without any surgical intervention.
- **Cast:** Above knee plaster cast is applied for 6 weeks. Depending on the type of fracture, above knee cast may be followed by below knee patellar bearing plaster cast or to a functional cast brace between 4th to 8th weeks.
  Indications:
  - Closed low energy fractures with acceptable alignment.
    - <5° of varus-valgus angulation.
    - <10° of anterior/posterior angulation
    - >50% cortical apposition
    - <1 cm shortening
    - <10° of rotational malalignment
  - Nonambulatory (i.e. paralyzed) patients or those who are unfit for surgery.

Surgical Treatment
Operative fixation is required in unstable fractures.
- **Open reduction and internal fixation:**
  Indications:
  - Associated intra-articular and shaft fractures
  - Unacceptable alignment with closed reduction and casting
  - Relative shortening
  - Segmental fractures
  - Comminuted fractures
  - Ipsilateral femoral and tibial fracture
  - Multiple trauma.
- **External fixation:**
  Indications: Often used in open fractures with significant bone and soft tissue loss.

Postoperative physiotherapy treatment: Table 39 shows postoperative physiotherapy treatment for distal tibial fracture.

■ TARSAL FRACTURE

Seven tarsal bones of foot are calcaneus, talus, cuboid, navicular, medial cuneiform, intermediate and lateral cuneiform. Tarsal

Table 39: Postoperative physiotherapy treatment protocol for distal tibial fracture.

	Precaution	ROM exercises	Strengthening exercises	Weight bearing
Week 0–4	Avoid PROM	AROM of MTP and knee joint	Isometric exercise for quadriceps, PF and DF	None
Weeks 4–6	Same as above	AROM of MTP, ankle and knee joint	Same as above	None
Weeks 6–8	Avoid high impact activities	Begin AROM, AAROM and gentle PROM exercise for ankle and subtalar joint	Begin gentle resistive exercise for DF, PF, invertors and evertors	PWB
Weeks 8–12	Avoid high impact activities	Complete AROM and PROM exercise for knee	Isometric, isotonic and progressive resisted exercises for DF, PF, invertors and evertors	Progress from TTWB to FWB

(PROM: passive range of motion; ROM: range of motion; AROM: active range of motion; MTP: metatarsophangeal; AAROM: active-assisted range of motion; PF: plantar flexion; DF: dorsiflexion; PWB: partial weight bearing; TTWB: toe touch weight bearing; FWB: full weight bearing)

fracture accounts for approximately 10% of all skeletal injuries.

Clinical Presentation
- Severe pain, swelling, tenderness and/or bruising of foot
- Limping
- Inability to bear weight on affected foot.

Calcaneal Fracture
Calcaneus is the largest tarsal bone. It is the most frequently fractured tarsal fracture. Calcaneal fracture accounts for approximately 60% of all tarsal fracture and about 1–2% of all skeletal injuries.

Mechanism of Injury

High energy impact on heel, such as in MVA or fall from height onto the heel due to axial loading.

Classification

On the basis of involvement of articular surfaces of calcaneum (Fig. 55):
- Extra-articular fracture
- Intra-articular fracture.

Extra-articular Fracture

About 25–30% of calcaneal fractures are extra articular. It includes all the fractures that do not involve the fracture of posterior facet.

Table 40: Classification of extra-articular calcaneal fracture.

Type	Description
A	Anterior calcaneal fracture
B	Mid calcaneal fracture
	Body
	Substentaculum
	Peroneal tubercle
	Lateral process
C	Posterior calcaneal fracture
	Posterior tuberosity
	Medial calcaneal tubercle

Classification of extra-articular fracture of calcaneus: Figure 56 and Table 40 show the classification of extra-articular fracture of calcaneus.

Intra-articular Fracture

About 70–75% of calcaneal fractures are intra-articular and result from axial loading.

Classification of intra-articular fracture of calcaneus: Sanders classification based on the number of fracture fragments in Figure 57 and Table 41.

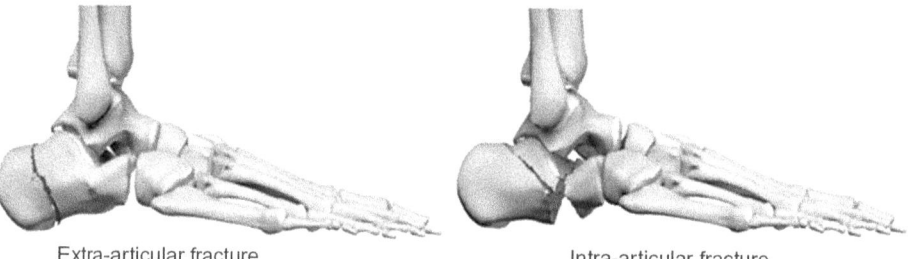

Extra-articular fracture   Intra-articular fracture

Fig. 55: Classification of calcaneal fracture on the basis of the involvement of articular surfaces of calcaneus.

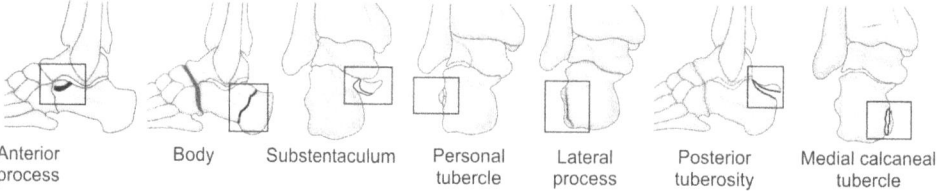

Anterior process   Body   Substentaculum   Personal tubercle   Lateral process   Posterior tuberosity   Medial calcaneal tubercle

Fig. 56: Types of extra-articular calcaneal fracture.

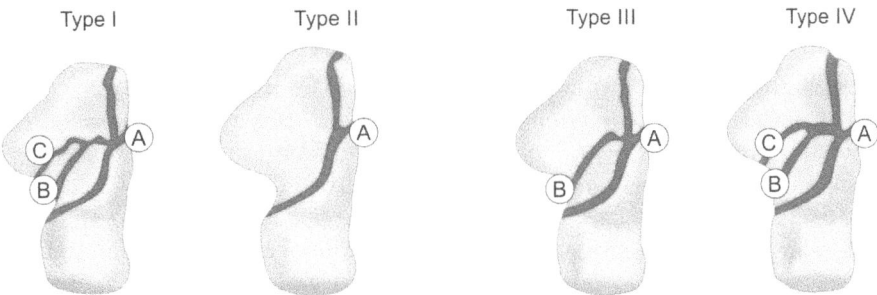

Fig. 57: Sanders classification of intra-articular calcaneal fractures based on the number of fracture fragments.

Table 41: Sanders classification of intra-articular calcaneal fractures.

Type	Description
I	All nondisplaced articular fractures, i.e. less than 2 mm of articular displacement
II	2 part fracture of posterior facet
III	3 part fracture of posterior facet
IV	4 or more part fracture of posterior facet with more than 2 mm of articular displacement, i.e. comminuted fracture

Complications

- **Foot compartment syndrome:** It more commonly occurs in calcaneal fracture due to associated massive soft tissue damage and edema.
- **Post-traumatic subtalar joint arthritis:** It occurs due to the degenerative changes associated with disrupted articular facets of subtalar joint.
- **Associated ligamentous and tendon injury:** Entrapment of tendons between fracture fragments may cause tendon injuries. Associated Achilles tendon injury disables the gastrocnemius-soleus complex which restricts the plantar flexion of ankle.
- **Heel fat pad syndrome (HFPS):** It is characterized by heel pain that occurs due to damage or disruption of the fatty pad that sits under the calcaneus. After massive trauma the ability of fat pad to absorb shock and giving cushioning effect to the heel bone diminished.

Fracture healing time: 8–12 weeks

Talus Fracture

Talus is the second most common fractured tarsal bone after calcaneus. Talus fracture accounts for around 5–10% of all tarsal fractures. It is also the second largest tarsal bone with more than half of its surface covered by articular cartilage.

Mechanism of Injury
- Fall from height causing axial load to plantar foot.
- Forced hyperdorsiflexion injury to foot or ankle.

Classification
Anatomical classification of talus fractures:
- Talar neck fracture
- Talar body fracture
- Talar head fracture
- Lateral process fracture
- Posterior process fracture.

Complications
- **Avascular necrosis/osteonecrosis:** AVN of talar body commonly occurs following fracture of talar neck because of loss of

blood supply to the lower part, i.e. body of talus.
- **Post-traumatic arthritis:** It results due to the collapse (due to AVN), malunion and poor blood supply of talus.
  - **Subtalar arthritis:** Commonly occurs after talar neck fractures.
  - **Tibiotalar arthritis:** Commonly occurs after talar body fractures.
- **Malunion:** Malalignment of talar neck is due to either malreduction or loss of reduction of bony fragments. Common deformity patterns include talar neck shortening, varus and dorsiflexion. Varus malunion of talar neck often cause loss of subtalar motion and foot eversion.

Fracture healing time: 8–12 weeks

Navicular Fracture

Navicular bone is the keystone of medial column of foot. It places an integral role in maintaining the medial longitudinal arch of foot.

Mechanism of Injury

According to the cause of injury navicular fracture can be broadly of three types:
1. **Avulsion fractures:** Caused by sudden contraction of muscles simultaneous with extreme movement of foot and usually associated with ligamentous injuries. Avulsion fractures accounts for approximately 50% of all acute navicular fractures. It includes:
   - **Cortical avulsion fracture:** Avulsed by dorsal talonavicular ligament in extreme plantarflexion/inversion or by anterior division of deltoid ligament in extreme eversion.
   - **Tuberosity avulsion fracture:** Caused by eversion with simultaneous PTT contraction.
2. **Traumatic fractures:** Navicular body fracture can be caused by:
   - Direct trauma like dropping of heavy object on foot
   - Indirect trauma like fall from height or MVA.
3. **Stress fracture:** These are chronic injuries caused by continuous and repetitive overload on the bone resulting in microfracture. They eventually becomes a true cortical fracture. They are more common in athletes and comprise around 35% of all stress fractures.

Classification

Sangeorzan Classification of Navicular Body Fracture

On the basis of plane of fracture and degree of comminution is given in Table 42.

Fracture healing time: 6 weeks–4 months

Cuboid Fracture

Cuboid is a tarsal bone that is located on the lateral aspect of midfoot. Isolated fracture of cuboid is very rare and commonly associated with other fractures and midfoot dislocations.

Compression fracture of cuboid is known as **nutcracker fracture**. It is called so because of compression/crushing of cuboid bone between calcaneus and fourth and fifth metatarsal during forced plantar flexion and abduction.

Mechanism of Injury

- **Direct injury:** Direct blow on the foot.
- **Indirect injury:** When axial torsional/twisting force applied to plantar flexed and abducted foot causing crushing of

Table 42: Sangeorzan classification of navicular body fracture.

Type	Desctiption
Type I	Transverse fracture with no dislocation (no associated deformity)
Type II	Oblique fracture with medial forefoot displacement (associated with adduction deformity)
Type III	Comminuted fracture with lateral foot displacement (associated with abduction deformity)

Table 43: OTA classification of cuboid fracture.

Type	Description
A	Extra-articular fracture
A1	Avulsion
A2	Coronal
A3	Comminuted, crush
B	Single joint articular (involving either calcaneocuboid or metatarsocuboid joint)
B1	Sagittal
B2	Horizontal
C	Multiarticular, comminuted (involving major joint surfaces)
C1	Nondisplaced
C2	Displaced

cuboid between calcaneus and 4th and 5th metatarsals called nutcracker fracture.
- **Stress fracture:** Due to chronic overuse injuries, such as excessive weight bearing activities like running, sprinting, jumping, etc.

Complications
- **Compartment syndrome** is an important acute complication of midfoot fractures in general.
- **Chronic dysfunction of the peroneus longus:** It occurs when the peroneal sulcus is damaged.

OTA classification of cuboid fracture is shown in Table 43.

Fracture healing time: 6 weeks–4 months

Postoperative physiotherapy treatment: Table 44 shows postoperative physiotherapy treatment for tarsal fracture.

■ METATARSAL FRACTURE

Metatarsal fractures are the most common traumatic foot injuries and accounts for approximately 5–6% of all skeletal injuries of the body.

Relative incidence of metatarsal bones fracture are:
- First metatarsal fracture: 5%
- Second metatarsal fracture: 12%
- Third metatarsal fracture: 14%
- Fourth metatarsal fracture: 13%
- Fifth metatarsal fracture: 56%
- Multiple metatarsal fractures: 15.6%

Clinical Presentation
- Immediate pain, swelling, tenderness and bruising over the foot.
- Pain intensifies on weight bearing and relieves on rest.
- Crooked or abnormal appearance of the toe.

Fracture of Fifth Metatarsal Bone (Fig. 58)

Fifth metatarsal bone fracture is most commonly occurring metatarsal fracture. Fifth metatarsal has unique blood supply and biomechanics than other four metatarsals. It has comparatively less soft tissue coverage and attachment of intrinsic muscles than others. It is also the most mobile metatarsal.

Mechanism of Injury
- **Avulsion injury:** This commonly occurs due to inversion injury after the break where the tendon continues to pull the tip of bone away from the rest of the metatarsal.
- **Stress fracture:** It results from chronic overuse injury, e.g. in runners. These are common in army persons due to repeated practice of march parade therefore also known as "march fracture". They mostly occur in midshaft region. Gradually it converts into a complete fracture. Second metatarsal is commonly affected but fifth metatarsal can also be affected.
- **Dancer fracture:** It is the fracture of shaft of metatarsal and commonly occurs due to twisting of foot during landing from jump. e.g. in ballet dancers. These fractures heal rapidly with immobilization without any surgical treatment.

Table 44: Postoperative physiotherapy treatment for tarsal fracture.

	Precaution	ROM exercises	Strengthening exercises	Weight bearing
Week 0–4	Avoid PROM	AROM of IP and MTP joints	Isometric exercises for ankle, PF, DF, evertors and invertors in cast	NWB
Weeks 4–6	Same as above	• Same as above • Gentle AROM for subtalar and ankle joint if out of cast	Same as above	NWB or PWB with assistive device depends on the fracture type
Weeks 6–8	Avoid aggressive PROM	AROM, AAROM and gentle PROM exercise to ankle and subtalar joint if out of cast	Isometric and isotonic exercises for ankle and subtalar joint if not in cast	PWB if not treated with ORIF
Weeks 8–12	Avoid high impact activity	AROM, AAROM and PROM exercise for ankle and subtalar joint	Isometric, isotonic and progressive resisted exercises for PF, DF, evertors, invertors, long flexors and extensors of toes	PWB to FWB with or without assistive device

(PROM: passive range of motion; ROM: range of motion; AROM: active range of motion; IP: interphalangeal; MTP: metatarsophalangel; AAROM: active-assisted range of motion; PF: plantar flexion; DF: dorsiflexion; NWB: no weight bearing; PWB: partial weight bearing; ORIF: open reduction and internal fixation; FWB: full weight bearing)

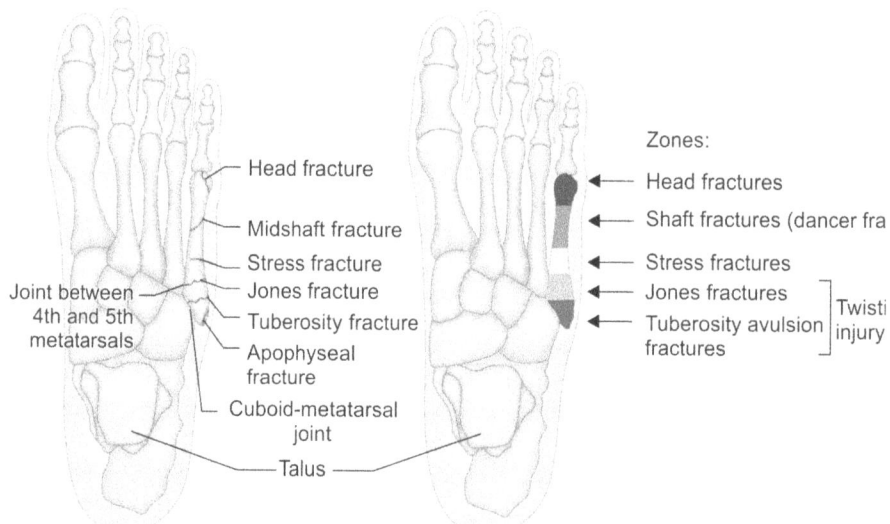

Fig. 58: Zones of fifth metatarsal fracture.

- **Jones fractures:** Fracture in metadiaphyseal region, i.e. junction between the base of metatarsal and shaft is known as "jones fractures". This zone is relatively avascular which increases the chances of nonunion. It can either be a stress fracture on an acute break.

Fracture of First to Third Metatarsal Bone

First metatarsal fracture most commonly occurs in children of less than 4 years.

Mechanism of Injury

Acute injury: It is usually caused by direct forceful trauma, such as dropping of something heavy on foot, kicking of foot against hard object or any sports related injury. First, second and fifth metatarsal are commonly injured in sports.

Complications
- **Nonunion:** Fractures in proximal diaphysis i.e. up to 1.5 cm distal to tuberosity are at significantly higher risk for delayed or nonunion because of the disruption of the blood supply after the fracture.
- **Delayed healing or refracture:** High arched foot puts extra pressure on fifth metatarsal that affects the healing process.
- **Foot compartment syndrome:** It commonly occurs in high impact injuries, such as MVA or heavy crush injuries.
- **Neurovascular injury:** It may be due to increased pressure because of edema or direct injury to neurovascular structures.
- **Postfracture stiffness of ankle and foot:** Due to prolonged immobilization required for the treatment of fracture.
- **Malunion:** It may occur due to the malalignment of the fracture fragments and continuous movement of the foot during weight bearing.

Fracture Healing Time
- **First and fifth metatarsal fractures:** 6–8 weeks
- **Second, third and fourth metatarsal fractures:** 4–6 weeks.

Management

Nonsurgical Treatment
- **Closed reduction and cast immobilization:** Close reduction and short leg walking cast are applied.

Indications:
- Nondisplaced fractures
- Minimally displaced fractures including stress fractures.

Surgical Treatment
- **Closed reduction and percutaneous pinning:** Intramedullary K-wire fixation is done and postsurgically the foot is immobilized in nonweight bearing short leg cast for 2–3 weeks until the pins are removed.
  Indications: Closed, displaced or angulated metatarsal shaft fractures.
- **Open reduction and internal fixation:** Intramedullary K-wire is used to maintain the reduction and foot is immobilized in the short leg cast for 2–3 weeks.
  Indications: Open, displaced or angulated metatarsal shaft fractures.

VERTEBRAL FRACTURE

ATLAS FRACTURE (JEFFERSON FRACTURE) (FIG. 59)

Burst fracture of C1 (atlas) is known as Jefferson fracture. In this both anterior and posterior arch fractures and the occipital condyles are forced into the lateral masses of C1.

Mechanism of Injury

It is caused by axial loading.
- Diving into shallow water when the head strikes at the bottom of the pool and transmits the force to the cervical spine.
- Falling onto the head from height.
- In MVA, when the head is thrown forcefully against the windshield that produce both hyperextension and compression at cervical spine.

Classification

Table 45 and Figure 60 shows the Jefferson classification and its types.

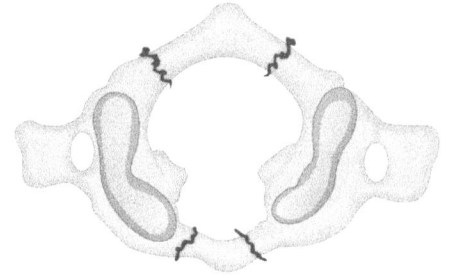
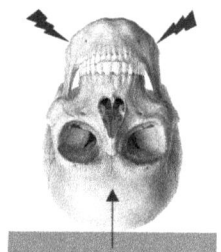

Burst (Jefferson) fracture   Axial loading

Fig. 59: Atlas fracture (Jefferson fracture) and its mechanism of injury.

Table 45: Jefferson classification of C1 fracture.

Type	Description
I	Posterior arch fracture
II	Anterior arch fracture
III	Both anterior and posterior arch fracture (burst fracture)
IV	Lateral mass of C1 fracture

Associated Injuries

- Approximately 33% of burst fractures are associated with C2 fracture
- About 50% cases are associated with cervical spine injuries
- Concurrent head injuries occurs in 25–50% of young children
- **Vertebral basilar artery injury (VBI):** Having symptoms of vertigo, blurred vision and nystagmus.
- **Cranial nerve injury:** Cranial nerve lesions of 6th to 12th and neuropraxia of suboccipital and greater occipital nerve may be associated.

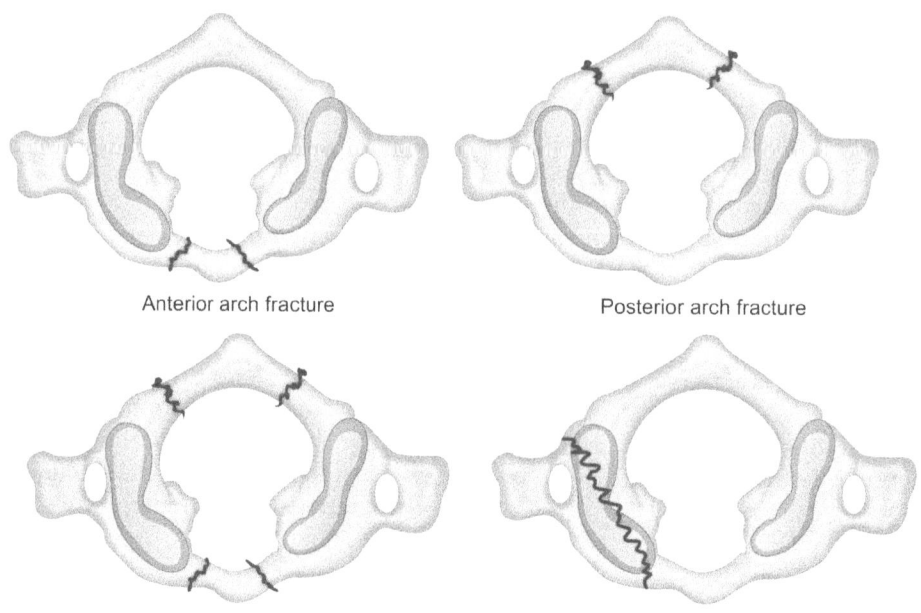

Fig. 60: Types of Jefferson fractures.

Fractures and Dislocations

Postoperative physiotherapy treatment: Table 46 shows postoperative physiotherapy treatment for atlas fracture.

■ AXIS FRACTURE

Hangman's Fracture

Scheider et al. introduced the hangman term on the basis of occurrence of these fractures in hanged criminals. It is a fracture that involves the pars interarticularis or pedicles of C2 on both the sides resulting in the separation of C2 body from its posterior element. This is the most frequent fracture of cervical spine.

Mechanism of Injury

It is a result of hyperextension and distraction or hyperextension and compression.

- **Motor vehicle accidents:** Motor vehicle collisions in which the patient's chest hit by the steering wheel and head launches forward and is stopped by the windshield (Fig. 61).

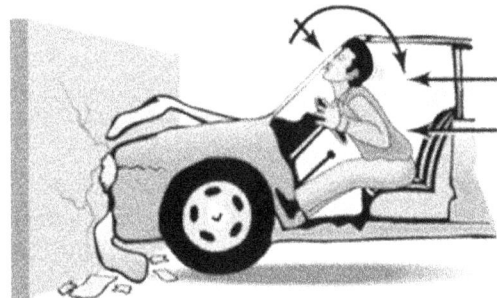

Fig. 61: Motor vehicle accidents.

Table 46: Postoperative physiotherapy treatment for atlas fracture.

	Precaution	ROM exercises	Strengthening exercises	Weight bearing
Week 0–2	Avoid PROM	• No ROM in closed reduction treatment • Gentle AROM and PROM for MTP and IP joints when treated with ORIF	No strengthening exercise	• NWB in first and fifth metatarsal fracture • WBAT in stable fractures of metatarsals
Weeks 2–4	Avoid PROM	• No ROM in first metatarsal and Jones fracture • AROM for MTP and IP joints in other metatarsal fractures	• Same as above • Isometric exercises for ankle muscles	Same as above
Weeks 4–6	Avoid PROM	• No ROM in first metatarsal and Jones fracture • Full AROM for MTP and IP joints in other stable metatarsal fractures	Isometric and isotonic exercises to ankle muscles (i.e. PF, DF, evertors and invertors)	NWB to PWB in first and fifth metatarsal fracture
Weeks 6–8	No high impact activities	AROM, AAROM and gentle PROM for MTP, IP and ankle joints	• Same as above • Begin resistance exercise for ankle muscles • Isometric and isotonic exercises for long toes flexors and extensors	Progress from PWB to FWB
Weeks 8–12	Same as above	AROM, AAROM and PROM for MTP, IP and ankle joints	Resistance exercise for long toes flexors and extensors	FWB

(PROM: passive range of motion; ROM: range of motion; AROM: active range of motion; MTP: metatarsophalangeal; IP: interphalangeal; AAROM: active-assisted range of motion; PF: plantarflexion; DF: dorsiflexion; NWB: non-weight bearing; WBAT: weight bearing as tolerated; PWB: partial weight bearing; FWB: full weight bearing)

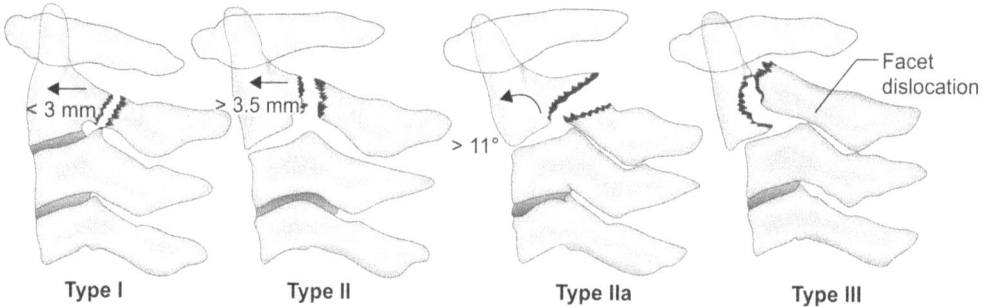

Fig. 62: Levine and Edwards classification of Hangman's fracture.

- In judicial hanging, the mechanism is hyperextension with distraction and is fatal.
- Sports activities, such as a forceful hit while playing football or rugby.

Classification
Figure 62 and Table 47 shows Levine and Edwards classification of Hangman's fracture and its types.

Odontoid Fracture
It is the fracture through the odontoid process of C2 spine and also known as peg or dens fracture. It accounts for around 15% of all cervical spine fractures.

Mechanism of Injury
It commonly occurs due to the combination of cervical flexion or extension with rotation.
- Motor vehicle accident
- Fall from height.

Classification
Figure 63 and Table 48 shows the Anderson D'alonzo classification of odontoid fracture and its types and description.

Diagnosis
Radiographs Findings
- **Open mouth odontoid view:** It shows asymmetry of spaces between dens and lateral masses of C1. Distance greater than 6 mm indicates ligamentous injury.
- **Lateral view:** Prevertebral soft tissue swelling anterior to C1 and predate space

Table 47: Levine and Edward classification.

Type	Description
I	Fracture with < 3 mm anteroposterior deviation No angular deviation
II	Fracture with > 3 mm anteroposterior deviation Significant angular deviation Disruption of posterior longitudinal ligament
IIa	Fracture line is horizontal/oblique (instead of vertical) Significant angular deviation without anterior translation
III	Type I with bilateral facet joint dislocation

(distance between anterior tubercle of C1 and dens) of more than 3 mm indicates the transverse ligament injury.

CT Scan and MRI
CT scan demonstrates the number of fractures, their locations and degree of displacement of fragments.

MRI demonstrates local soft tissue and ligamentous injury.

Expected fracture healing time: 8–16 weeks

Management
Nonsurgical Treatment
- **Hard collar/halo immobilization:** The spine is immobilized for 6–12 weeks.
  Indications: Stable fractures with intact transverse ligament.

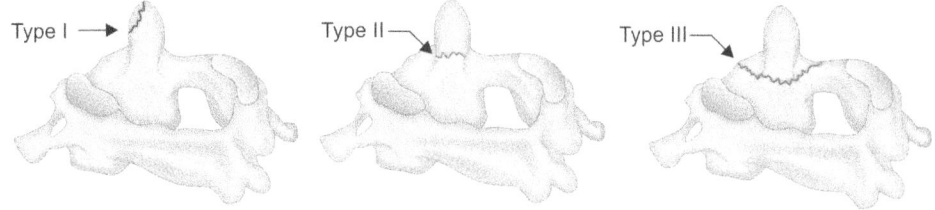

Fig. 63: Anderson D'alonzo classification of odontoid fracture.

Table 48: Anderson D'alonzo classification.

Type	Description
I	Oblique avulsion of tip of dens
II	Fracture at base of dens in transverse plane
III	Fracture extends down into the body of C2 and considered unstable fracture

Surgical Treatment
- **Open reduction and posterior spine fusion:**
  Indications:
  - Unstable fractures
  - Failure of closed reduction.

Postoperative physiotherapy treatment: Table 49 shows postoperative physiotherapy treatment for axis fracture.

■ LOWER CERVICAL VERTEBRAE FRACTURE

Cervical spine is more receptive to get injured because of higher mobility with relatively small vertebral bodies and supports the head that is heavy and acts as a lever.

Lower cervical fractures are more common in adults because the fulcrum of movement is at C5/6 whereas in children the fulcrum is at C2/3 that predisposes them to upper cervical fractures.

Mechanism of Injury
- Four major mechanisms of injury are: Flexion, extension, rotational and shearing. Each fracture is associated with certain patterns of fracture.
- Direct trauma or axial loading.

Table 49: Postoperative physiotherapy treatment for axis fracture.

	Precaution	ROM exercises	Strengthening exercises	Weight bearing
Week 0–4	Avoid overhead movement of UE	Gentle AROM for UE and LE	• Isometric exercise for postural muscles, i.e. abdominals, gluteus and quads, etc. • Gentle strengthening exercise for UE and LE	WB with assistive device
Weeks 4–8	Maintain cervical immobilization	AROM for UE and LE	Same as above	WBAT with assistive device to FWB
Weeks 8–12	No jerky movement at cervical spine	Gentle AROM for cervical spine	Isometric exercise for cervical spine	FWB
Weeks 12–16	No contact sports	AROM and gentle PROM for cervical spine	Isometric exercise for cervical spine	FWB

(UE: upper extremity; ROM: range of motion; AROM: active range of motion; LE: lower extremity; PROM: passive range of motion; WB: weight bearing; WBAT: weight bearing as tolerated; FWB: full weight bearing)

Classification

Allen and Ferguson Classification of Subaxial Spine Injuries

On the basis of mechanism of injury. Table 50 shows Allen and Ferguson classification.

Usually bones fails in flexion and ligament fails in extension.

■ THORACOLUMBAR VERTEBRAE FRACTURE

Vertebral column is divided by Denis into 3 vertical parallel columns (Fig. 64 and Table 51) on the basis of biomechanical studies related to the stability following traumatic injury. Instability occurs due to injury of 2 contiguous columns (e.g. anterior and middle column or middle and posterior column) or all 3 columns.

Denis Classification of Spinal Trauma

According to Denis' system, spinal traumas are classified to **Minor** and **Major** injury, based on their potential risks to cause instability.

Tables 52 and 53 show the Denis classification of spinal trauma with major and minor injuries.

Compression Fracture

Caused by forward or lateral flexion. It is a failure of the anterior column. The middle column is intact and acts as a hinge. There may be partial failure of posterior column when the compression exceeds over 50% of vertebral height or 20° of angulation.

There are 4 subtypes of compression fractures which are shown in Figure 65 and Table 54.

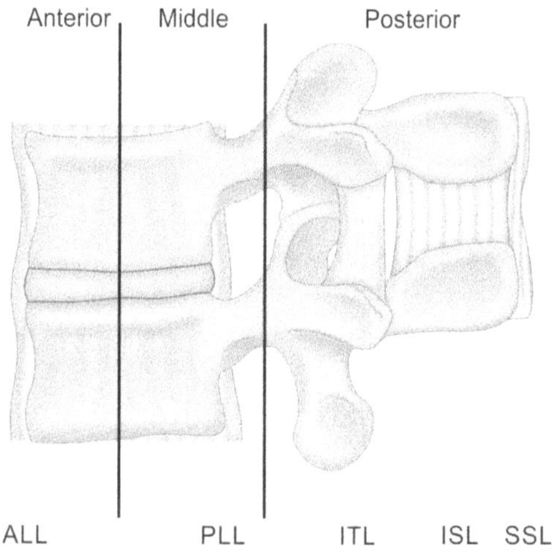

Table 50: Allen and Ferguson classification (of subaxial spine injuries).

S.No.	Mechanism of injury	Injured structures
1.	Distractive flexion	Posterior ligament tear
		Hyperflexion sprain
		Bilateral facet dislocation
		Unilateral facet dislocation
2.	Compressive flexion	Anterior vertebral body fracture
		Wedge compression fracture
		Flexion teardrop
3.	Distractive extension	Anterior ligament tear
		Hyperextension sprain
		Hyperextension teardrop
		Hyperextension dislocation
4.	Compressive extension	Posterior element fracture
		Unilateral or bilateral laminar
		Lateral mass or spinous process fracture
5.	Axial compression	Vertebral body burst fracture

Contd...

Contd...

S.No.	Mechanism of injury	Injured structures
6.	Lateral bending	Uncinate process fracture
		Unilateral vertebral fracture
		Posterior element fracture
7.	Clay-shoveler fracture	Isolated spinous process fracture of C7 (C6-T1)

Fig. 64: Denis' three column theory.

Table 51: Vertebral column given by Denis.

Anterior column	Middle column	Posterior column
Anterior longitudinal ligament (ALL)	Posterior longitudinal ligament (PLL)	Structures posterior to PLL
Anterior 2/3rd of vertebral body	Posterior 1/3rd of vertebral body	Pedicles
Anterior 2/3rd of intervertebral disc (annulus fibrosus)	Posterior 1/3rd of intervertebral disc (annulus fibrosus)	Facet joints and articular processes
		Ligamentum flavum
		Neural arch and interconnecting ligaments, i.e. intertransverse, interspinous and supraspinous ligaments

Table 52: Denis classification of spinal trauma.

Major injuries	Minor injuries
Compression fracture	Transverse process fracture
Burst fracture	Articular process fracture
Seat belt fracture	Pars interarticularis fracture
Fracture-dislocation	Spinous process fracture

Table 53: Major injuries of spinal trauma.

Type	Mechanism of injury	Columns involved
Compression	Flexion	Anterior column compression with/without posterior column distraction
Anterior	Anterior flexion	
Lateral	Lateral flexion	
Burst		Anterior and middle column compression with/without posterior column distraction
A	Axial load	
B	Axial load with flexion	
C	Axial load with flexion	
D	Axial load with rotation	
E	Axial load with lateral flexion	
Seat belt	Flexion distraction	Anterior column intact or distracted with middle and posterior column distraction
Fracture-dislocation		Any column can be affected (alone or in combination)
Flexion rotation	Flexion rotation	
Shear	Shear (A-P, P-A)	
Flexion distraction	Flexion distraction	

Burst Fracture

Caused by axial loading. It causes failure of both anterior and middle columns originating at the level of one or both end plates of same vertebra.

There are 5 subtypes of burst fractures which are shown in Figure 66 and Table 55.

Seat Belt Type Injury

Occurs due to the combination of flexion with axis of rotation just anterior to vertebral col-

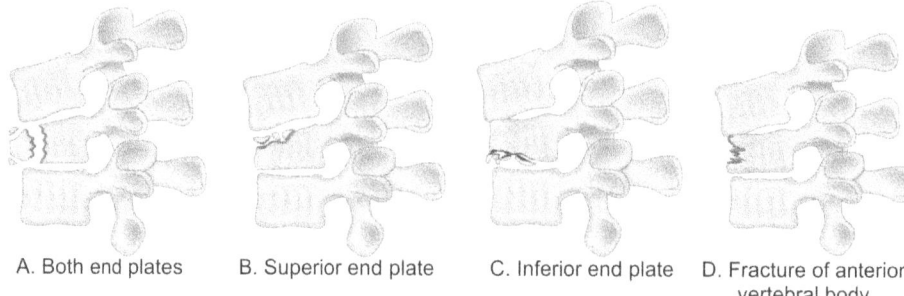

Fig. 65: Compression fracture.

Table 54: Subtypes of compression fracture.

Type	Description
A	Involvement of both end plates
B	Involvement of superior end plate
C	Involvement of inferior end plate
D	Fracture of anterior vertebral body without involvement of end plates.

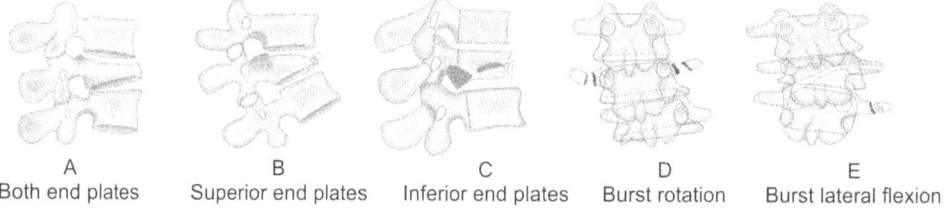

Fig. 66: Burst fracture.

Table 55: Types of burst fracture.

Type	Description
A	Fracture of both end plates Bone is retropulsed into the canal
B	Fracture of superior end plate: Occurs due to combination of axial load with flexion
C	Fracture of inferior end plate
D	Burst rotation: Occurs due to combination of axial load with rotation.
E	Burst lateral flexion: It differs from lateral compression fracture as it present an increase of interpediculated distance on anteroposterior roentgenogram.

umn and distraction begins from posteriorly that eventually directs anteriorly. In these both the posterior and middle column fails. The anterior column may be spared partially or completely that functions like a hinge. In this spine is mainly unstable in flexion.

There are 2 subtypes of seat belt injury (Fig. 67):

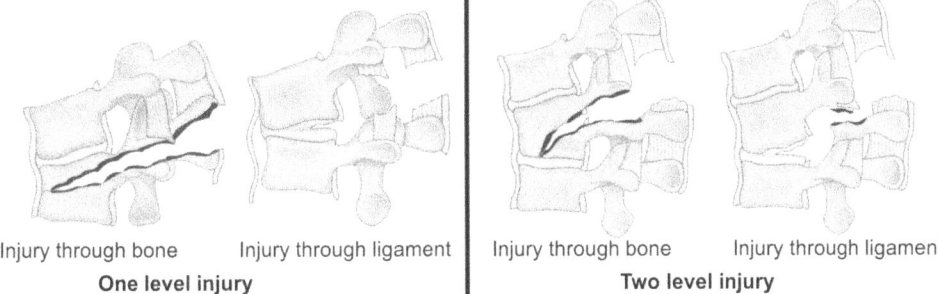

Injury through bone   Injury through ligament | Injury through bone   Injury through ligament
One level injury   **Two level injury**

Fig. 67: Seat belt type injury

- **One level injury:** A simple chance fracture going through bone or a ligamentous disruption passing through ligamentous complex and intervertebral disc.
- **Two level injury:** Middle column is ruptured either through bone or disc.

Fracture-Dislocations

Failure of all the 3 columns under compression, tension, rotation or shear.

There are 3 subtypes of fracture-dislocations based on the mechanism of injury.

- **Flexion-rotation type fracture-dislocation (Fig. 68):** Complete disruption of posterior and middle column occurs due to tension and rotation, whereas anterior column may also be damaged due to compression and rotation.
- **Flexion distraction type fracture-dislocation (Fig. 69):** Disruption of posterior and middle columns along with the tear of anterior annulus fibrosus and stripping of anterior longitudinal ligament during the subluxation or dislocation.
- **Shear type fracture-dislocation (Fig. 70):** Results from extension type of mechanism in which anterior longitudinal ligament is disrupted and upper segment translates anteriorly or posteriorly over the top of inferior segment. It has 2 subtypes:
  1. **Posteroanterior shear:** The upper vertebral segment shear off forward over the top of lower segment. In this fracture of the posterior arch of last one or two vertebrae of upper segment occurs in translation causing a floating posterior arch. The risk of complete paralysis is relatively high in this type of fracture.

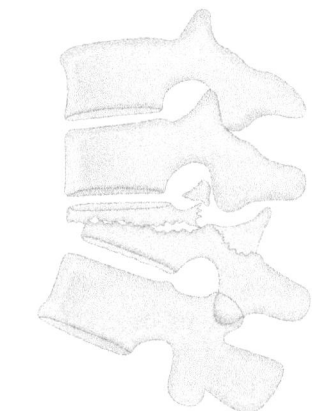

Fig. 68: Flexion rotation type of fracture-dislocation.

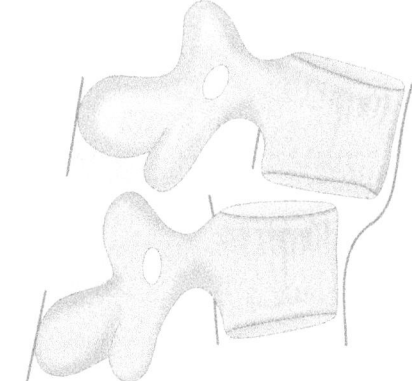

Fig. 69: Flexion distraction type of fracture-dislocation.

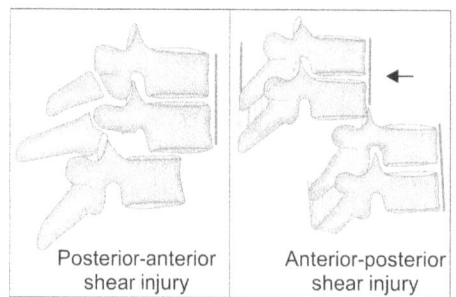

Fig. 70: Shear type of fracture dislocation.

Posterior-anterior shear injury | Anterior-posterior shear injury

2. **Anteroposterior shear:** The upper segment shear off posteriorly over the top of lower segment.

Management

Nonsurgical Treatment
- **Orthotics or body cast:** Orthosis is applied for 6–12 weeks depending on the degree of instability.
  Indications: Most of the thoracic and thoracolumbar fractures especially burst and compression fractures are treated non-operatively when there is no neurological injury.

Surgical Treatment
Instrumentation/Arthrodesis
Indications:
- Progressive neurologic deficits
- Myelomalacia
- Gross spinal instability.

Postoperative physiotherapy treatment: Table 56 shows postoperative physiotherapy treatment protocol for thoracolumbar vertebrae fracture.

■ MANAGEMENT OF UNSTABLE VERTEBRAL FRACTURES

Unstable vertebral fractures frequently associated with spinal cord injuries. Therefore, the comprehensive treatment and rehabilitation of vertebral fractures entirely depends on the level of lesion and extent of spinal cord damage and accordingly the rehabilitation program is planned and implemented.

The spinal column consists of 33 vertebrae that include 7 cervical, 12 thoracic, 5 lumbar, 5 sacral and 4 coccygeal vertebrae. Correspondingly the spinal cord also has

Table 56: Postoperative physiotherapy treatment for thoracolumbar vertebrae fracture.

	Precaution	ROM exercises	Strengthening exercises	Weight bearing
Week 0–4	Avoid spinal flexion, rotation and sit ups	Gentle AROM of UE and LE	♦ Isometric exercises for postural muscles, i.e. abdominals, gluteus and quads, etc. ♦ Gentle strengthening exercises for UE and LE	WB with assistive device
Weeks 4–8	♦ Same as above ♦ Avoid PROM for TL spine	AROM of TL spine for stable compression fracture at the end of 6 weeks	Same as above	WBAT with assistive device to FWB
Weeks 8–12	Avoid PROM of TL spine	Gentle AROM for TL spine of flexion, extension, lateral flexion and rotatory movements	Isometric exercise and gentle strengthening exercise for trunk and paraspinal muscles once fusion is achieved	FWB
Weeks 12–16	No contact sports	AROM and gentle PROM for cervical spine	Isometric exercise for cervical spine	FWB

(PROM: passive range of motion; TL: thoracolumbar; ROM: range of motion; AROM: active range of motion; UE: upper extremity; LE: lower extremity; WB: weight bearing; WBAT: weight bearing as tolerated; FWB: full weight bearing)

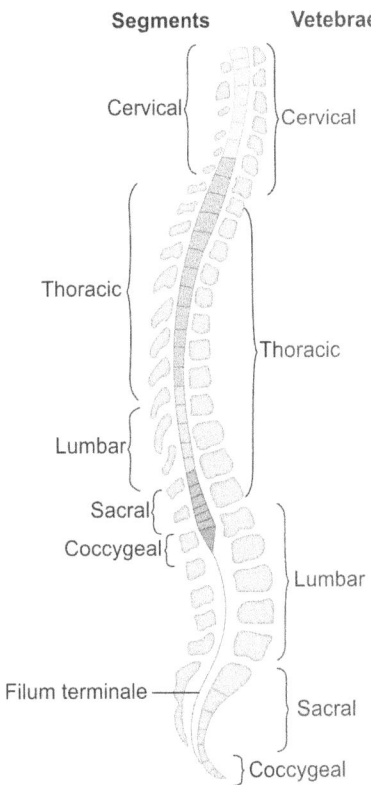

Fig. 71: Spinal and vertebral segments

segmented levels which are marked by the spinal roots emerges from it. Spinal cord consist of 31 segments that include 8 cervical, 12 thoracic, 5 lumbar, 5 sacral and 1 coccygeal. As the length of spinal cord i.e. 45 cm is comparatively smaller than the total length of vertebral column, i.e. 65 cm, the spinal segments are short and crowded particularly in the lower part of cord. Hence, the spinal and vertebral segments do not lie at the same level and the spinal segments always lie above the numerically corresponding vertebra (Fig. 71).

31 pairs of spinal nerve roots emerge from the sides of spinal cord which are named after the vertebra it exits from. There are 8 cervical, 12 thoracic, 5 lumbar, 5 sacral and 1 coccygeal nerve roots. The cervical nerve roots exit the vertebral canal above the corresponding vertebrae except the eighth that emerges between 7th cervical and 1st thoracic vertebrae. The remaining spinal nerve roots emerge below the corresponding vertebrae.

Relation of Spinal Cord and Vertebral Segments (Fig. 72)

- **Rough calculation to obtain a relation between the spinal cord and vertebral segments:**
  - C1–C4 vertebrae correspond to same spinal segmental level, i.e. C1–C4.
  - From C4–T3 vertebrae add 1 to determine the spinal segmental level, i.e. C5–T4.
  - From T3–T6 vertebrae add 2 to determine the spinal segmental level, i.e. T5–T8.
  - From T6–T9 vertebrae add 3 to determine the spinal segmental level, i.e. T9–T12.
  - T10–T12 vertebrae have whole lumbar segments.
  - L1 vertebra has whole sacral and coccygeal segments.
  - Spinal cord tapers at L2 vertebral level.
  - Beyond L2 is the cauda equina.

- **Exact relation of spinal cord and vertebral segments:**
  - C1–C2 spinal cord segments correspond to C1–C2 cervical vertebrae.
  - C3–C8 spinal cord segments lies between C3–C7 vertebral levels.
  - T1–T2 spinal cord segments correspond to T1–T2 vertebral levels.
  - T3–T12 spinal cord segments lies between T3–T8 vertebral levels.
  - Lumbar spinal cord segments lies between T9–T11 vertebral levels.
  - Sacral spinal cord segments lies between T12–L1.
  - Tip of spinal cord lies at L2 vertebral level.
  - Below L2 vertebra, only bunch of spinal roots are present known as cauda equina. Cauda equina consists of roots

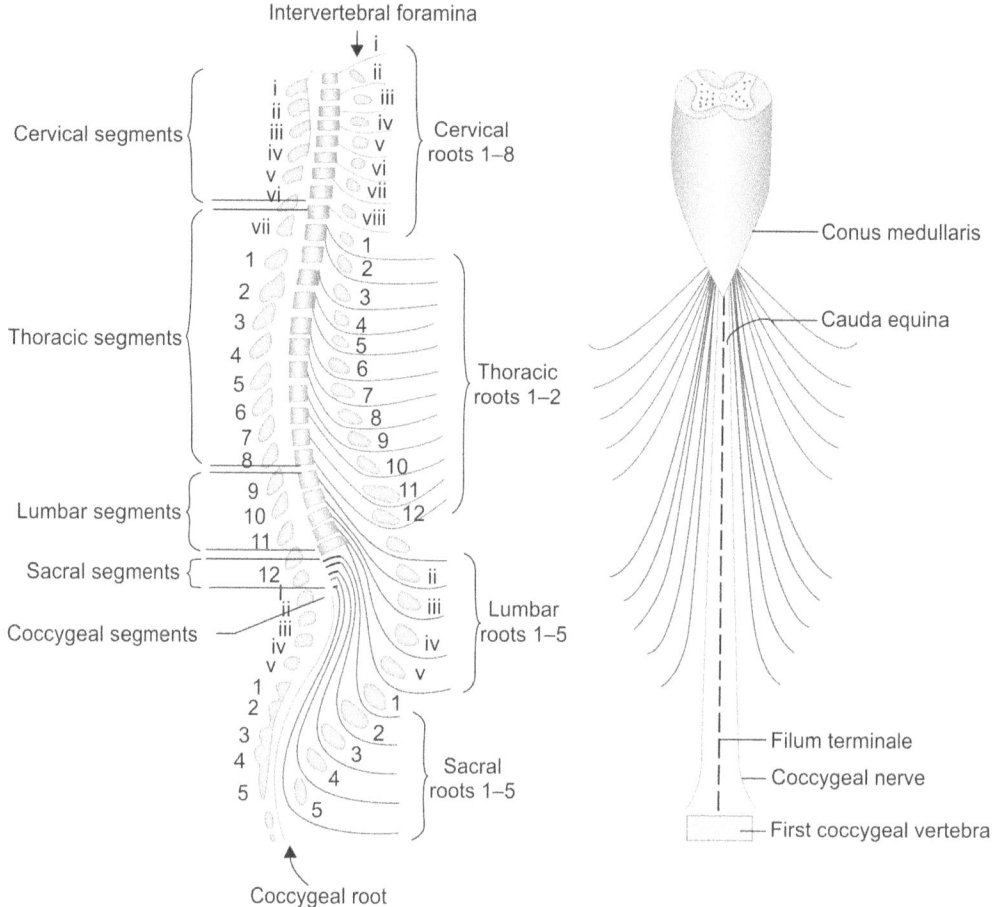

Fig. 72: Relation of spinal cord and vertebral segments.

of lower four pairs of lumbar, five pairs of sacral and one pair of coccygeal nerve.

The sensory motor deficiencies caused after unstable fractures entirely depends on the level of involvement of spinal cord segment. This spinal cord segment involvement could be roughly estimated by the corresponding vertebrae fracture.

The detailed evaluation of sensory motor impairment is done by using the region wise comprehensive neurological examination (Table 57).

Rough Estimation of Functional Impairments at Different Vertebral Level Fracture

- **Injury above C4 vertebral level:** All the functions including breathing are severely affected. So the patient may require ventilator for proper respiration.
- **Injury above T1 vertebral level:** Loss of trunk and both upper and lower extremity functions known as quadriplegia.
- **Injury below T1 vertebral level:** Loss of trunk and lower extremity functions. The upper extremity functions are spared.

Table 57: Spinal cord injury levels and motor functions.

Spinal segment	Motor functions	Impairment after injury
C1, C2	Neck flexion/extension	Loss of all the functions including breathing
C3	Neck side flexion	Loss of all the functions including breathing
C4	Shoulder elevation Supply the diaphragm	Loss of all the functions including breathing
C5	Shoulder abduction	Loss of all functions of upper limb, trunk control and ambulation
C6	Elbow flexion and wrist extension	Same as above except shoulder movements
C7	Elbow extension and wrist flexion	Same as above except shoulder movements
C8	Finger flexion, thumb extension and ulnar deviation	Loss of hand movements and grip along with trunk control and ambulation
T1	Finger abduction and adduction	Loss of fine hand movement along with trunk control and ambulation
T1–T6	Intercostal and trunk above waist	Loss of trunk control and ambulation
T7–L1	Abdominal muscles	Same as above
L1, L2	Hip flexion	Loss of bladder and bowel control along with walking disability
L3	Knee extension	Loss of bladder and bowel control along with walking disability
L4	Ankle dorsiflexion	Loss of bladder and bowel control along with walking disability
L5	1st metatarsal extension	Loss of bladder and bowel control along with walking disability
S1	Ankle plantar flexion, eversion and hip extension	Loss of bladder and bowel control along with walking disability
S2	Knee flexion	Loss of bladder and bowel control along with walking disability
S3, S4	Anal wink	Only loss of bladder and bowel control

- **Injury below T9 vertebral level:** Trunk and abdominal control are spared and have loss of lower extremity function known as paraplegia.

FRACTURES NOMENCLATURE

- **Aviator fracture:** Fracture of neck of talus.
- **Banana fracture:** Complete, horizontally oriented pathological fracture of deformed bone affected by Paget disease.
- **Bankart fracture:** Fracture of anterior glenoid associated with anterior shoulder dislocation.
- **Barton fracture:** Intra-articular fracture of distal radius with radiocarpal joint dislocation.
- **Bennett fracture:** Noncomminuted, intra-articular fracture of base of first metacarpal.
- **Bosworth fracture:** Fracture of distal fibula with posterior dislocation of proximal fibula.
- **Boxer fracture:** Fracture of neck of fifth metacarpal.
- **Bumper fracture:** Compression fracture of lateral tibial plateau.

- **Chance fracture/Seat belt fracture:** Horizontal fracture through spinous process or vertebral body with mild or no compression of vertebral body.
- **Chauffeur fracture/Hutchinson fracture:** Oblique fracture of radial styloid.
- **Chisel fracture:** Incomplete fracture of head of radius.
- **Chepart fracture:** Fracture dislocation through talonavicular and calcaneocuboid joints.
- **Clay Shoveller's fracture:** Fracture of spinous process of C6, C7 or T1.
- **Colles fracture/Pouteau fracture:** Fracture of distal radius with dorsal displacement and angulation of distal fragment.
- **Cotton fracture/Trimalleolar fracture of ankle:** Fracture of both malleoli and posterior lip of tibia.
- **Dashboard fracture:** Fracture of posterior rim of acetabulum.
- **Die-punch fracture:** Intra-articular fracture of lunate fossa of distal radius.
- **Dupuytren's fracture:** Bimalleolar fracture of ankle along with the rupture of distal tibiofibular ligaments and lateral displacement of talus.
- **Duverney fracture:** Isolated fracture of one iliac wing.
- **Essex–Lopresti fracture:** Comminuted fracture of radial head with disruption of interosseous membrane and subluxation of radioulnar joint.
- **Galeazzi fracture/Piedmont fracture:** Fracture of shaft of radius with distal radioulnar joint dislocation.
- **Gosselin fracture:** V-shaped fracture of distal tibia extending into the tibial plafond.
- **Hangman fracture:** Fracture through the pedicles of C2 with anterolisthesis of C2 over C3.
- **Hill-Sachs fracture:** Compression fracture of posterolateral head of humerus associated with anterior dislocation of shoulder.
- **Hoffa fracture:** Posterior tangential fracture of one (usually lateral) or both femoral condyles.
- **Holstein-Lewis fracture:** Spiral fracture of distal third of humerus (commonly associated with neuropraxia of radial nerve).
- **Holdsworth fracture:** Unstable spinal fracture–dislocation at thoracolumbar junction.
- **Jefferson fracture:** Burst fracture of C1 vertebra.
- **Jones fracture/Robert Jones fracture:** Fracture of base of 5th metatarsal bone.
- **Lead pipe fracture:** Combination of greenstick and buckle fracture, i.e. incomplete transverse greenstick fracture of one side of cortex and torus fracture of the opposite side of cortex.
- **Le Fort facial fractures:** Series of facial fractures.
- **Le Fort ankle fracture/Wagstaffe–Le Fort fracture:** Avulsion fracture of medial aspect of distal fibula due to avulsion of anterior tibiofibular ligament attachment.
- **Lisfranc fracture:** Fracture dislocation of midfoot.
- **Maisonneuve fracture:** Spiral fracture of proximal fibula.
- **Malgaigne fracture:** Vertical pelvic fracture through both pubic rami and ilium or sacroiliac joint with vertical displacement.
- **March fracture:** Stress fracture of metatarsal shaft.
- **Monteggia fracture:** Fracture of proximal ulna with dislocation of radial head.
- **Moore's fracture:** Fracture of distal radius associated with ulnar dislocation and entrapment of styloid process under annular ligament.
- **Nightstick fracture:** Transverse fracture of midshaft of ulna.
- **Nursemaid fracture:** Dislocation of radial head.

- **Pipkin fracture-dislocation:** Posterior dislocation of hip with avulsion fracture of fragment of femoral head by ligamentum teres.
- **Posadas' fracture:** Transcondylar humeral fracture with the displacement of distal fragment anteriorly and dislocation of radius and ulna from the bicondylar fragment.
- **Pott's fracture:** Bimalleolar fracture of ankle with rupture of deltoid ligament and lateral subluxation of talus.
- **Reverse Barton fracture:** Intra-articular distal radial fracture with volar displacement.
- **Rolando fracture:** Intra-articular comminuted fracture of the base of first metacarpal.
- **Runner's fracture:** Stress fracture of distal fibula 3–8 cm above the lateral malleolus.
- **Salter-Harris fracture:** Fracture involving a growth plate.
- **Segond fracture:** Avulsion fracture of lateral tibial plateau with anterior cruciate ligament tear.
- **Shepherd fracture:** Fracture of lateral tubercle of posterior process of talus.
- **Smith fracture/Goyrand fracture:** Fracture of distal radius with volar displacement of distal fracture fragment.
- **Stieda fracture/Pellegrini-Stieda disease:** Avulsion fracture of medial femoral condyle at the origin of medial collateral ligament.
- **Straddle fracture:** Bilateral fracture of all pubic rami.
- **Tillaux fracture:** Avulsion fracture of anterolateral margin of distal tibia.
- **Toddler's fracture:** Undisplaced oblique fracture of distal tibia in children under 8 years old.
- **Torus fracture:** Impaction fracture of childhood as the bone buckles instead of fracturing completely
- **Trough sign/fracture:** Fracture of anteromedial aspect of humeral head.
- **Wagon wheel fracture:** Separation of distal femoral epiphysis from metaphysis in a child.
- **Walther's fracture:** Ischioacetabular fracture that passes through the pubic rami and extend towards the sacroiliac joint.

DISLOCATIONS

- **Joint dislocation:** A complete separation of two articulating bony surfaces is known as joint dislocation.
- **Subluxation:** A partial or incomplete dislocation is known as subluxation.

SHOULDER DISLOCATION

It refers to the dislocation of glenohumeral joint. In this, head of humerus forcibly moves out of the glenoid fossa.

Shoulder subluxation is the partial dislocation of the humerus from glenoid fossa.

Classification of Shoulder Dislocation (Fig. 73)

- **Anterior dislocation:** Forward displacement of head of humerus when it lies anterior to the glenoid fossa. This is the most common type of shoulder dislocation that comprises of more than 95% of cases. Subtypes of anterior dislocation of shoulder (Fig. 74):
  - **Subcoracoid dislocation:** When head of humerus lies anterior to glenoid fossa and inferior to coracoid process.
  - **Subglenoid dislocation:** When head of humerus lay anteroinferior to glenoid fossa.
  - **Subclavicular dislocation:** When head of humerus lies anterior to glenoid fossa and medial to coracoid process or inferior to clavicle.
  - **Intrathoracic dislocation:** When the head of humerus lay anteromedial to glenoid fossa between the ribs.

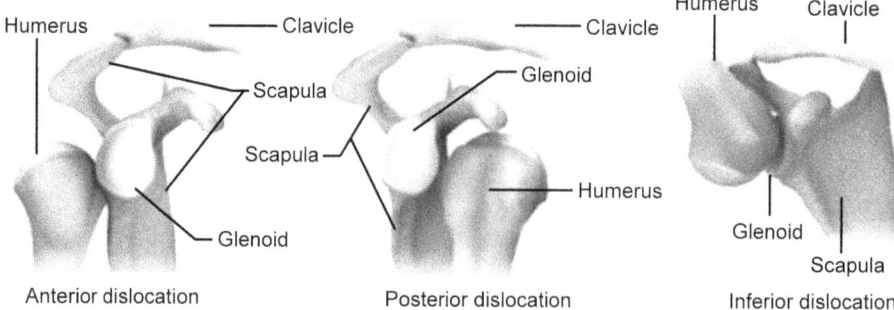

Fig. 73: Classificaiton of shoulder dislocation.

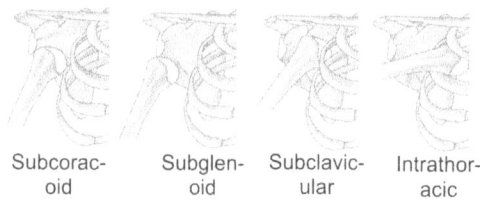

Fig. 74: Subtypes of anterior dislocation.

Causes:
- Commonly results from combined abduction, extension and external rotation of shoulder.
- In young people, it is usually sports related injury like overhead throwing of balls.
- In elderly, it can even be caused by fall on an outstretched arm.

- **Posterior dislocation:** Backward displacement of head of humerus when it lies posterior to the glenoid fossa. It accounts for around 2-4% of all shoulder dislocations.

  Subtypes of posterior dislocation
  - **Subacromial dislocation:** When the head of humerus lies beneath the acromion. It is most common type that comprises 98% of posterior dislocation.
  - **Subglenoid dislocation:** When the head of humerus lies beneath the glenoid.
  - **Subspinous dislocation:** When the head of humerus lies medial to acromion and beneath the spine of scapula.

Causes:
- Severe internal rotation and adduction of shoulder.
- Commonly related to seizures and electric shock.
- Fall on an outstretched arm
- Blow to the front of the shoulder.

- **Inferior dislocation:** Displacement of head of humerus downwards that lies just beneath the glenoid fossa. This is the rarest type that occurs in less than 1% of all shoulder dislocations. This condition is also known as "Luxatio Erecta" because the arm appears to held upward or behind the head permanently. This dislocation has greater risk of complications due to associated vascular, neurological, tendon and ligament injuries.

Causes:
- Hyperabduction of arm that forces the humeral head against the acromion.
- Violent downward jerk or movement of arm.

Clinical Presentation
- Severe pain in shoulder.
- Restricted movement of shoulder.
- Distortion of shoulder contour:
  - In anterior dislocation, side silhouette of shoulder has an abnormal square shaped appearance instead of sloping and rounded contour.

- In posterior dislocation, the front of shoulder looks abnormally flat.
- **Bruising or abrasion** over shoulder may occur due to impact injury.
- **A hard knob** under the skin near the shoulder.

Diagnosis: On Examination

- **Attitude of limb:** Patients keeps the limb in particular attitude:
  - **In anterior dislocation:** Arm is held in slight (10-20°) abduction and external rotation. The patient bends forward and supports the affected limb with the contralateral hand.
  - **In posterior dislocation:** Arm is held in adduction and internal rotation along the side of body and the arm is often bent at elbow joint.
  - **In inferior dislocation:** Arm is held in fully abduction with elbow supported behind or over the head.
- **Contour of shoulder:**
  - **In anterior dislocation:** Shoulder normal contour is lost, glenoid is empty and humeral head can be palpated anteriorly. Deltoid and acromion prominence shifts posteriorly and laterally.
  - **In posterior dislocation:** Squaring of shoulder occurs with prominent coracoid process and prominent head can be palpated posteriorly.
  - **In inferior dislocation:** Head of humerus can be palpated on the lateral chest wall.

Complications

- **Anatomical lesions:**
  - **Bankart's lesion:** Avulsion of anteroinferior glenoid labrum with rupture of joint capsule and inferior glenohumeral ligament injury.
  - **Hill-Sachs lesion:** An indentation fracture on posterolateral humeral head caused by the impaction of soft base of humeral head against the relatively hard anterior glenoid. It occurs in around 35-40% cases of anterior dislocations.
- **Associated fractures:** Approximately 30% of shoulder dislocations are associated with other fractures like greater tuberosity, glenoid rim, clavicle or acromion fracture.
- **Rotator cuff injury:** Approximately 40-50% cases have associated with rotator cuff injury more often in elderly.
- **Recurrent dislocation of shoulder joint:** Severe or repeated shoulder dislocation make the joint instable that predispose it to re-injure and dislocate easily.
- **Nerve damage:** Usually, the circumflex axillary nerve is injured in around 3% cases of anteroinferior dislocation that results in numbness, tingling, paresthesia in the lateral aspect of upper arm and weakness of deltoid muscles.
- **Rare complications:** More commonly occurs in inferior shoulder dislocation during initial dislocation or during the reduction of the dislocation.
  - Axillary artery and brachial plexus injury.

Expected Recovery Time
- Closed reduction: 6-8 weeks
- Open/surgical reduction: 12-16 weeks

Management

Nonsurgical Treatment
- Acute reduction and immobilization for 4 to 6 weeks
  - In anterior and posterior dislocation shoulder is immobilized in 10-20° external rotation with elbow at side.
- **Indications:**
  - Inactive elderly patients
  - In absence of acute traumatic rotator cuff injury.

Surgical Treatment
Arthroscopy or open repair
Indications: Active younger patients.
Postoperative physiotherapy treatment: Table 58 shows postoperative physiotherapy treatment for shoulder dislocation.

Table 58: Postoperative physiotherapy protocol for shoulder dislocation.

	Precaution	ROM exercises	Strengthening exercises
Week 0–2	No shoulder movement	• Shoulder is immobilized in adduction and IR • AROM exercises for wrist and finger	Isometric strengthening exercise for deltoid, biceps and triceps
Weeks 2–4	Avoid combination of abduction/ER of shoulder	• AROM exercises for elbow • Gentle pendular exercises of shoulder in flexion, extension • Relaxed passive abduction of shoulder up to 45° with arm in IR • Relaxed passive ER of shoulder with arm in adduction by the side of body	Isometric and gentle isotonic resistance of shoulder musculature
Weeks 4–6	Avoid abduction and external rotation combination at 90° shoulder abduction	Progress ER to 60° and 90° abduction according to patient tolerance	Resistive strengthening exercises to rotator cuff muscles, parascapular muscle, deltoid and major muscle groups of UE
Weeks 6–10	Avoid wide grip or overhead strengthening exercises, e.g. bench press or military press	Full AROM and PROM exercise for shoulder in all planes	• Progressive resisted exercises for shoulder muscles • UE proprioceptive exercises

(ER: external rotation; ROM: range of motion; IR: internal rotation; AROM: active range of motion; PROM: passive range of motion; UE: upper extremity)

■ ELBOW DISLOCATION

Elbow is a hinge joint that consists of three bones named humerus, radius and ulna. Elbow dislocation occurs when the lower end of humerus loses its contact with the upper ends of forearm bones, i.e. radius and ulna. It is the second most common major joint dislocation following the dislocation of shoulder.

Elbow dislocation may be partial or complete. In complete dislocation, joint surfaces of humerus and forearm bones are completely separated whereas in partial dislocation also known as subluxation the joint surfaces are not completely separated.

Mechanism of Injury

Elbow is relatively a stable joint therefore a sufficient force is required to dislocate the joint.

- **FOOSH:** When the force is transmitted through the forearm to the elbow that pushes the elbow out of its socket.
- **Sports activity:** Commonly in sports like gymnastics, cycling, roller blading or skateboarding.
- **Sideswipe injury:** In MVA, when the subject has elbow out of the window. The direct impact causes a severe fracture-dislocation of elbow.

Classification (Fig. 75)

On the basis of the position of radius and ulna in relation to the humerus:
- **Posterior elbow dislocation:** Having 2 subtypes:
  - Posteromedial elbow dislocation
  - Posterolateral elbow dislocation
- Anterior elbow dislocation
- Medial elbow dislocation
- Lateral elbow dislocation
- Divergent elbow dislocation.

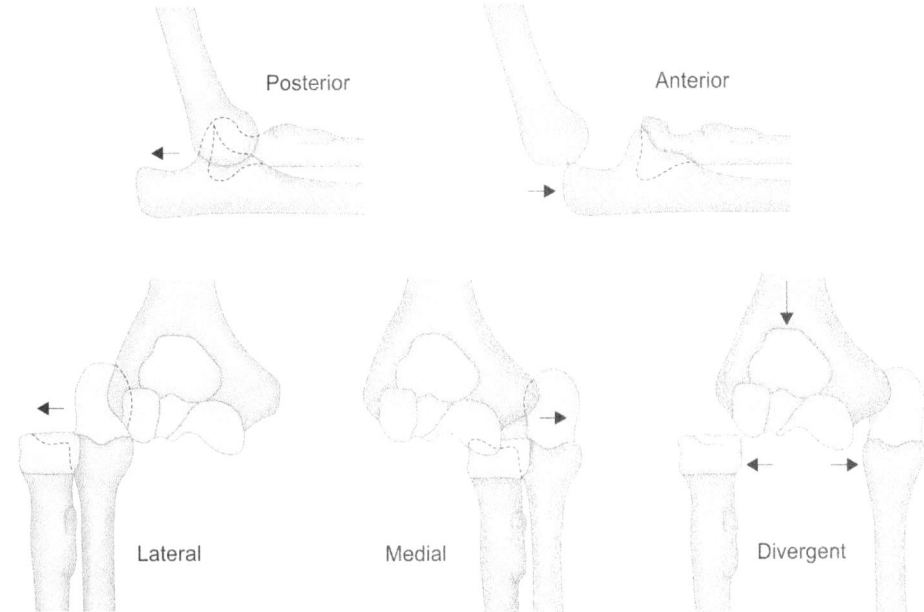

Fig. 75: Classification of elbow dislocation.

Classification on the Basis of Associated Injuries

The two types of elbow dislocation are:
1. **Simple elbow dislocation:** Dislocation without any associated fracture.
2. **Complex elbow dislocation:** Dislocation associated with fracture.

Clinical Presentation

- Severe pain, swelling and bruising in and around the elbow joint.
- Pain and inability to move elbow.
- Deformed appearance of arm.
- Contralateral limb supports the affected limb to prevent the movement at elbow.

Physical Examination

- Signs of associated injury to neurovascular structures should be checked.
  - For blood vessel:
    - Radial pulse should be checked below the thumb at the base of the wrist
    - Press on the tips of the fingers and check for the color of nail beds. They should blanch (turn white) and then return to a normal pink color within 3 seconds.
  - For nerve injury: Different nerve function should be checked.
    - **Radial nerve function:** Patient is asked to extend the wrist as if he is saying "STOP".
    - **Median nerve function: Okay test:** Patient is asked to touch the tips of index finger and thumb.
    - **Ulnar nerve function:** Patient is asked to spread the fingers.
- **Observation of the contour and attitude of arm:** Patient used to support the affected limb with the sound limb to prevent any movement at the joint.
- **Sensory function:** Sensation of forearm and hand for any numbness should be checked.
- **ROM of elbow:** Passive movement of elbow will be painful, especially extension and supination.

- Presence of compartment syndrome should be examined.

Complications
- **Heterotrophic ossification:** Anteriorly it forms between the brachialis muscle and joint capsule and posteriorly it forms between the triceps muscles and joint capsule. Since the risk is increased with the presence of associated bony and soft tissue injuries, the forcible manipulation or passive stretching should be avoided that may results in extensive soft tissue injuries.
- **Contracture or joint stiffness:** Prolonged immobilization commonly results in loss of terminal extension of elbow.
- **Vascular injury:** Brachial artery is the most commonly injured artery because of its proximity to the joint.
- **Nerve injury:** Median, ulnar, radial and anterior interosseous nerves are more vulnerable to get injured in elbow dislocation.
- **Joint instability or recurrent dislocation:** Joint instability increases due to associated collateral ligament injury. Coronoid process and radial head fracture further predispose the joint to dislocate which is also known as terrible triad of elbow.
- **Compartment syndrome:** It may results from massive swelling due to soft tissue injury. Therefore, postreduction therapy must include elevation and avoidance of hyperflexion of elbow.

Expected healing time: 4-6 weeks

Management

Nonsurgical Treatment
- **Closed reduction and immobilization:** After reduction the elbow is immobilized in posterior mold splint with at least 90° flexion and appropriate forearm rotation for 1-3 weeks followed by the use of extensor block brace for 3-4 weeks.
  The appropriate position of forearm rotation is determined by the injured structure:
  - **When LCL is disrupted:** Elbow is more stable in pronation.
  - **When MCL is disrupted:** Elbow is more stable in supination.

  Indications:
  - Acute simple stable dislocations.
  - Recurrent instability after simple dislocations.

Surgical Treatment
- **ORIF with repair of injured ligaments:**
  Indications:
  - Acute complex elbow dislocations, i.e. associated fracture of coronoid, radial head, and olecranon.
  - Persistent instability after reduction.
  - Entrapped soft tissue or osteochondral fragments.
  - When closed reduction is not possible.

Postoperative physiotherapy treatment: Table 59 shows postoperative physiotherapy treatment for elbow dislocation.

■ HIP DISLOCATION

Hip dislocation occurs when the head of femur moves out of the socket of acetabulum. Hip dislocations in younger individuals are relatively rare accounting for only 5% cases of all dislocations.

Classification
On the basis of the position of femoral head:
- **Posterior dislocation (Fig. 76):** When the head of femur is pushed backwards. It comprises around 90% case of hip dislocation.
  Causes: Axial loading on femur with the hip in flexion and adduction, e.g. dashboard injury (axial load through flexed knee).
- **Anterior dislocation (Fig. 77):** When the head of femur slips in forward direction.
  Causes: Hip in abduction and external rotation.
  It is further classified in two types:
  1. **Superior dislocation:** Hip extension results in superior dislocation.

Fractures and Dislocations

Table 59: Postoperative physiotherapy protocol for elbow dislocation.

	Precaution	ROM exercises	Strengthening exercises
Week 0–2	• Elbow immobilized in splint/brace as needed • No lifting/pushing/pulling	• AROM/PROM or shoulder, wrist, and hand • Gentle PROM exercise for elbow	• Grip strengthening exercises • Isometric exercises for deltoid, biceps, triceps
Weeks 2–4	Splint is removed	AROM, PROM of elbow flexion, extension	Isotonic exercises to elbow, forearm, wrist and hand muscles
Weeks 4–6	No heavy lifting and pushing activities	AROM to AAROM for elbow including flexion, extension	Resistive strengthening exercise to elbow muscles. Closed chain exercises for UE
Weeks 6–10	No heavy lifting and pushing activities	Full AROM and PROM exercise for elbow	Progressive resisted exercises for elbow muscles

(ROM: range of motion; AROM: active range of motion; PROM: passive range of motion; AAROM: active-assisted range of motion; UE: upper extremity)

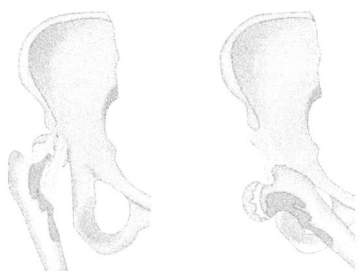

Fig. 76: Posterior dislocation.

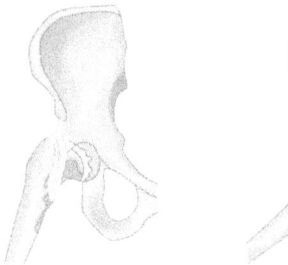

Fig. 77: Anterior dislocation.

2. **Inferior dislocation:** Hip flexion results in inferior dislocation.

On the basis of associated injured structures:
- **Simple hip dislocation:** Dislocation without any associated fracture.
- **Complex hip dislocation:** Dislocation associated with acetabulum or proximal femur fracture.

Mechanism of Injury
- **Motor vehicle collision:** It is the most common cause of traumatic hip dislocations. Also known as dashboard injury. It occurs when the knee hits against the dashboard in a collision and the force pushes the femur backward and drives the head of femur out of the hip socket.
- Fall from significant height.
- **Sports injuries:** High-risk contact sports like football, soccer, rugby, etc.

Clinical Presentation
- Severe pain, bruising and/or swelling in and around the hip joint.
- Inability to move the limb.
- Visible deformity of the hip joint.
- Affected limb appears shorter than the other limb.

Physical Examination
Attitute of Limb
- **In posterior dislocation:** Hip and leg in slight flexion, adduction and internally rotated.
- **In anterior dislocation:** Hip and leg in flexion, abduction and externally rotated.

Complications
- **Post-traumatic arthritis:** Associated injury to the joint cartilage increases the risk of developing arthritis.
- **Avascular necrosis:** It occurs in around 40% of cases. Temporary or permanent disruption of blood supply results in the necrosis of femoral head.
- **Sciatic nerve injury:** It occurs in approximately 8-20% of hip dislocation. It is usually caused by stretching of nerve from posteriorly dislocated head or from a displaced fracture fragment.
- **Recurrent hip dislocation:** It occurs in less than 2% cases due to the injury of supporting capsule, labrum, cartilage and ligaments.

Expected healing time: 8-12 weeks

Management
Nonsurgical Treatment
Closed reduction within 6 hours: Closed reduction is followed with protected weight bearing for 4-6 weeks.
  Indications: Acute simple anterior and posterior dislocation.

Surgical Treatment
Open reduction, ORIF or arthroscopy:
  Indication:
  - Associated fracture of acetabulum, femoral head or neck.
  - Irreducible dislocation
  - Massive intra-articular injuries to cartilage, capsule and labrum
  - Radiographic evidence of incarcerated fragment.

Postoperative physiotherapy treatment: Table 60 shows postoperative physiotherapy treatment for hip dislocation.

■ PATELLAR DISLOCATION (FIG. 78)

Complete displacement of patella from its normal position, i.e. patellofemoral groove is known as patellar dislocation.

It mostly occurs in females, frequently in the second and third decades of life. According to the studies approximately 30-72% of patellar dislocations are sports related and around 28-39% cases are associated with osteochondral fractures.

An unstable patella may dislocate in any direction (proximal, medial, superior or inferior) however lateral dislocation is the most common location of patella dislocation.

Types of Patellar Dislocation
- **Acute dislocation:** It occurs in response to trauma.
- **Recurrent dislocation:** It occurs as recurrent isolated episodes of subluxation in response to trauma. It is commonly associated with malalignment of lower limb, patella alta, ligament laxity, lateral soft tissue contracture, muscular imbalance.
- **Habitual patellar dislocation:** It is painless dislocation of patella that occurs during each flexion movement. It usually occurs due to tight lateral structures, such as tightness of ITB and vastus lateralis.
- **Congenital dislocation:** It is an irreducible dislocation present since birth and associated with lateral placement of entire quadriceps mechanism.

Mechanism of Injury
In acute dislocation:
- Powerful quadriceps contraction with sudden flexion and internal rotation of femur relative to knee (i.e. external rotation of tibia) while the foot is planted on the ground.
- Direct trauma to patella with knee in flexion.

Anatomical Risk Factors for Patellar Instability
- Increased Q angle (due to pes planus, genu valgum, external tibial torsion, excessive femoral neck anteversion or internal femoral torsion) leads to the lateralization of tibial tuberosity.

Fractures and Dislocations

Table 60: Postoperative physiotherapy treatment protocol for hip dislocation.

	Precaution	ROM exercises	Strengthening exercises	Weight bearing
Week 0–6	• Avoid terminal hip extension, adduction and ER • Sleep supine with one pillow under knee and one pillow between knees • Avoid WB exercises	• Supine ROM only • Hip flexion 10°–90° (heel slides–active and passive) • Hip—IR 5°, ER 5° • No abduction/adduction	Isometric exercise for glutei, quads Ankle pumps	TTWB with two crutches
Weeks 6–12	Avoid end range movement and combination movement at hip joint	• Gentle gravity—eliminated hip ROM exercises (pain-free), increase range as comfort allows • Supine abduction and adduction	Isometric exercises for glutei, quadriceps and hamstrings • Isometric abduction and adduction	PWB with two crutches
Weeks 12–16	Avoid overstressing the hip joint and femoral head	• Antigravity hip ROM exercises and progress • Standing hip flexion, abduction, adduction and extension	• Resistance ROM (bduction, adduction, extension) • No hip flexor strengthening until week 16	FWB
Weeks 16–20	None	Complete AROM and PROM exercise for hip	Progressive Resisted exercises for hip (abduction, adduction, extension and flexion)	FWB

(ER: external rotation; WB: weight bearing; ROM: range of motion; AROM: active range of motion; PROM: passive range of motion; TTWB: toe touch weight bearing; PWB: partial weight bearing; FWB: full weight bearing)

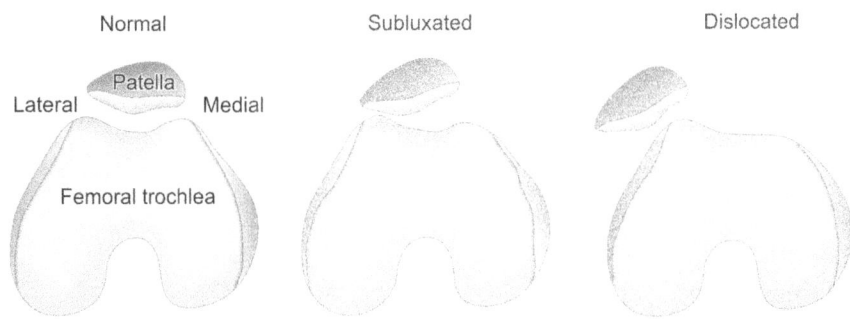

Fig. 78: Subluxed and dislocated patella.

- Genu recurvatum
- Patella alta (high riding patella)
- Excessive lateral patellar tilt
- Trochlear dysplasia or hypoplasia
- Patellar dysplasia or hypoplasia
- Vastus medialis weakness or atrophy
- Overpull of lateral structures (iliotibial band or vastus lateralis)
- Generalized ligamentous laxity (Ehlers-Danlos syndrome).

Clinical Presentation
- Severe pain, swelling and/or tenderness around the patella.
- Feeling of instability or giving way during weight bearing.
- Inability to extend the knee.
- Creaking or cracking sounds on knee movement.
- Deformed appearance of knee: Visible translation of patella.
- Hearing of popping sound when the patella dislocates.

Physical Examination
- **Contour of knee:** Examination of the anterior defect, laterally deviated patella and swelling around the patella.
- **Palpation:** Tenderness on medial joint line in partially flexed knee.
- **Neurovascular examination** distal to patella.
- **Special test:** Apprehension test is used to evaluate the lateral patellar instability.
  - **Apprehension test:** The therapist gently and slowly pushes the patella laterally. Presence of the signs of apprehension or reflex quadriceps contraction indicates the presence of lateral instability of patella (Fig. 79).

Management
Nonsurgical Treatment
- **Closed reduction and physical therapy:** After closed reduction the knee immobilizes in above plaster cast or cylinder splint for 2–3 weeks followed by physical therapy.

Indications:
- First time patellar dislocation without any loose bodies or intra-articular damage.
- Habitual dislocation.

Surgical Treatment
The goal of surgery is to repair the knee damage associated with patellar dislocation and to correct the primary anatomical anomaly. According to the condition, the surgeon may reconstruct a damaged ligament, release tight surrounding structures that might be pulling the knee off track or make changes to the bone alignment of femur or tibia.

Surgical options are:
- Medial patellofemoral ligament (MPFL) reconstruction or repair
- Lateral release
- Trochleoplasty
- Medialization of tibial tuberosity
- Medial capsular plication.

Indications:
- Serious ligament tear (MPFL).
- Recurrent patellar dislocation.
- Not responding to conservative treatment.
- Presence of anatomical abnormalities.
- Osteochondral fractures.

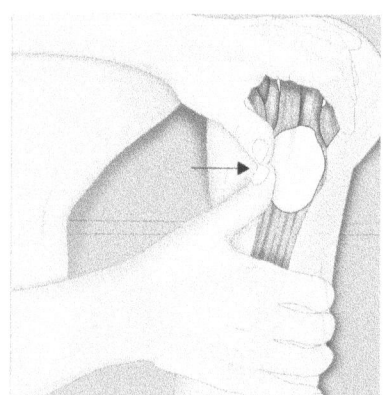

Fig. 79: Apprehension test for patellar dislocation.

Complications
- Residual instability/recurrent dislocation
- Patellofemoral arthrosis
- Anterior knee pain
- Restricted knee ROM
- Hemarthrosis
- Patellar fracture
- Secondary osteoarthritis.

Physiotherapy treatment: Tables 61 and 62 show conservative and postoperative physiotherapy treatment for patellar dislocation.

Table 61: Conservative physiotherapy treatment for patellar dislocation.

	Precaution	ROM exercises	Strengthening exercises	Weight bearing
Week 0–4	Brace in full extension at all times	PROM exercise for knee 0–45° in brace	Isometric exercise for quadriceps and hamstring	WBAT in hinged brace
Weeks 4–6	Discontinue the hinged brace and advance to patellar stabilization brace when the quads control is adequate	• Gentle patellar mobilization • PROM, AAROM, and AROM with brace off • Full knee extension and 0–115° of knee flexion.	PRE for hamstrings	FWB
Weeks 6–8		• AROM, AAROM and PROM exercise • Full knee extension and 0–125° knee flexion	• PRE of quads • Proprioceptive training bilateral stance	FWB
Weeks 8–12	None	Complete AROM and PROM exercises for knee	Plyometric and agility training	FWB

(ROM: range of motion; PROM: passive range of motion; AAROM: active-assisted range of motion; AROM: active range of motion; PRE: progressive resistance exercise; WBAT: weight bearing as tolerated; FWB: full weight bearing)

Table 62: Postoperative physiotherapy treatment for patellar dislocation.

	Precaution	ROM exercises	Strengthening exercises	Weight bearing
Week 0–1	Brace in full extension at all times	• PROM of knee 0–30° in brace.	Isometric exercise for quadriceps and hamstring	WBAT with brace locked in extension
Weeks 2–4	Same as above	• PROM of knee 0–60° by 2nd week • PROM of knee 0–90° by 4th week • AROM, AAROM of knee	• PRE for quads and hams • PRE for hamstrings, hip adduction and abduction	Same as above
Weeks 4–6	Wean off brace	• Gentle patellar mobilizations • PROM of knee 0–105° • AROM, AAROM for knee	• Same as above • Proprioceptive training bilateral stance	FWB or FWBAT using assistive device
Weeks 6–8	None	• Complete AROM and PROM exercise of knee	• Plyometric and agility training	FWB

(ROM: range of motion; PROM: passive range of motion; AROM: active range of motion; AAROM: active-assisted range of motion; PRE: progressive resistance exercise; WBAT: weight bearing as tolerated; FWB: full weight bearing)

CHAPTER 3

Deformities

HIP DEFORMITIES

■ COXA VARA

Coxa vara is a hip deformity in which femoral neck – shaft angle (i.e. angle of inclination) is less than 120° (Figs. 1A and B).

Epidemiology

- Occurrence is equal in males to females
- Bilateral involvement is observed in one-third of patients.

Etiology

Exact etiology of developmental coxa vara is not known, although there are many possible theories. The most popular theory that proposed by Dylkkanes in 1960, states that defect in endochondral ossification of medial part of femoral neck is the cause of deformity. During early developmental years of child, bending or fracture of femoral neck occurs due to stress forces applied during learning process of weight bearing, i.e. crawling or standing. With continued weight bearing it collapses and results in varus and retroversion shift. Gradually this leads to varus, retroversion shortening and bowing of shaft.

Classification of Coxa Vara

- **Congenital coxa vara (CCV):** CCV is present at birth and caused by osteo-chondrodysplasia of femoral neck. It is also known as infantile or cervical coxa vara.
- **Acquired coxa vara:** It occurs secondary to some underlying cause, such as:
  - Slipped capital femoral epiphysis
  - Pathological bone disorder, e.g. fibrous dysplasia, osteogenesis imperfect
  - Avascular necrosis of femoral epiphysis, e.g. Legg-Calvé-Perthes disease
  - Metabolic bone diseases, e.g. Paget's disease, rickets, etc.
  - Bone infection, i.e. osteomyelitis of femoral neck
  - Developmental—progressive, usually present between 2–6 years
  - Post-traumatic, e.g. intertrochanteric fracture.

Clinical Presentations

- Pain, stiffness and flexion contracture in affected hip
- Child stands with hip adducted, leg medially rotated and foot everted, i.e. pronation at subtalar joint and pelvis is tilted down on affected side
- Hip abduction and medial rotation is limited (abduction is restricted due to

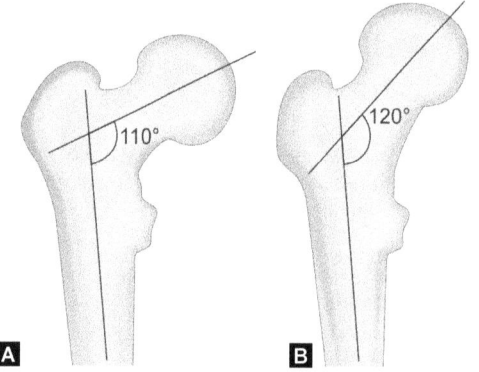

Figs. 1A and B: A. Coxa vara; B. Normal.

impingement of superior portion of femoral neck or greater trochanter or hip abductor contracture)
- **Gait:** Painless limp is present
  Trendelenburg gait in unilateral involvement
  Waddling gait in bilateral involvement
- Shortening of affected limb
- Commonly associated with hyperlordosis or scoliosis.

Biomechanics

Coxa vara leads to ipsilateral limb shortening which shifts weight-bearing area of the hip more superiorly and laterally to femoral head resulting in abductor contracture on the affected side. Moment arm acting on hip abductors is increased that reduces the demand on hip abductors resulting in their weakness (Fig. 2).

Diagnosis: X-Ray Findings

- Increased Hilgenreiner epiphyseal (HE) angle: It is angle between a Hilgenreiner line (horizontal line connecting the triradiate cartilage) and the line drawn parallel to capital femoral physis. Normally it is less than 30° (Fig. 3).
- Decreased femoral anteversion.

Other X-Ray Findings (Fig. 4)

- Decrease of femoral neck shaft angle, i.e. less than 120°.
- Short and flat femoral head.
- More vertical oriented physeal plate.
- Coxa brevis—short neck with overgrown trochanter

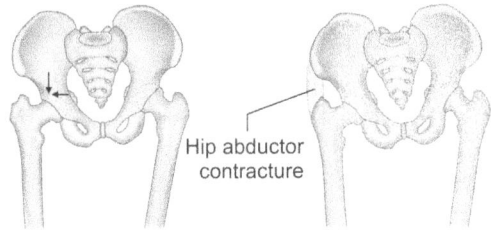

Fig. 2: Coxa vara of hip demonstrating abductor contracture.

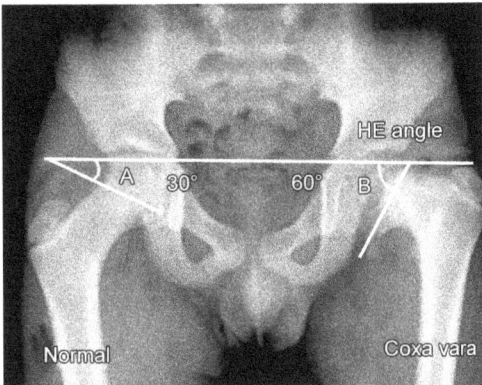

Fig. 3: Hilgenreiner epiphyseal angle.

- Abnormal bony fragment inferolateral to physeal plate that contained in inverted Y shaped lucency.

Physical Examination

- Limb length discrepancy, i.e. shortening of affected limb (usually less than 2.5 cm)
- **Gait:** Trendelenburg test positive in unilateral involvement and waddling gait in bilateral involvement.
- Greater trochanter of affected side is more elevated and prominent.
- Limited medial rotation and abduction of affected hip joint.
- Commonly associated with compensatory lordosis or scoliosis.
- Presence of anterior pelvic tilt in bilateral involvement.
- Excessive lordosis, limited abduction, mild hip flexion contracture, and limited hip extension may occur concomitantly in bilateral involvement.
- Patient may also have excessive femoral retroversion and decreased anteversion, so patient will walk with toe-out gait to restore stability (Fig. 5).

Complications

- Hip subluxation
- Acetabular dysplasia
- Degenerative arthritis of hip joint
- In bilateral cases increased lordosis.

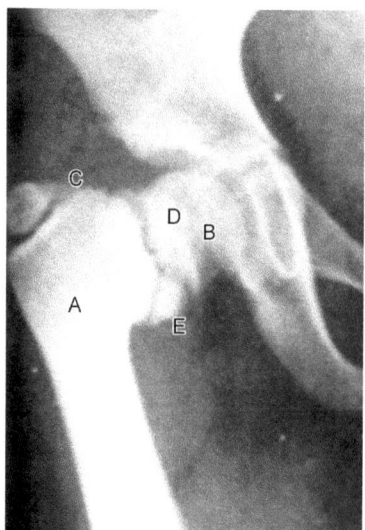

Fig. 4: X-ray findings of coxa vara.

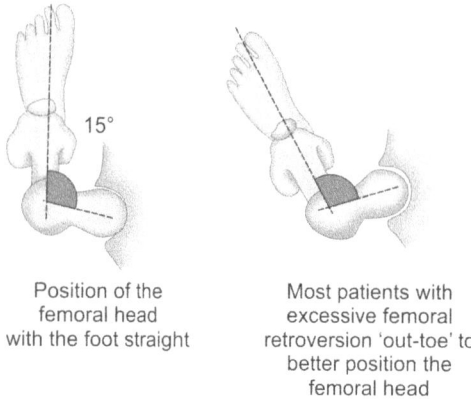

Fig. 5: Excessive femoral retroversion.

Management

Non-surgical Treatment

Indications
- Hilgenreiner's epiphyseal angle <45.
- When the deformity is non-progressive.
- Neck shaft angle approaches normal.
- About 20% cases correct spontaneously without surgery.

Conservative Treatment
- Indicated in early adolescent cases when it occurs due to slipped epiphyseal. In detected early cases, complete bed rest is advised to relieve strain on epiphysis.
- Traction is applied in abduction for about 4-6 weeks to obtain joint reduction.
- Following this, patient is fitted with weight relieving caliper or plaster retained for 12-18 months.
- Stretching of hip adductor and lateral rotator muscles may be needed.

Surgical Treatment

Indications
- Progressive varus deformity.
- Presence of painful limp.
- Presence of Trendelenburg gait.
- Unilateral progressive shortening.
- Associated with leg length discrepancy.
- Neck shaft angle <110°.
- HE angle >60°.

Surgical Techniques

Corrective valgus derotation osteotomy (CVDO): Valgus osteotomy reduces deformity, normalizes neck shaft angle, improves gluteal forces, improves joint congruency, increases limb length to reduce limb length discrepancy along with the correction of rotational deformities of femur.

Deformities

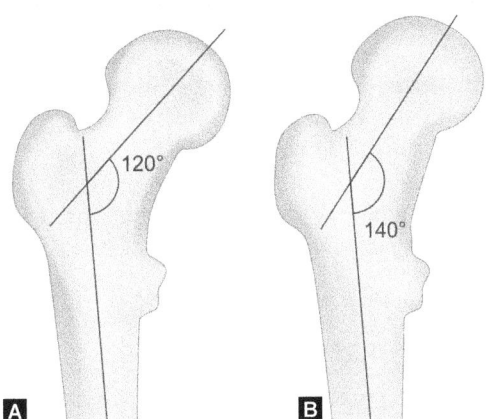

Figs. 6A and B: A. Normal; B. Coxa valga.

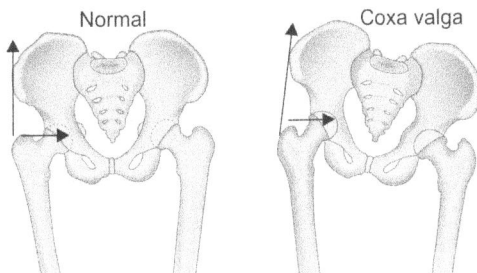

Fig. 7: Adductor tightness with upward pelvic obliquity in coxa valga.

◼ COXA VALGA

Coxa valga is a hip deformity in which femoral neck—shaft angle is more than 120° (Figs. 6A and B).

But it is quite rare as compared to coxa vara.

Classification

- **Congenital coxa valga:** It is present since birth.
- **Acquired coxa valga:** It occurs secondary to some underlying cause includes
  - Slipped femoral capital epiphysis.
  - Skeletal dysplasia: Turner syndrome.
  - Post-traumatic: Femoral fractures.
  - Metabolic bone disease: Rickets, Paget's disease, etc.
  - Secondary to knee deformity: Genu valgum.
  - Bone infection: Osteomyelitis of hip bone.
  - Neuromuscular disorders: Cerebral palsy.

Etiology

Most common cause of progressive coxa valga is cerebral palsy along with other neuromuscular disorders. Increased muscular pull on femoral head due to spasticity and abnormal forces eventually cause subluxation or dislocation of femoral head.

Physiological Coxa Valgum

Normal femoral neck shaft angle at birth is 150° that progressively decrease to 115–120° due to gradual weight bearing in children at the age of 2–3 years.

Clinical Presentation

- Limb length discrepancy—affected limb becomes long
- Trendelenburg gait in unilateral involvement
- Adductor tightness with upward pelvic obliquity and weakness of the abductors also on the affected side (Fig. 7)
- Altered pelvic mechanics may cause back pain or sacroiliac joint dysfunction.

Physical Examination

- Limb length discrepancy present—affected limb is long.
- Trendelenburg test positive.
- Usually associated with femoral increased anteversion, so patient will walk with toe-in gait to restore stability (Fig. 8).
- Increased internal rotation of hip joint.
- Posterior pelvic tilt.
- Greater trochanter is at lower level.

Diagnosis

X-ray findings: Increased neck shaft angle than 120° (Fig. 9).

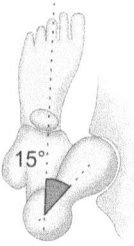
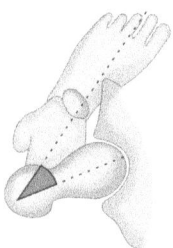

| Position of the femoral head with the foot straight | Most patients with excessive femoral anteversion 'in-toe' to better position the femoral head |

Fig. 8: Excessive femoral anteversion.

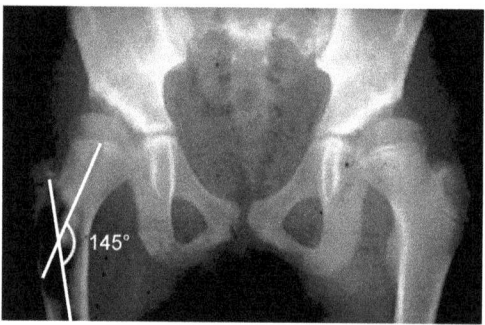

Fig. 9: Increased femoral angle of inclination in coxa valga.

Treatment

Conservative Treatment

Indicated for mild symptomatic coxa valga.
- **Stretching exercises:** Stretching of adductor muscles of affected side.
- **Strengthening exercises:** Strengthening of abductor muscles of the same side.
- Patients should be taught to keep neutral positioning of pelvis to eliminate the limp.
- Foot-drill exercise should be given to correct feet position.
- General leg exercises should also be practiced.
- Patient should avoid performing exercises in standing position in initial stage.
- Shoe lift of unaffected side is advised to equalize leg length discrepancy.

Surgical Treatment

Severe cases are treated with osteotomy to correct leg-length difference and to restore normal mechanics.

Varus derotation osteotomy: This surgical technique is commonly used to treat coxa valga in which rotational correction for anteversion is also considered.

KNEE DEFORMITIES

■ GENU VARUM

Lateral angulation of leg over thigh at knee joint is termed as **genu varum** or **bow legs** (Fig. 10). Usually it is bilateral.

Etiology

- Physiological or developmental genu varum.
- Early weight bearing, especially in children who are heavy and fatty.
- Metabolic bone diseases, such as rickets or osteomalacia, Paget's disease (osteitis deformans).
- Skeletal dysplasias.
- Disorder which causes distorted epiphyseal growth, such as Blount's disease.
- Post-traumatic: Fracture of lower part of femur or upper part of tibia with malunion.
- Osteoarthritis: More common in elderly females.

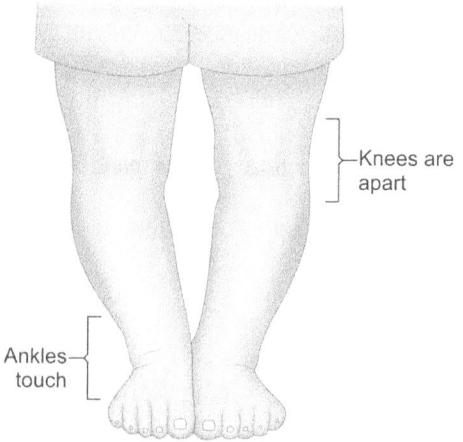

Fig. 10: Genu varum or bow legs.

Deformities

Physiological Genu Varum (Fig. 11)

Uterine space during gestational period, forces the lower extremity of fetus to lie in "Buddha" position, i.e. hip and knee flexion and medial rotation of tibia. This position causes the contracture of medial knee capsule and posterior oblique ligament. Presence of residual tightness of capsular/ligamentous contracture leads to varying amount of bow-leggedness at onset of walking. Over the course of time these contractures stretch and spontaneous resolution of this "physiologic" bowing is seen.

Normally all newborns are born bow legged and at around 6–12 months genu varum reached to its maximum. Gradually the bowing improves when infant begins to walk, i.e. at around 18–24 months and by the age of 3 to 4 years, bowing has corrected and the legs typically regained a normal appearance.

Pathological Changes

Bones

Shaft of femur, tibia and fibula are all curved outward.

Muscles and Ligaments

- Ligaments on outer side of knee are lengthened and those on inner side shortened.
- Muscles of outer side of thigh and leg, i.e. biceps femoris and peronei are stretched while the muscles on inner side, i.e. adductors are shortened.

Clinical Presentations

- Usually asymptomatic in children.
- Knees do not touch each other when standing with feet together (ankles touching)
- Adult may feel some discomfort on inner aspect of knee due to excess compressive force on the medial side.
- Inversion of feet while standing or walking.
- Limp may be present.
- Difficulty in carrying activities of daily living.
- Difficulty in cross leg sitting.

Diagnosis

Physical Examination

- **Q angle:** It is formed between a line drawn from ASIS to central patella and the line tibial tubercle to central patella.
  Normal Q angle is 14° in males and 17° in females. In genu varum Q angle is decreased (Fig. 12).
- **Femoral intercondylar distance:** Distance between the femoral medial condyles is measured by placing the medial

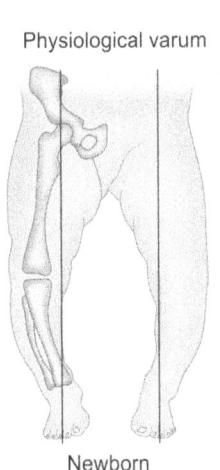
Physiological varum
Newborn

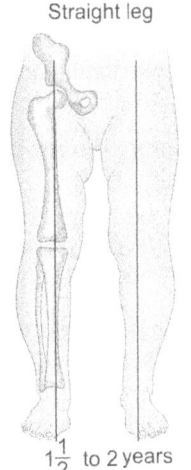
Straight leg
1½ to 2 years

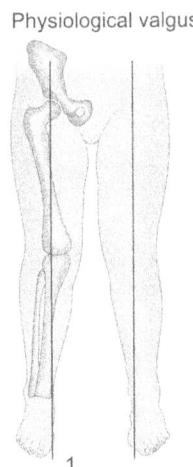
Physiological valgus
2½ years

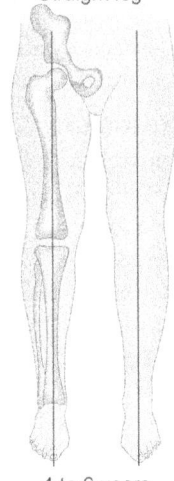
Straight leg
4 to 6 years

Fig. 11: Physiological evolution of leg alignment at various ages (genu varum).

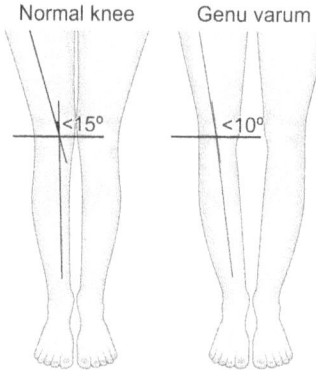

Fig. 12: Decreased Q angle in genu varum.

malleolus of both sides in contact with each other (in supine or standing position). Greater than 6 cm is considered to be abnormal.
- **Gait:** Waddling gait present in case of bilateral involvement.
- **Limb length measurement:** In unilateral case the involved limb is shorter.

Complications
- Osteoarthritis of knee: Genu varum may cause osteoarthritis due to abnormal amount of stress on knee joint, i.e. line of gravity falls further medial to knee joint than usual, putting more stress on the medial compartment of the knee.
- Chronic cases may lead to pain and inflammation in other joints of lower extremity also due to uneven loading and altered biomechanics.

Treatment

Conservative Treatment
In physiological genu varum, no actual treatment is required as the condition resolves itself by the age of 2 years while in borderline cases, regular follow up after every 6 months is mandatory.

To resolve pathologic genu varum:
- Knee brace: It act as compartmental unloader. Correction of early deformity is done by dynamic bracing or splints. Valgus orthosis for knee is needed to place valgus stress on the knee, to decrease natural varus moment and lower the stress on the medial tibiofemoral joint.
- Shoe modification—elevation of outer border of shoe or lateral heel wedge.
- In defined metabolic conditions, such as rickets and osteomalacia—vitamin D and calcium intake is advisable.

Physiotherapy Management
- **Avoid or minimize weight bearing activities** with knee flexion and reduce body weight to reduce joint loading.
- **Electrotherapeutic modalities:** To reduce joint effusion and pain. High voltage pulsed galvanic stimulation (HVPGS), interferential therapy, strong faradic electrical stimulation or TENS can be used.
- When knee movements are limited in capsular pattern—joint traction, capsular stretching, soft tissue massage, mobilization techniques, etc. are useful to stretch the tight capsule.
- **Stretching exercises:** Stretching is reported to be effective on prevention of musculoskletal damage, to increase the connective tissues around the joints and to improve the motor performance and in rehabilitating musculoskeletal system. Stretching of hamstrings, hip adductors are performed for reduction of pain and re-orientation of joint.
- **Strengthening exercises:** Strengthening of hip abductors, gluteus muscles quadriceps and hamstrings are used to deload the joint and provide joint protection.

Surgical Treatment

Indications
- When it persists beyond 4 years of age
- Unilateral presentation
- Progressive worsening of curvature.

Surgical Techniques
- Stapling of outer aspect of knee when child is within the growth period.
- **Tibial osteotomy:** Cutting a wedge of bone from outer portion of tibia. It is performed after attaining the skeletal maturity.

- **Total knee replacement surgeries:** Advised in very advanced cases of knee osteoarthritis caused by genu varum.

GENU VALGUM

Inward or medial angulation of leg over thigh at knee joint is termed as **genu valgum** or **knock knee** (Fig. 13).

Etiology

- Metabolic bone disease—rickets
- Muscular and ligaments weakness in adolescents
- Muscular paralysis of semimembranosus, semitendinosus
- Post-traumatic: Fractures and injuries involving the knee joint
- Secondary to coxa vara, flat foot, knee osteoarthritis or spinal curvatures.

Normal Physiology (Fig. 14)

Most children are bowlegged from birth to around 1-1½ years then knock knees until the age of 2½ to 4 years. Gradually the knees become straighten by the age of 6 to 7 years.

Pathological Changes

Two degree of deformities:
1. **Bony changes**: Medial condyle of femur is hypertrophied and lengthened. The pressure on outer side is intensified.
   - Shaft of the femur or tibia may be curved: Lower third of femur or upper third of tibia may be curved with inward convexity.
2. **Ligamentous and muscular changes**: Shortening of lateral ligament and stretching of medial ligaments.
   - Semimembranosus, sartorius and vastus medialis becomes elongated.
   - Tendon of biceps femoris and iliotibial band of fascia becomes contracted.

Stability of knee joint is affected due to these muscular and ligamentous imbalance and further leads to following biomechanical changes.

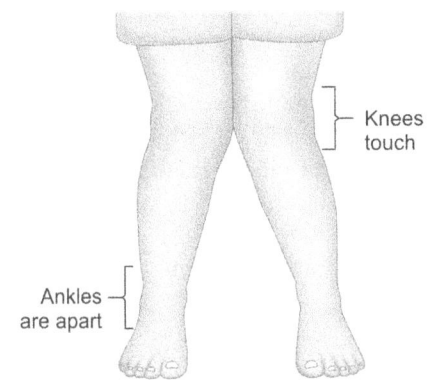

Fig. 13: Genu valgum of knock knee.

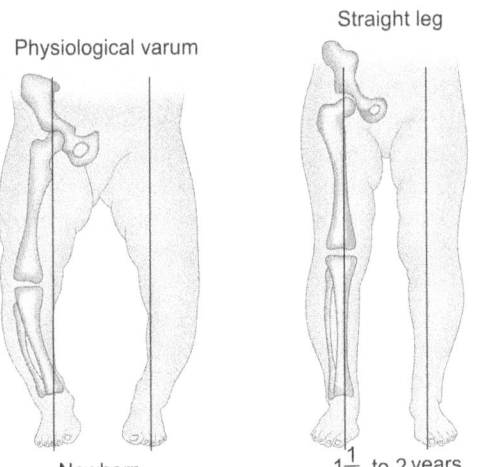 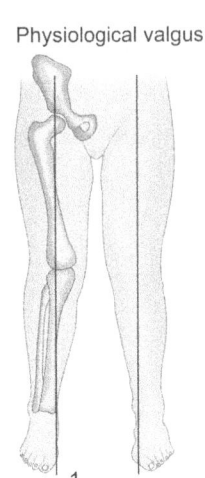 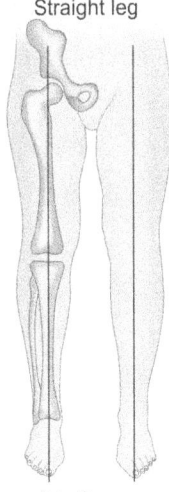

Fig. 14: Physiological variation of leg alignment at different ages (genu valgum).

- Increase mobility at knee joint.
- **Increased Q angle:** Patella may displace or dislocated outwards due to increase in lateral force on the patella.
- Tibia is rotated outwards on femur by contracted biceps femoris tendon.
- Femur may be rotated inwards.

Clinical Presentation
- Often associated with flatfoot deformity.
- Knees touch each other while standing.
- Leg curved inwardly.
- While standing, when feet placed together, the knees become crossed.
- Gait is clumsy and uncertain because of weakness of ligaments and instability of joints and because of the tendency of knees to cross.
- Premature fatigue with activity.

Complications
- Chondromalacia patella—patellar subluxation and abnormal tracking of patella
- Flat feet
- Shin splint/medial tibial stress syndrome
- **Scoliosis:** In case unilateral involvement.

Diagnostic

Physical Examination
- **Q angle:** In genu valgum Q angle is increased (Fig. 15).
- **Intermalleolar distance:** Distance between the medial malleolus is measured by placing knees together in standing or supine position. Intermalleolar distance of ≥3.5 inches (9 cm) between feet is abnormal.

Management
Genu valgum may be classified into 2 classes:

Class I: Genu valgum with Negligible Bony Changes

Conservative Treatment
- **Observation of deformity:** In case of physiological genu valgum in children of less than 6 years age and when Q angle is <15°.
- Children who are weak and have rickets: Rest and avoidance of weight bearing activities adviced.
- Bracing: Used in progressive physiological genu valgum
  - Lateral single bar KAFO
  - Shoe modification—elevation of inner border of shoe or medial heel wedge.
  - Although there is no such clinical evidence that shows the efficacy of shoe modification or splint.

Physiotherapy Treatment
- **Massage:** It is given to improve circulation and soften the structures on outer side of thigh.
- **Stretching Exercise:** Stretching to iliotibial band, biceps femoris and to lateral ligaments of knee.
- **Passive movements** of lower extremity to maintain the mobility of joints.
- In bilateral cases, ankle may be tied and strapped together or sandbag being placed between knees and left the patient in this position for 10 minutes.
- **Active movements:** To maintain the stability of knee.
- **Strengthening exercise:** Helps to realign and stabilize the knees. Strengthening of lengthened muscles, e.g. vastus medialis, quadratus femoris, gracilis, sartorius and semitendinosus.

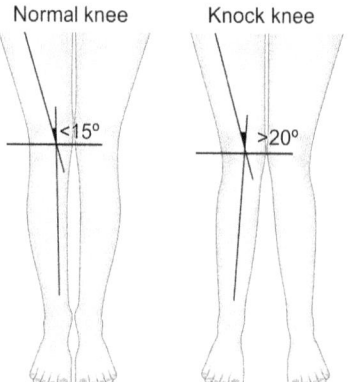

Fig. 15: Increased Q angle in genu valgum.

Class II: Genu Valgum with Marked Bony Changes

Surgical Treatment

Indications
- Age > 7 years
- Unilateral problem, i.e. asymmetry of leg.
- Intermalleolar distance > 9 cm.
- Associated symptoms: Marked pain, limp and joint instability affecting functional ability.

Surgical Techniques
- **Osteotomy:** Excision of a wedge of bone from medial side of distal femur or proximal tibia.
- **Osteoclasis:** It consists of fracture of lower end of femur or slight displacement of its lower epiphysis. This procedure is rarely performed nowadays.

FOOT DEFORMITIES

PES CAVUS

Pes cavus is the presence of extraordinary high plantar longitudinal arch, i.e. forefoot is plantar flexed in relation to rearfoot. It is also known as hollow foot or claw foot. In pes cavus, the foot is relatively inflexible and it is much less common than pes planus (Figs. 16A and B).

Etiology
- **Progressive neuromuscular disorders:** Friedreich's ataxia, syringomyelia, muscular dystrophy, etc.
- **Nonprogressive neurological disorders:** Poliomyelitis, cerebral palsy
- **Congenital disorders:** Idiopathic cavus foot, spina bifida, congenital talipes equinovarus, arthrogryposis, etc.

- **Post traumatic:** Compartment syndrome, crush injury, peroneal nerve injury, severe burn, etc.

Clinical Presentation
- **Pain:**
  - Pain in sole of foot because of pressure on metatarsal heads, that may radiates into dorsum of foot and up the front of leg.
  - Lateral foot pain due to increase weight bearing on lateral foot.
  - Metatarsalgia: Pain and inflammation at MTP joint.
- Painful callosities may be present at MTP joint, on lateral side or heel of the foot due to uneven weight distribution.
- Discomfort or fatigue on standing or walking.
- Ankle joint instability: Due to supination of foot, adduction of forefoot and varus of hind foot.
- Lack of coordination.
- Increased plantar arch, prominent and painful metatarsal heads, shortened foot length along with various deformities of toes, e.g. hammer toes, claw toes (Fig. 17).

Causes of Acquired Pes Cavus
- Paralysis or weakness of lumbricals and interossei muscles of foot.
- Paralysis of long flexors of toes, enabling the foot to be drawn into strong dorsiflexion

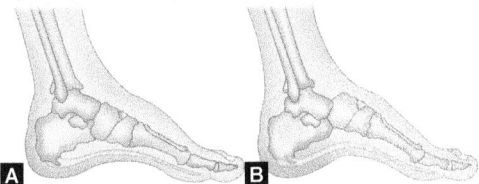

Figs. 16A and B: A. Normal foot; B. Pes cavus.

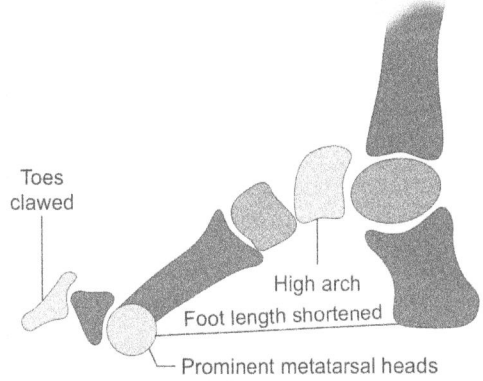

Fig. 17: Skeletal structure in pes cavus.

by unopposed anterior tibial muscles. Calcaneus is directed upwards and tarsus is angulated.
- Boots, shoes or socks which are too short and therefore cramp the foot.

Biomechanism

- **Paralysis of long flexors:** Unopposed pull of anterior tibial muscles raises the anterior part of calcaneus and forefoot drops at midtarsal joint. The anterior transverse arch is depressed by strain put on it and in time becomes convex. The toes are hyperextended at MTP joint, partly because of pull of long extensors and partly because of lowering of MT heads. The first phalanx points upwards and distal phalanx becomes flexed.
- **Paralysis of lumbricals and interossei:** In this, changes occur in reverse order. Normally lumbricals and interossei act synergically during the action of long flexors, to prevent flexion of IP joint during contraction of long flexors in walking. If this synergism action is lost, long flexors are unopposed and toes become clawed. Proximal phalanx exerts pressure on MT heads, forcing them down. In this stage transverse arch drops and angle of forefoot is altered.

Diagnosis: X-ray Findings

Calcaneal pitch angle: The angle formed between a horizontal line and a line passes from the base of heel and inferior cortex of calcaneus. Normal calcaneal pitch angle is 20°. In pes cavus calcaneal pitch angle is increased, i.e. more than 20° (Fig. 18).

Lateral talar-1st metatarsal angle (Meary's angle) (Fig. 19): The angle formed between the longitudinal axis of talus and first metatarsal in lateral view of radiograph in weight bearing position. Normally these two midline axis are in line with each other

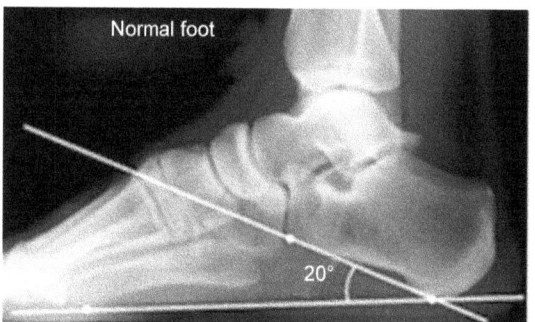
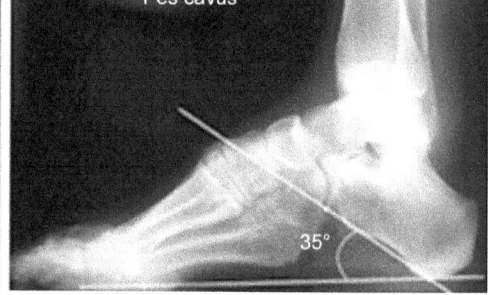

Fig. 18: Calcaneal pitch angle in normal and claw foot.

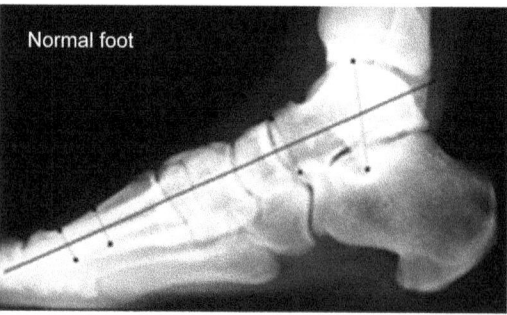
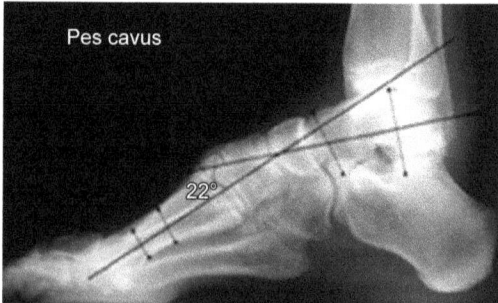

Fig. 19: Meary's angle in normal and claw foot.

Deformities

and the Meary's angle is 0°. Whereas in pes cavus the angle is more than 4° with upward convexity.

Physical Examination
- **Observation**
  - Observe the increase arch of foot.
  - Callosities may present below the MT heads.
  - Presence of hammer toes or claw toes.
  - Shortening of length of foot.
  - Footwear evaluation: Collapse of shoes on lateral side.
  - Gait: Walking with hindfoot inversion and forefoot varus in stance phase.
  - Gait: The foot remains kept in hindfoot inversion and forefoot varus throughout the stance phase.
- **Palpation**
  - Tenderness on lateral aspect or sole of foot or under MTP joint.
  - Palpate the presence of callus or corn on most affected region of foot.
- **Flexibility:** Look for plantar fascia and Achilles tendon tightness.
- Muscle strength of foot muscles.
- Balance and coordination test.
- PROM of foot and ankle to check the mobility.
- Neurological examination to assess any underlying pathology.
- **Footprint test (Stahl index) (Fig. 20):** Conventionally in normal footprint, forefoot is joined by hind foot by a strip that is approximately half the width of the forefoot. However, this strip is thinner or may be absent in cavus foot.
- **Coleman block test:** It assesses the flexibity of subtalar joint. Test is performed by asking the patient to stand on 1 inch thick block, with the heel and lateral border of foot on the block. While first, second and third metatarsal are allowed to hanged freely in plantar flexion and pronation. If correction of heel varus occurs on weight bearing, the subtalar joint is considered to be flexible.

Management

Physiotherapy Treatment
- **Therapeutic modalities:** Such as ultrasound, TENS or IFT are used to decrease associated pain and inflammation.
- Stretching exercises: Stretching of plantar fascia, Achilles tendon and calf muscles.
- Strengthening exercise: Strengthening of long flexors and intrinsic muscles of foot depends on the cause of pes cavus.
- Faradic foot bath helps to reduce pain and inflammation along with the strengthening of intrinsic foot muscles.
- Resisted toe extension to prevent clawing of toes.
- **Footwear modification:** To reduce and redistribute the loading of plantar pressure.
  - Lateral wedge to correct varus deformity.
  - Extra depth shoes helps to offload bony prominences and prevent rubbing of toes.

Surgical Treatment
- **Soft tissue reconstruction:** Indicated for flexible deformities.
  - Plantar fascia release
  - Steindler stripping
  - Lambrinudi's operation
  - Gracaeu and Brahms procedure
  - Tendon transfer: Jones suspension, Hibbs suspension, Tibialis posterior transfer, Peroneus transfer.

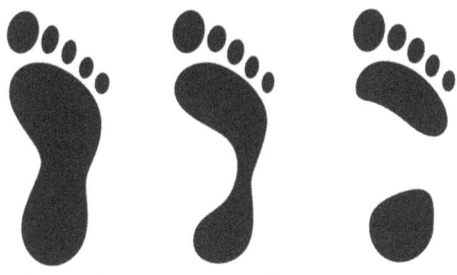

Fig. 20: Footprint test of pes cavus.

- **Osseous procedure:**
  - Triple arthrodesis
  - Dwyer calcaneal osteotomy
  - DFWO metatarsal (Dorsiflexory wedge osteotomy)
  - Digital reduction.

■ PES PLANUS

It is a term applied to a variation in normal contour of foot in which longitudinal arch is reduced or collapsed and the medial border of foot comes close to or in contact with the ground (Figs. 21A and B).

Etiology

- **Physiological flat foot:** Very common in toddlers if they are overweight or have lax joints. Presence of physiological foot is normal up to the age of 3 years.
- **Pathological flat foot:**
  - **Congenital flat foot:** Present at or around birth. Due to any structural/bony anomalies, e.g. coalition of tarsal bone, equinus deformity, tibial abnormalities or rotational deformities.
  - **Ligamentous laxity:** e.g. Marfan's syndrome, Down's syndrome, Ehlers-Danlos syndrome or familial.
  - **Acquired flat foot:** It may occur due to following causes:
    - Due to general muscle hypotonicity from chronic general illness.
    - **Occupational:** Excessive fatigue or strain of muscle in occupation which involve prolonged standing or walking.
    - **Obesity:** Heavier body weight results in higher plantar pressure, with largest effect on longitudinal arch and MT heads.
    - Posterior tibial tendon dysfunction.
    - Achilles tendon contracture.
- Other less common causes of acquired flat foot are:
  - **Traumatic flat foot:** Direct or indirect foot injury, e.g. crush injury of foot, in and around ankle joint, fracture of bones of lower limb resulting in malalignment.
  - **Paralytic flat foot:** Selective paralysis of postural muscles of foot as occurs in poliomyelitis.
  - **Inflammatory flat foot:** Occurs from inflammation and infiltration of ligament and plantar fascia of foot following acute rheumatism or rheumatoid arthritis.

Clinical presentations: Depends on age of onset and underlying causes.

Clinical presentation in children: Condition is usually asymptomatic but may cause:
- Foot pain, ankle pain or lower leg pain
- Outward tilting of heel.

Clinical presentation in adults
- Fatigue and pain in feet after unaccustomed strain such as prolonged standing, weight bearing or wearing of heavy shoes.
- Pain is usually bilateral and commonly extends from medial border of foot and across its dorsum.
- Calf pain may also present.
- As condition progresses:
  - Foot arches may disappear completely.
  - Feet becoming turning out.
  - Toe pointing outwards, i.e. pronation of foot, abduction of forefoot and valgus of hind foot (Fig. 22).
  - Gait becomes awkward, stiff and without spring.
- In advanced cases osteoarthritis of small joints of feet may develop.

Complications of flat foot:
- Inflammation and pain in ligaments of sole of feet

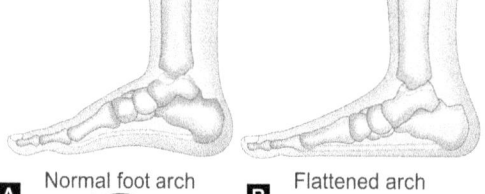

Figs. 21A and B: A. Normal foot; B. Pes planus.

Deformities

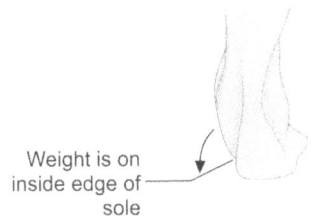

Fig. 22: Pronation of foot.

- Achilles and posterior tibial tendonitis
- Stress fracture in lower leg
- Bunion
- Calluses.

Diagnosis

X-ray Findings

Calcaneal pitch angle: Calcaneal pitch angle is decreased, i.e. less than 20° in pes planus. (Fig. 23).

Lateral talar-1st metatarsal angle (Meary's angle) (Fig. 24): Meary's angle is more than 4° with downward convexity in pes planus.

Physical Examination
- **Observation**
  - Swelling and tenderness
  - Look for abnormal callosities.
  - Look for ligament laxity.
  - Footwear evaluation—collapse of shoes on medial side.
- **Palpation**
  - Tenderness on medial aspect of foot
  - Palpate the presence of callus or corn on most affected region of foot
  - Look for ligament laxity.
- Muscle strength of foot muscles
- Balance and coordination test.
- **Footprint test (Stahl index) (Fig. 25):** In footprint of flat foot, the strip that join the forefoot with hindfoot is comparatively broader or of same width of forefoot.
- **Special Test**
  - **Test for tibialis posterior dysfunction syndrome:** Patient cannot be able to perform single limb heel raise.

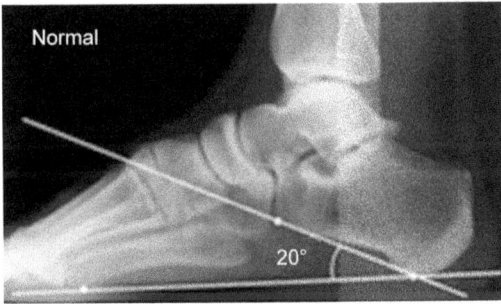 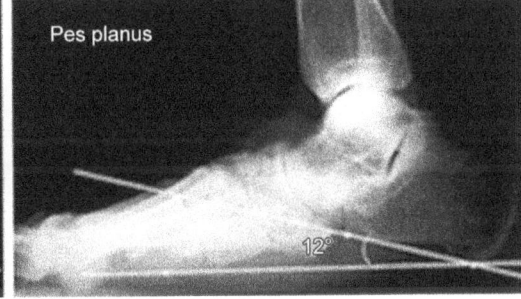

Fig. 23: Calcaneal pitch angle in normal and flat foot.

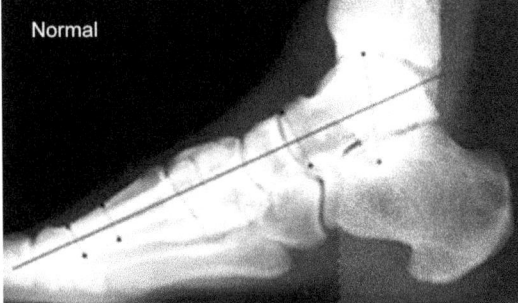 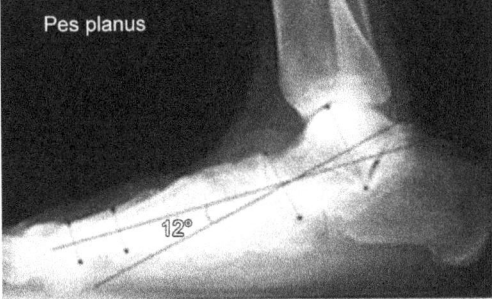

Fig. 24: Meary's angle in normal and flat foot.

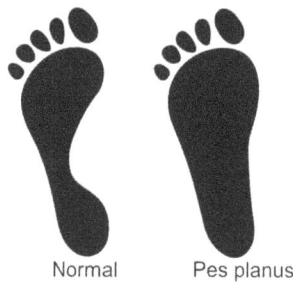

Fig. 25: Foot print test of pes planus.

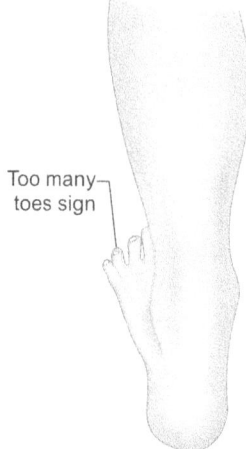

Fig. 26: Too many toes sign.

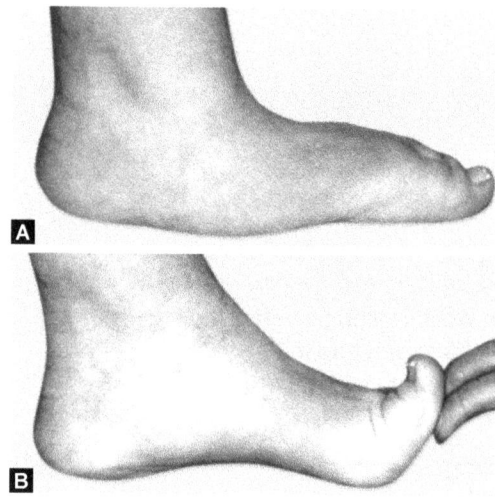

Figs. 27A and B: Jack test.

- **Too many toes sign (Fig. 26):** Patient appears to have more than normal toes when viewed from behind because of over pronation or abduction of forefoot and flattening of medial longitudinal arch that causes splaying of forefoot.
- **Test for Achilles tendon contracture:** Patient places the knee to be assessed in flexion. Therapist stabilizes the foot in dorsiflexion. Test is considered to be positive when gradual extension of knee causes plantarflexion of foot.
- **To differentiate between rigid and flexible flat foot:**
  - **Jack test/Hubscher's maneuver (Figs. 27A and B):** Patient is in standing position. Therapist passively dorsiflexes the great toe and observe whether the convexity of foot arch is increased or not. Increase in the arch of foot determines the flexible foot whereas in rigid foot, arch of foot remains the same.
  - **Standing tip toe test (Figs. 28A and B):** In flexible foot the arch will increase or reappear when standing on toes but in rigid flatfoot it remains same.

Management

Conservative Treatment

- Indicated for flexible flatfoot.
- **Faradic foot bath:** To improve blood circulation and strength of foot muscles.
- **Strengthening exercises:** Strengthening of intrinsic foot muscles or tibialis posterior muscle depend on the cause.
- **Stretching exercises:** Stretching of tibialis posterior (i.e. tendo Achilles)
- **Footwear modifications:**
  - Medial arch support
  - Extended heel cup
  - Wedge placed behind heel to prevent it turning and rolling
  - Outside iron and inside Y or T strap on lower end of tibia.

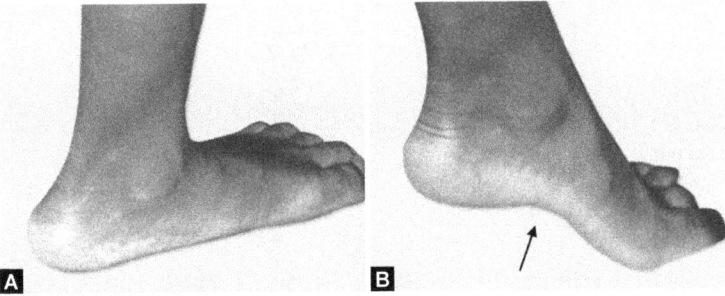

Figs. 28A and B: Standing tip toe test.

Surgical Treatment
- Heel cord lengthening
- Lengthening of lateral column
- Calcaneal osteotomy
- Triple arthrodesis

Indications
- Cerebral palsy
- Painful rigid flat foot
- Painful flexible flat foot

Contraindications
- Hypermobile joints.
- In adults, if feet are asymptomatic.

SPINAL DEFORMITIES

■ SCOLIOSIS

It is an abnormal lateral curvature or angulations of spine. It may be accompanied by rotation of affected vertebra on a vertical axis, the bodies of vertebra rotates towards the convexity of curve (Fig. 29).

Etiology
- **Nonstructural/functional/temporary scoliosis:** Vertebra is normal and curvature occurs as a result of other problems.
  - **Postural scoliosis:** Often associated with poor muscular development due to poor posture.
  - **Sciatic scoliosis:** Occurs in lumbar region secondary to irritative lesion such as prolapsed intervertebral disk (PIVD) or spinal cord tumors.
  - **Compensatory scoliosis:** It is a compensatory mechanism to maintain the trunk vertical when pelvis is tilted laterally due to limb length discrepancy or fixed adduction or abduction deformity at one hip joint.
- **Structural/permanent scoliosis:** Caused by vertebral anomalies.
  - **Idiopathic scoliosis:** It is classified according to the age of onset:
    - **Infantile scoliosis:** 0–3 years.
    - **Juvenile scoliosis:** 4–9 years.
    - **Adolescent scoliosis:** 10–18 years.
    - **Adult:** > 18 years.
      Adolescent scoliosis comprises approximately 80% of all idiopathic scoliosis cases.
  - **Congenital scoliosis (Fig. 30):** Due to congenital deformity of vertebrae:
    - **Wedge vertebra:** Partial unilateral failure of vertebral formation
    - **Hemi vertebra:** Complete unilateral failure of vertebral formation
    - **Congenital bar:** Unilateral failure of segmentation
    - **Block vertebra:** Bilateral failure of segmentation
  - **Neuromuscular scoliosis:** Usually secondary to
    - Poliomyelitis
    - Neurofibromatosis
    - Syringomyelia
    - Friedreich ataxia
    - Lower motor neuron disease

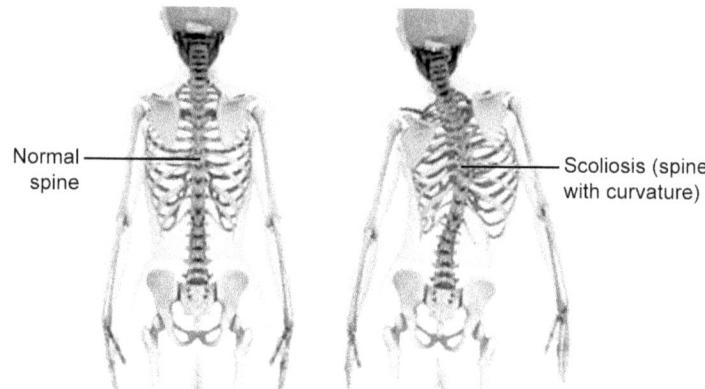

Fig. 29: Normal and scoliotic spine.

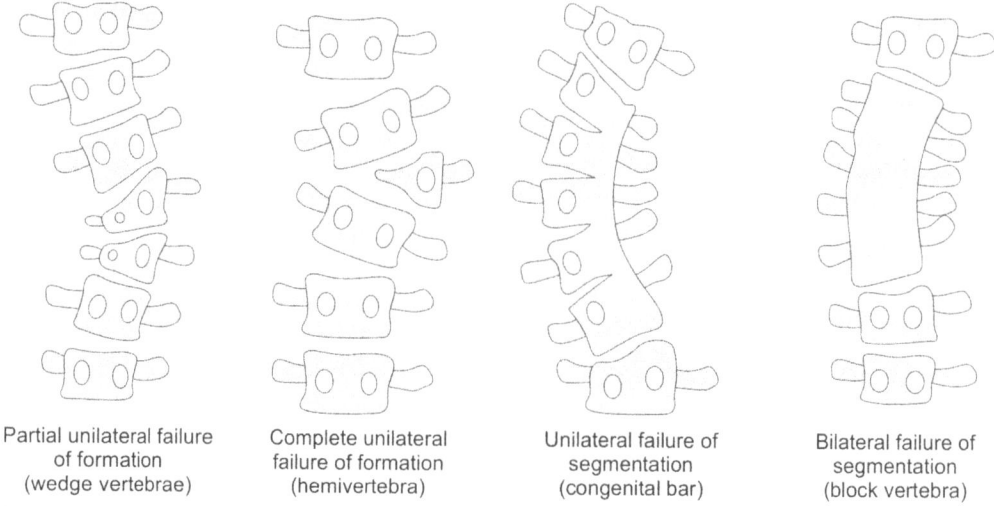

Fig. 30: Congenital deformities of vertebrae.

- Cerebral palsy
- Muscular dystrophy
- **Traumatic scoliosis:** Occurs due to
  - Fracture of spine
  - Surgical operation such as thoracoplasty
  - Irradiation
- **Other causes:**
  - Rickets
  - Osteomalacia
  - Juvenile rheumatoid arthritis
  - Marfan's syndrome
  - Hyperparathyroidism.

Common Types of Curves

There are four common patterns of scoliosis curves:

1. **Right thoracic scoliosis:** When major curve is towards the right side in thoracic region.
2. **Right thoracolumbar scoliosis:** When major curve is towards right side in both lower thoracic and lumbar region, i.e. starting in thoracic and ending in lumbar region. This is commonly known as C curve.

3. **Left lumbar scoliosis:** When major curve is towards left side in lumbar region, i.e. starting and ending in lumbar region.
4. **Double major scoliosis:** It is a double sided curve with right thoracic curve and left lumbar curve. This is commonly known as S curve.

Clinical Presentation

- **Clothes fit awkwardly or hang unevenly.**
- **Sideways curvature observed while in bathing suit or changing clothes.**
- **Gait:** Extra compensation is required to maintain balance for uneven hips and legs that can lead to early fatigability of muscles.
- **Reduced range of motion:** Rotational spinal deformity increases rigidity that reduces the spinal flexibility.
- **Labored breathing:** Excess spinal rotation at thoracic region leads to crowding of rib cage on concave side results in decreased space available for lungs. This can compromise lungs function and make breathing more difficult.
- **Cardiovascular problems:** Similarly, reduced space for heart can hamper its blood pumping ability.
- **Back pain:** Back pain occurs because of paravertebral muscles spasm, local inflammation around strained muscles and degenerative changes in intervertebral discs and facets joint due to uneven loading.
- **Lower self-esteem:** Patient may suffer from psychological stress and depression because of noticeable spinal changes or spinal brace that may be uncomfortable or limit activity.

Diagnosis

Imaging Studies

X-ray: X-ray findings are needed to measure the degree of curvature and confirm the diagnosis.

There are 3 important factors that should be taken into consideration:

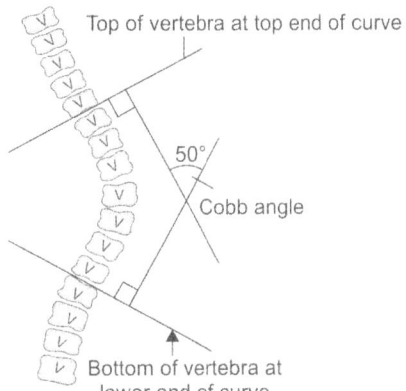

Fig. 31: Cobb's angle.

1. **Lateral curvature measurement (Fig. 31):** One of the sensitive method to measure lateral curvature of spine is through Cobb's angle. It is an angle formed by the intersection of two perpendicular lines drawn over the two horizontal lines which are marked from the superior and inferior border of superior and inferior end vertebrae respectively. End vertebra is the vertebra that maximally tilts towards concave side of curvature.

   Normally Cobb's angle is less than 10°. More than 10° of Cobb's angle is considered to be scoliosis. Classification of scoliosis according to severity of curvature:
   - Mild scoliosis: 10°–20°
   - Moderate scoliosis: 20°–50°
   - Severe scoliosis: >50°

2. **Axial rotation assessment:** Lateral curvature of spine is usually associated with rotation of vertebrae along the vertical axis. This abnormal spinal rotation progressively affects the rotation of rib along with rigidity of curve.
   - **Displacement of pedicle:** Degree of rotation of vertebra is measured at apex of curve by looking at the relation of pedicle to midline (Fig. 32).

3. **Skeletal maturity:** Spinal vertebral ossification is oftenly estimated by the Risser sign. It is an indirect method to measure the skeletal maturity by using the radiographical stages

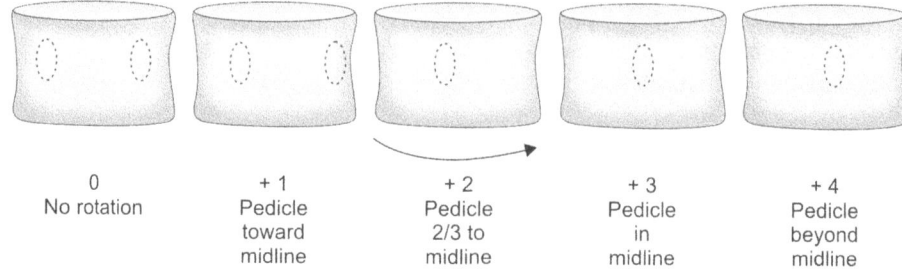

Fig. 32: Measurement of degree of vertebral rotation.

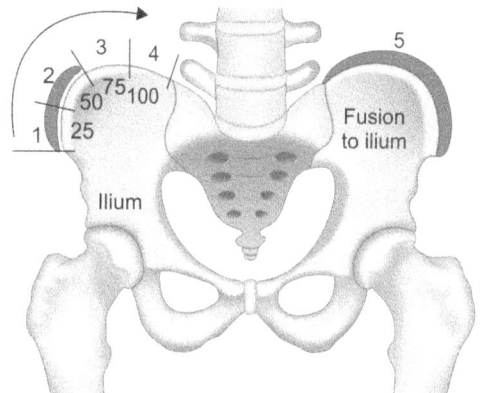

Fig. 33: Risser grades.

Table 1: Risser grades.

Stage	Description
Stage 0	No ossification center at the level of iliac crest apophysis
Stage 1	Apophysis of less than 25% of iliac crest
Stage 2	Apophysis of more than 25-50% of iliac crest
Stage 3	Apophysis of more than 50-75% of iliac crest
Stage 4	Apophysis of more than 75% of iliac crest
Stage 5	Complete ossification and fusion of iliac crest apophysis

of ossification and fusion of apophysis of iliac crest (Table 1 and Fig. 33).

Scoliotic curve progressively increases until the subject attains skeletal maturity. Therefore it is very critical to plan treatment in children and teens before the attainment of complete skeletal maturity.

Physical Examination

- Check for disparity (Fig. 34)
  - Ear levels and contour of neck to check cervical curvature.
  - Shoulder level to check cervicodorsal or high dorsal curve: Elevated shoulder on convex side.
  - Scapular level: Shifting of vertebral border of scapula away from midline along with higher scapular and eversion of inferior angle on convex side indicates the involvement of thoracic curve.
  - Position of arms and waistline:
    - Arm on convex side hangs close to body
    - Waistline more prominent on concave side.
  - Thorax (Fig. 35)
    - Ribs crowded on concave side and apart on convex side.

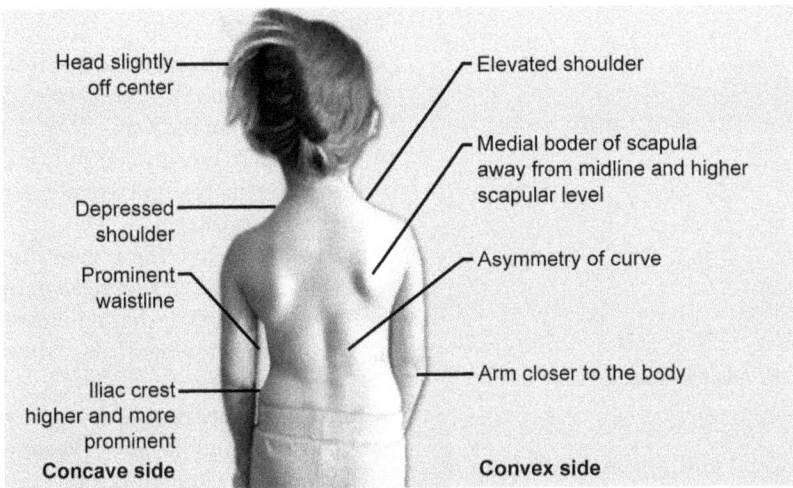

Fig. 34: Symptoms of scoliosis.

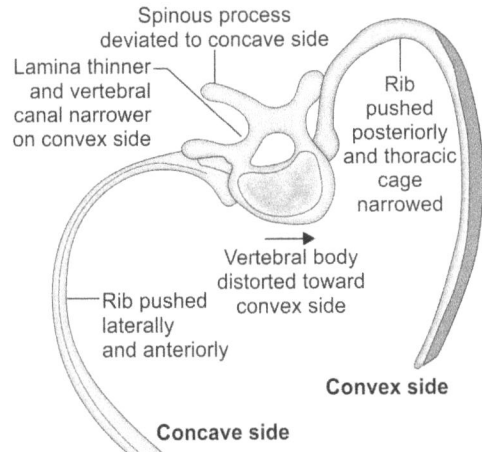

Fig. 35: Distorsion of vertebra and ribs in thoracic scoliosis.

- Ribs bulge backward on convex side and appear flattened on concave side.
- Hips: Hips and pelvis are higher on concave side.
- Pelvis
  - Forward rotation of pelvis on concave side.
  - Iliac crest prominent and higher on concave side.
  - Gluteal fold higher on concave side.
- Knees: Observe the level of patella.
- Feet:
  - Even distribution of body weight is examined.
  - Any deformities in feet and toes.
- **Respiratory status:** should be examined for scoliosis of thoracic region.
  - Vital capacity and chest expansion (normal = 2–5 inches) decreases in scoliosis.
- **Rib hump:** In thoracic scoliosis, rib hump is measured with scoliometer/inclinometer.
- **Spinal ROM:** All the spinal movements including flexion, extension, side bending and rotation.
  - **Adam forward bending test (Figs. 36A and B):** To determine the presence of scoliosis and also to distinguish functional and structural scoliosis. Patient is asked to perform 90° spinal flexion with knees straight, feet together and stretches the arm towards ground. Examiner looks along the horizontal plane of spine and observe the abnormalities if present. Asymmetry present in scoliosis are:
    - Elevation of one sided shoulder blade.
    - Rib hump, i.e. elevation of rib cage on one side.

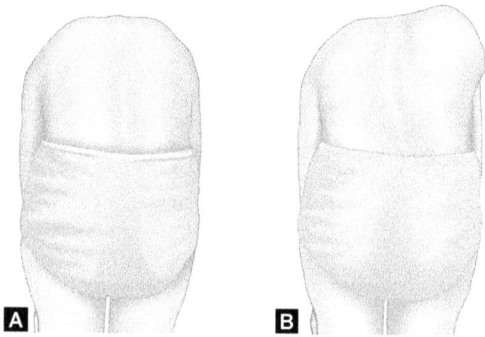

Figs. 36A and B: Adam forward bending test.

- Elevated and prominent hip on one side.
- Uneven appearance of waist
- Tilting of body towards one side.
- Appearance of one leg shorter than the other.

Normal spine without any scoliotic curve is symmetrically straight. This test can only be applicable for thoracic scoliosis and not for lumbar scoliosis because of non-involvement of rib rotation.

- **Differentiation between structural and functional scoliosis**: In functional scoliosis, characteristics of scoliosis becomes more apparent on spinal forward flexion. However in structural scoliosis, scoliotic deformity remains same as in standing position.
- **Scoliometer to measure spine rotation (Fig. 37):** Scoliosis is used to measure the angle of trunk rotation (ATR). It is also named as scoliometer. It is placed flat over the back in forward bending position where the asymmetry looks maximal.

As a general rule, ≥ 5° of asymmetrical trunk rotation (ATR), subject should schedule for follow-up examination or referred for exact diagnosis. X-ray imaging is needed to measure the degree of curve and confirm scoliosis.

Management

Factors to determine choice of treatment:
- **Gender:** Females are more commonly involved than males.
- **Location of curve:** Centrally located curve are more likely to get worsen than upper or lower based curves.
- **Curve severity:** The severe the curve, the greater the risk of progression over time.
- **Type of curve:** S-shaped curves are more prone to get worse over time than the C-shaped curve.
- **Skeletal maturity:** Risk of curve progression is negligible after the attainment of complete skeletal maturity.
- Braces are more effective while bones are still growing.

Conservative Treatment

Indicated in mild postural curve, i.e. when curve is less than 40°: Muscle imbalance due to elongated and stretched muscle on convex side and shortened musculature on opposite side, i.e. concave side. Patient encountered with different problems such as backache, shallow breathing, sciatica, headache, muscle spasm and insomnia. Aim of conservative treatment is to reduce symptoms along with correction of curve.

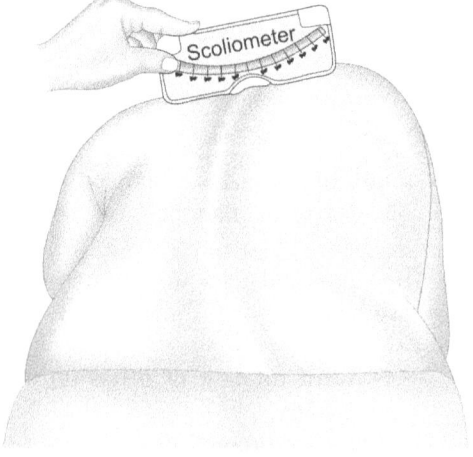

Fig. 37: Scoliometer for measuring angle of trunk rotation.

Physiotherapy Treatment
- **Observation**: In mild scoliosis, i.e. < 20° regular observation after every 4-6 months is necessary.
- **Spinal brace**: Braces are intended to minimize the progression of curve to an acceptable level.
  Indications:
  - When spinal curve is below 40° and greater than 20°.
  - More than 25-30° curve in skeletally immature subjects.
  - Progresses at least 5° during 4-6 months period.
    - Milwaukee brace: It can be used for treating any curve in spine.
    - Thoracolumbosacral orthosis (TLSO): It is used when the apex of curve is at or below seventh thoracic vertebra.

  Action of braces:
  - Provides 3-point force system to correct or prevent progression of deformity.
  - Stabilizes weak or injured structures.
  - Controls back pain by limiting motion and unload disc, vertebra and other spinal structures by compressing the abdomen.

  Two types of scoliosis bracing:
  1. Full time bracing: These are prescribed to be worn all the time, i.e. for 16-23 hours per day except during bathing, exercising and skin care.
  2. Night time bracing: These are to be worn during night for at least 8 hours.

  Full time bracing is recommended for curve of at least 35° whereas either of spinal bracing can be used for curves of less than 35°.

  Brace should be worn until the patient attains complete skeletal maturity. Careful fitting and continued adjustment of brace optimizes the correction of curve. Regular intermittent radiographs, i.e. after every 4-6 months are necessary for monitoring possible progression of curve.

- **Active correction:** Self corrective postural attitudes should be recommended. Patient should avoid habitual positions or activities that could increase the curvature.
- **Passive correction:**
  - Hanging: Unequal hanging, i.e. hanging using one hand (of concave side).
  - Hanging in head suspension apparatus.
  - Axial skeletal traction (manual traction).
- **Electrical stimulation:** As the muscles on convex side are stretched and weak and the muscles on concave side are tight and strong, electrodes should be placed over convex side of spine. Electrical stimulation is given to stimulate weak muscles to increase the ability to contract and pull the spine in normal vertical position.
- **General body relaxation techniques:** Used to relax shortened muscle that aid in active correction of posture by self-awareness.
- **Massage therapy:** Deep tissue massage over tight muscles should be given to improve posture, reduce muscular pain, elongate tightened areas, increase flexibility and facilitate healing due to increased blood flow. It must not be given on overstretched muscles covering the rib cage.
- **Active ROM of spine:** To improve the mobility of spine, i.e. spinal flexion, extension, side flexion or rotation.
- **Strengthening exercises**: Strengthening of quadratus lumborum, gluteus medius on convex side and lumbar erector and multifidus muscle on concave side in lumbar region. In thoracic region, strengthening of trapezius medius, trapezius distalis and serratus anterior muscles of convex side and rhomboideus muscles of concave side should be done.
- **Stretching exercises**: Stretching of soft tissues on concave side, hip flexors and hamstring, should be done as these structures have tendency to shorten due to pelvic tilt.

- **Deep breathing exercises:** As scoliosis has a rotational component. It causes the crowding of ribs on concave side of thoracic region that may progressively lead to respiratory dysfunction and postural deviation. Deep breathing exercises helps to improve respiratory function, abdominal core muscle strength and counteract the progression of scoliosis.
- **Pelvic tilting exercises:** Lateral pelvic tilt or pelvic obliquity towards one side due to functionally shortened leg or tightened torso musculature may lead to scoliosis. Therefore lateral pelvic tilt exercises may be helpful to correct functional scoliosis caused by functional leg length difference. Anterior and posterior pelvic tilt exercises may be helpful to reduce the symptoms in scoliosis caused by impingement of nerves emerging from spine.
- **Core strengthening exercises:** Core muscles are designed to protect the spine by creating a sturdy rod that limits excessive movement in any direction. Therefore core muscles strengthening is necessary to correct postural deviation and improve functional ability.

Surgery

Indications
- Skeletally mature patient with curve more than 45°
- Persistent progression of curve
- Severe back or radicular pain
- Progressive respiratory dysfunction
- Psychological inability to accept spinal brace
- Severe cosmetic postural alterations
- Curve progression with coronal or sagittal plane imbalance.

Spinal fusion is achieved by operating on spine and fixed with spinal instrumentation.

Surgical interventions for idiopathic scoliosis:
- **Spinal fusion:** It is a surgical technique that fuses two or more adjacent vertebrae to prevent any movements between the fused vertebrae. It is also known as spondylodesis and most commonly performed for scoliosis in adolescents or young adults.
- **Growing system/spinal instrumentation:** In this technique, rods are anchored to the spine to correct or maintain spinal curvature. Rods are lengthened after every 6–12 months to keep up the spinal growth of growing child. On reaching the skeletal maturity spinal fusion is performed. This procedure is selected to delay the spinal fusion.
- **Fusionless surgery:** In this procedure, constant pressure is applied on convex side of curve to slow or stop the growth on convex side while allowing the normal growth on concave side of spine. Continuous growth of spine in this manner reduces the lateral curvature of spine and makes it straighter.

■ KYPHOSIS

Kyphosis is an abnormal increase in posterior curvature of dorsal spine (Fig. 38).

Kyphosis stems from the Greek term "kyphos," meaning a hump, and is also known as a Dowager's hump, hunchback, round back, or humpback.

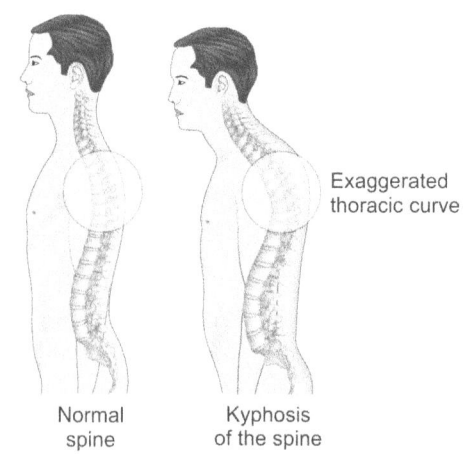

Fig. 38: Kyphosis.

Classification

- **Postural kyphosis:** It is the most common type of kyphosis that is caused by poor posture. Girls are more affected than boys. It is usually presented by smooth exaggerated curve which can be easily corrected or managed.
- **Structural kyphosis:** Caused by some structural abnormalities, i.e. abnormality affecting the bones, intervertebral discs, ligaments, nerves or muscles. It may require surgical intervention.
  - **Scheuermann's disease:** It is a juvenile (between 12-14 years) thoracic kyphosis measuring more than 40☐ results from abnormal bone growth and development such as wedging of 3 or more adjacent vertebra. Possible causes are vascular necrosis of vertebral ring apophysis, endocrinopathy, stress injury to vertebral, genetic, osteopenia, malnutrition.
  - **Congenital kyphosis:** Present since birth. It occurs due to defect in vertebral formation.
  - **Neuromuscular kyphosis:** Occurs in neuromuscular conditions such as cerebral palsy, spina bifida, muscle dystrophy, spinal cord injury.
  - **Traumatic kyphosis:** Occurs due to burst or compression fracture of vertebra.
  - **Nutritional kyphosis:** Occurs due to some nutritional deficiency like calcium or vitamin D deficiency that softens the bones and results in curving of spine.
  - **Gibbus deformity:** It is a form of structural kyphosis which occurs as a sequel to tuberculosis. In this deformity, an abrupt sharply angled posterior curve is present.

Potential Muscle Impairment (Fig. 39)

Faulty upper quadrant posture leads to an imbalance in length and strength of scapular and glenohumeral musculature known as upper cross syndrome.

- Tightness or decreased flexibility of anterior thoracic muscles (intercostal muscles), upper extremity muscles originating in the thorax (pectoralis major and minor, lattismus dorsi and serratus anterior muscles), muscles of cervical spine and head that attached to scapula (levator scapulae and upper trapezius).
- Stretching and weakness of thoracic erector spinae and scapular retractor muscles (rhomboids and middle trapezius). Progressively exaggerate thoracic kyphosis leads to compensatory lumbar lordosis to maintain the stability of spine that results in lower cross syndrome.
- Tightness or decreased flexibility of lumbar erectors, hip flexors and hamstring muscles.
- Stretching and weakness of abdominals and gluteal muscles.

Clinical Presentation

- Hunched forward posture
- Back pain with movement
- Fatigue
- Loss of height
- Tenderness and stiffness in spine
- Forward head posture

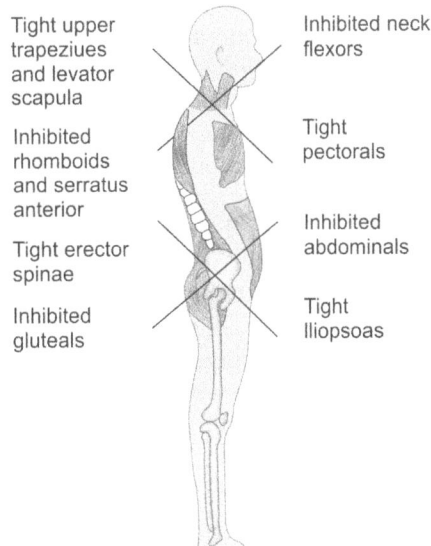

Fig. 39: Upper and lower cross syndrome.

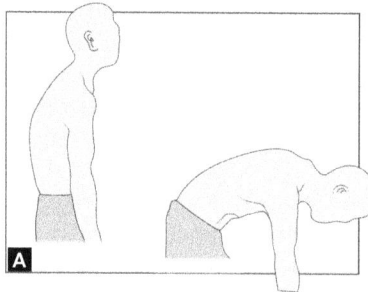 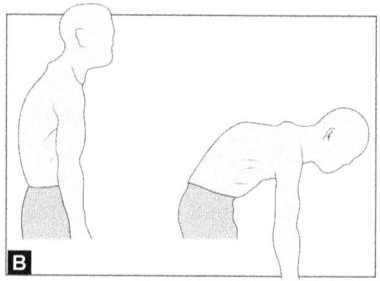

Figs. 40A and B: Adam's forward bending test. A. Postural kyphosis; B. Scheuermann's kyphosis.

- Radiating pain in legs or other neurological symptoms such as paresthesia, weakness, loss of bowel and bladder function due to compression of spinal cord.
- Chest pain or dyspnea may present in chronic cases due to compression of lungs.

Physical Examination

- Normal thoracic kyphosis is 35–40°. More than 40° is considered to be hyperkyphosis.
- Normal lumbar lordosis is 55–65°.
- Lumbar lordosis should be around 30° more than the thoracic kyphosis.
- Mild scoliosis is present in around 30% of kyphotic patients.
- **Palpation:** Palpation of spine for any tenderness or stiffness.
- **Observation:**
  - Posture
    - Increased kyphotic curve
    - Protracted scapula (stopping shoulders)
    - Forward head posture
    - Increased cervical lordosis
    - Increased lumbar lordosis with protuberant abdomen
    - Presence of anterior pelvic tilt.
- **Neurological examination:** Sensation, reflex, and bowel and bladder function should be examined.
- **Muscle tightness:** Commonly hamstring and pectoralis muscle tightness is present.
- **ROM:** Examination of AROM and PROM of spine.
- **Manual muscle test:** Commonly muscle weakness present in upper back extensors and abdominals.
- **Adam's forward bending test (Figs. 40A and B):** This test is used to distinguish postural and structural kyphosis. In postural kyphosis the curve is smooth and disappears on bending position while in structural kyphosis the curvature becomes more prominent.
- **Spinal hyperextension test:** To determine the rigidity of curve. Findings are same as in forward bending test. On hyperextension of back functional kyphotic curve disappears whereas structural or rigid kyphotic curve becomes more prominent.

X-ray Evaluation

- In rare conditions mild scoliosis with minimal vertebral rotation is also present.
- **Cobb's angle (Fig. 41):** Thoracic kyphosis > 40°.
  - **Mild kyphosis:** 40–50°
  - **Moderate kyphosis:** 50–75°
  - **Severe kyphosis:** >75°
- Presence of following features (Fig. 42):
  - More than 5° of anterior wedging of 3 consecutive vertebral bodies at the apex of deformity
  - Uneven end plates
  - Narrowing of intervertebral disc space
  - Schmorl's nodes
  - Hyperlordosis of lumbar vertebra.

Deformities

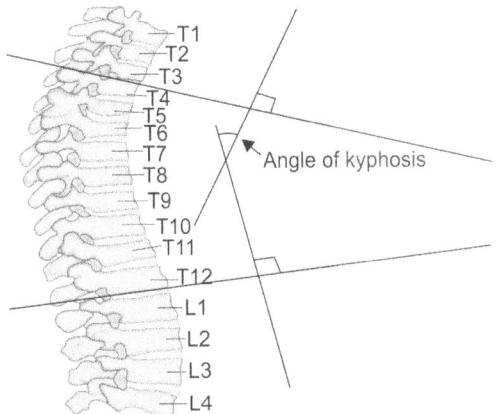

Fig. 41: Cobb's angle of kyphosis.

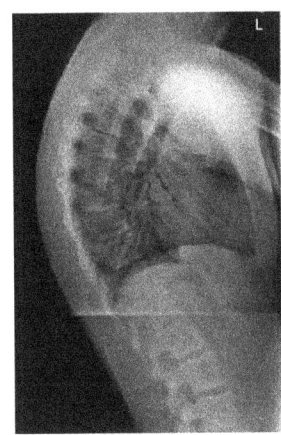

Fig. 42: X-ray findings of kyphosis.

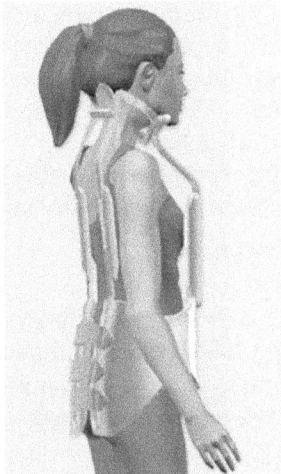

Fig. 43: Milwaukee brace.

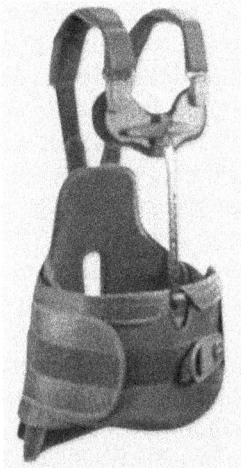

Fig. 44: Taylor brace.

Management

Physiotherapy Treatment

Indicated in mild and moderate thoracic kyphosis.
- **Brace:** Brace should be worn until complete skeletal maturity is achieved.
  - **Milwaukee brace (Fig. 43):** Milwaukee brace is used when apical vertebra is at or above T7 level.
  - **Taylor brace/thoracolumbosacral orthosis (TLSO) (Fig. 44):** TLSO is used when apical vertebra is below T7 level.

Initially bracing is done for full time, radiographs should be repeated after every 3–4 months.

Therapeutic Exercises

- **Strengthening exercises:** Secondary hyper lumbar lordosis occurs to compensate increased thoracic kyphosis, this further causes lower crossed syndrome (LCS). In LCS, inhibition and lengthening of abdominal muscle occurs because of associated anterior pelvic tilt that moves the lower attachment of abdominal downwards and increases its distance from the upper attachment. All this leads to stretching and weakening of abdominals. Consecutively excessive lordosis due to LCS facilitates lumbar erectors that reciprocally inhibit abdominals and cause further weakness of abdominals.

- **Abdominal strengthening exercises:** One should avoid traditional crunches and sits up, i.e. upper abdominal exercises because these exercises reinforce the excessive thoracic kyphosis. These exercise cause the contraction of abdominals in such a way that flexes the upper spine and movement of rib towards the hips that results in the undesirable progress of thoracic kyphosis. Therefore direct oblique training should be done to complement abdominals as the obliques and abdominals work together to stabilize and move spine.
- **Strengthening of gluteal muscles:** As weak gluteal muscles are responsible for posterior pelvic tilt. It is necessary to strengthen gluteals to restore the neutral alignment of pelvis that further helps in correction of spinal posture.
- **Strengthening of thoracic erector spinae muscle:** Due to upper cross syndrome, thoracic erector spinae muscles become stretched and weak this leads to massive muscular imbalance. Therefore strengthening of thoracic erector spinae muscle should be done to restore the upright position.

■ **Stretching exercises:**
- **Release of abdominal muscles:** Inspite of being inhibited in thoracic hyperkyphosis, abdominals surprisingly may have some trigger points typically near its attachment to the ribs. This leads to abdominal dysfunction. Therefore, abdominal release technique may be effective in restoring abdominals function and improving thoracic spine mobility.
- **Release and stretching of lower erector spinae muscles:** Tight lower back muscles contribute to weakness of abdominals. Therefore myofascial release technique followed by static stretching may help to regain normal muscle length that further facilitates the normal posture of lower spine and abdominal function.
- **Stretching of hamstring muscles:** It plays a key role in maintaining the pelvic in neutral alignment.
- **Stretching of pectoralis muscles, latissmus dorsi, upper trapezius and levator scapulae muscle:** Tightness occurs in these muscles due to faulty upper quadrant posture in exaggerated thoracic kyphosis. Therefore stretching of these muscle helps to restore upright position along with improving the muscular imbalance.

■ **Breathing exercises:** It helps to restore and maintain the pulmonary function.

Surgical Treatment
Indications
- Kyphosis with >80° Cobb's angle in thoracic spine and >65° in thoracolumbar spine.
- Not controlled by non-operative methods.
- Significant sagittal imbalance.

Surgical Intervention
- Halo traction.
- Maintain the correction by bone graft.
- Spinal decompression and stabilization.
- Spinal instrumentation and fusion.

■ LORDOSIS

Lumbar hyperlordosis is an exaggerated lumbar curve. It is also known as swayback, saddle back, and hollow back (Figs. 45A and B).

Normal lordotic curve: 30–50° (L_1–L_5).

Etiology
- **Thoracic hyperkyphosis:** It may create a compensatory lordotic curve in lumbar region.

Deformities

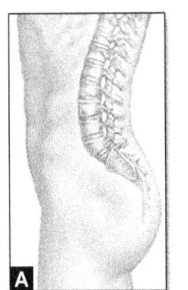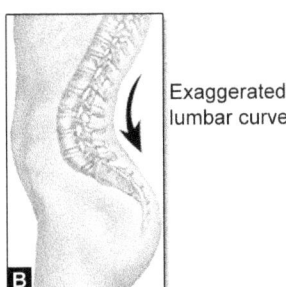

Figs. 45A and B: A. Normal spine; B. Lordosis of spine.

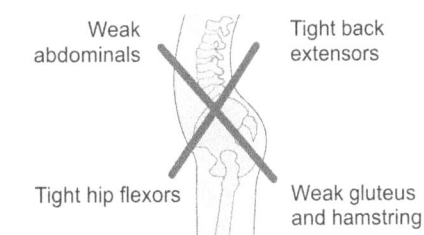

Fig. 46: Lower cross syndrome.

- **Achondroplasia** (bone growth disorder)
- **Vitamin D deficiency**, e.g. rickets
- **Obesity:** Obese subject tends to lean backward against protruding abdomen in order to improve balance.
- **Spondylolisthesis:** It is a spinal condition in which one vertebra slips over the adjacent vertebra. It commonly occurs in lumbar and lumbosacral region.
- **Posture:** Extended period of poor posture contribute to excessive lordotic curve.
- **Congenital disorders:** Defect in vertebral formation.
- **Wearing high-heeled shoes** for extended periods.
- **Core muscle weakness**, i.e. weakness of abdominals, hamstring etc.
- **Tightness** of hip flexors, erector spinae muscles.
- **Pregnancy.**

Pathophysiology

Lower cross syndrome (Fig. 46) is the condition of muscle imbalance in lower quadrant of body resulting in a faulty posture. Some of the muscles around the hip and spine become tight and others become stretched and weak.

A cross is formed by the intersection of two lines across the pelvis. One line passes from abdominals to gluteus and hamstring and other line from lower back extensors to hip flexors. Therefore it is named as crossed syndrome.

The muscles that become short and tight are back extensors, quadratus lumborum and hip flexors.

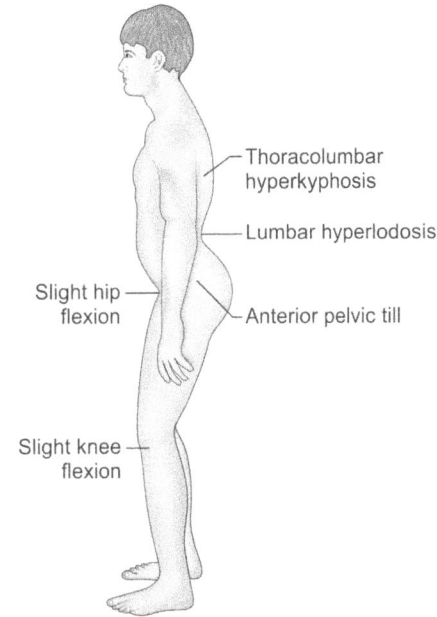

Fig. 47: Posture in lumbar hyperlordosis.

The muscles that become stretched and weak are abdominal muscles, i.e. internal and external oblique, rectus abdominus, hip extensors and gluteus maximus.

Clinical Presentation (Fig. 47)

- Exaggerated posture
- Buttocks protrude more than usual
- Lower back more inward than normal
- Mostly asymptomatic and painful
- Height loss of approximately 0.5–2.5 inches
- Low back pain in severe curve
- Bilateral referred pain in lower extremities
- ROM of spine might be reduced with a significant curvature.

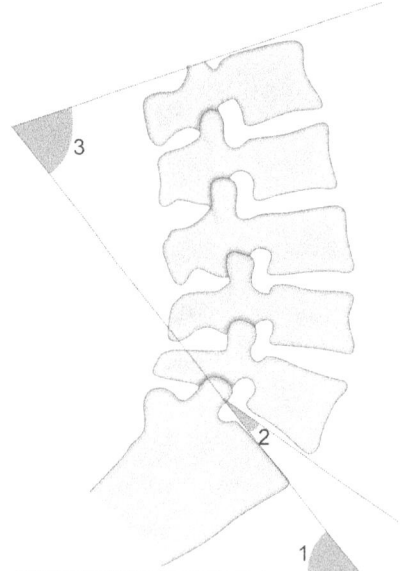

Fig. 48: Angle 1: Sacral inclination, Angle 2: Lumbosacral angle, Angle 3: Lumbar lordotic curve.

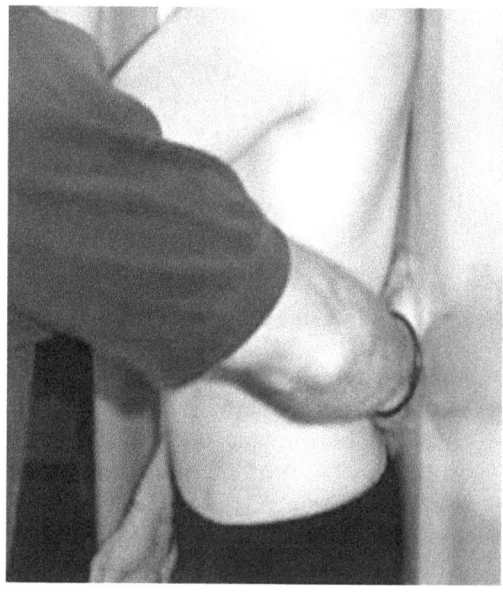

Fig. 49: Test to examine lumbar hyper lordosis.

Diagnosis: X-ray Findings (Fig. 48)

- **Sacral inclination:** The angle between the plane of upper surface of sacrum and the horizontal plane. Normal mean value is 50°.
- **Lumbosacral angle:** It is the angle formed between the lines passing from inferior endplate of L5 vertebra and superior endplate of sacrum. Normal mean value is 16°.
- **Lumbar lordotic curve:** Normal mean value of lumbar lordotic curve is between 30–50°. It is the angle formed between the lines passing from superior endplate of L1 vertebra and superior endplate of sacrum. Normal mean value is 70°.

Physical Examination (Fig. 49)

Test to examine exaggerated lumbar lordosis: Patient is asked to stand against wall. Therapist keeps hand with palm on wall and tries to slide it behind the lumbar region of patient to assess space between wall and lumbar spine.

In normal lordotic posture, therapist would only be able to slide the finger only. However in exaggerated lumbar lordosis the therapist would easily be able to slide the whole hand.

Preventive Measures

- Start a weight loss program.
- Take small breaks to get up and stretch during prolonged sitting.
- Periodically shift the weight from one foot to the other or from the heels to toes during prolonged standing.
- Use a pillow or rolled towel to support the lower back during sitting.
- Wear comfortable, low-heeled shoes.
- Sit with feet flat on the floor.

Management

Conservative Treatment

- **Braces:** Boston brace (Fig. 50).
  - Orthotic brace is generally used to treat lordosis when the spinal curve is >10° and <45°.

Deformities

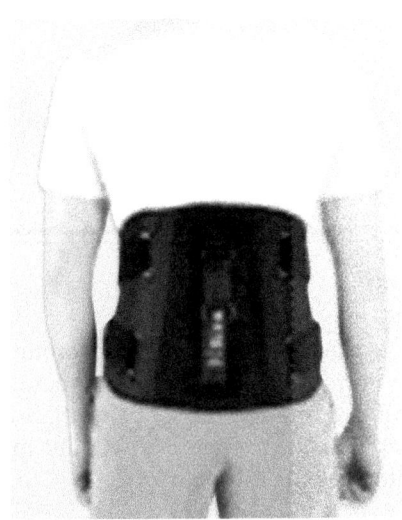

Fig. 50: Boston brace.

- These are prescribed to be worn all the time, i.e. for 16-23 hours per day except during bathing, exercising and skin care until subject attaints complete skeletal maturity.
- It controls progression of curve in adolescents.

Physiotherapy Treatment
- **Pain relieving modalities:** Used to decrease pain and associated muscle spasm.
  - Heating modalities, TENS, IFT, EMS, and IRR, US.
- **Strengthening exercises** for weak and stretched muscles.
  - Abdominal muscles like rectus abdominals, internal and external obliques.
  - Hip extensors like hamstring and gluteus maximus.
- **Stretching of short and tight muscles**
  - Trunk extensors like erector spinae and quadratus lumborum.
  - Hip flexors particularly iliopsoas muscle.
- **Spinal mobility exercises:** To maintain and improve the spinal mobility. AROM exercise of spinal flexion, extension, side flexion and rotation.

Surgical Treatment
Indications
- Severe cases with neurological involvement
- Not responding to non-surgical methods.

Surgical intervention: Spinal fusion.

CHAPTER 4

Peripheral Nerve Lesion

■ GENERAL INTRODUCTION OF PERIPHERAL NERVE LESION

Peripheral nerve lesion is the damage of nerves that connects brain and spinal cord to other parts of body characterized by loss of motor or sensory function.

Anatomy (Fig. 1)

Peripheral nerves: These nerves are located outside the brain and spinal cord that connects them to other areas of body such as muscles, skin, etc. Injury to a peripheral nerve interferes with the ability of brain to communicate with the area of the body supplied by that nerve.

Core structure of nerve is axon processes of sensory and motor neurons (i.e. nerve cell which consist of cell body, axons and dendrites). Large axons are covered by Schwann cells which form myelin sheath (it is a sheath of fat that wrap around an axon intermittently internal to endoneurium). Delicate connective tissue sheath around the individual axon with or without myelin sheath is called **endoneurium**.

↓

Group of axons bundled together to form fascicles. These fascicles are covered by a sheath called **perineurium**.

↓

Group of fascicles bundled together to form nerve. The nerve is covered by a sheath called **epineurium**.

Causes of Peripheral Nerve Lesion

- **Mechanical causes of peripheral nerve lesion:** Mechanical factors that usually cause mononeuropathy are
  - **Stretching/traction injury:** Around 8% elongation of nerve diminishes the nerve's microcirculation and 15% elongation disrupts the axons, e.g. stretch injury to suprascapular nerve, stinger or burner injury.
  - **Traumatic or crush injury:** In traumatic injuries, deformed nerve fibers cause local ischemia and increased vascular permeability that leads to endoneurial edema which in turn cause nerve dysfunction.
  - **Section/laceration injury:** These are sharp transection of nerve that disrupts the continuity of nerve. These are often caused by sharp wound by glass, firearms or knives.

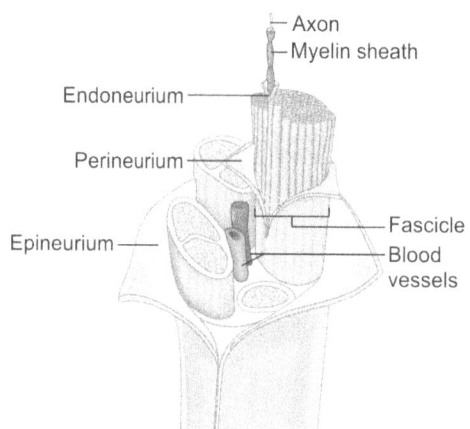

Fig. 1: Anatomy of peripheral nerve.

- **Entrapment injury:** This occurs due to prolonged compression on the nerve. Compression could be extrinsic or intrinsic
  - **Extrinsic compression** may occur through external influences at the anatomical bottleneck or any space occupying lesions in the vicinity of nerve, e.g. carpal tunnel syndrome, tarsal tunnel syndrome, etc.
  - **Intrinsic compression** mainly caused by nerve tumor.
- **Non-mechanical causes of peripheral neuropathy:** Non-mechanical factors usually cause polyneuropathy
  - Idiopathic inflammatory demyelinating process, e.g. Guillain-Barre syndrome, etc.
  - Metabolic and nutritional disturbances e.g. diabetes, hypothyroidism, uremia, liver disease, vitamin B12 deficiency etc.
  - Infections, e.g. AIDS, leprosy, diphtheria, sarcoidosis, sepsis and multiorgan failure, etc.
  - Vasculitis, e.g. polyarteritis nodosa (PAN), systemic lupus erythematosus (SLE), rheumatoid arthritis (RA), etc.
  - Paraneoplastic and paraproteinemic syndromes, e.g. cancer, paraproteinemias, amyloidosis, etc.
  - Drugs, e.g. hydralazine, isoniazid, phenytoin, pyridoxine, vincristine and toxins, e.g. alcohol, organophosphates, arsenic, lead, thallium, etc.
  - Hereditary diseases, e.g. porphyria, Krabbe's disease, Refsum's disease, Fabry's disease, etc.

Clinical Manifestation

Depending on the type of nerve involvement which could be sensory, motor and autonomic or mixed nerve.
- **Motor changes**
  - Muscle wasting, muscle atrophy or flaccid paresis of muscle(s) innervated by the affected nerve.
  - Loss of reflexes, e.g. loss of knee reflex in femoral nerve injury, loss of biceps reflex in musculocutaneous nerve injury, etc.
  - Joint contracture or deformity may occur in chronic cases of nerve injury due to muscle imbalance.
- **Sensory changes:** Sensory symptoms may vary on the basis of type of injury.
  - Loss of superficial sensation, e.g. pain, touch, temperature.
  - Loss of deep sensation e.g. proprioception (vibration sense, joint position sense and kinesthesia) and stereognosis, graphesthesia, touch localization, etc.
  - Abnormal sensation in area supplied by the damaged nerve like paresthesia, tingling or burning sensation.
- **Vasomotor disturbances**
  - Area supplied by the damaged nerve become pale and dry with crust formations.
  - Anhydrosis—diminished sweating.

In this chapter, we will study mononeuropathy which are caused by mechanical factors.

■ MONONEUROPATHY

Mononeuropathy is the damage to a single nerve characterized by sensory and motor disturbances in the area supplied by the affected nerve.

Classification of Nerve Lesion

Two main classifications of nerve lesions are Seddon's classification and Sunderland's classification. First classification was given by Seddon in 1943 that is predominantly based on the scale of injury. He classified the injuries into 3 categories—neuropraxia, axonotmesis and neurotmesis. Later in 1978, the classification was further expanded by Sunderland who subdivides the neurotmesis into 3 additional grades.

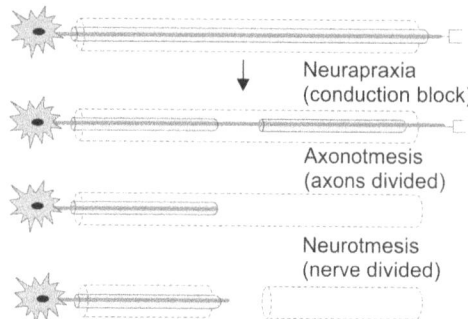

Fig. 2: Seddon's classification of nerve injury.

Seddon's Classification

This classification is useful in understanding the anatomical basis of injuries (Fig. 2 and Table 1).

Grade 1: Neuropraxia
- Local nerve compression
- Reversible conduction block with intact axon and preserved supportive structures i.e. without Wallerian degeneration.
- Recovery prognosis is excellent.
- Recovery—around 6–8 weeks.

Grade 2: Axonotmesis
- Disruption of axon and myelin sheath results in conduction block with Wallerian degeneration that usually occurs after 1–2 weeks.
- Intact endoneurium.
- Regeneration rate: about 1.5–3 mm/day.
- Recovery—weeks to months.

Grade 3: Neurotmesis
- Complete nerve division with disruption of endoneurium.
- No recovery without surgical repair.

Sunderland Classification

This classification gives additional information that is useful in treatment and prognosis of injury (Table 2).

Grade 1: Neuropraxia
- Reversible conduction block.
- Intact axon without Wallerian degeneration.

Grade 2: Axonotmesis
- Disrupted axon and myelin sheath leads to conduction block with Wallerian degeneration that occurs after 1–2 weeks.
- Intact endoneurium.

Grade 3: Neurotmesis with preservation of perineurium: Disrupted endoneurium.

Grade 4: Neurotmesis with preservation of epineurium.

Grade 5: Neurotmesis with complete transection of nerve.

Peripheral Nerve Regeneration Process (Fig. 3)

Peripheral nerve injury instantly evoked the migration of phagocytes, Schwann cells

Table 1: Seddon classification.

Grade	Myelin	Axon	Endoneurium	Wallerian degeneration	Reversible
I	Disrupted	Intact	Intact	No	Reversible
II	Disrupted	Disrupted	Intact	Yes	Reversible
III	Disrupted	Disrupted	Disrupted	Yes	Irreversible

Table 2: Sunderland classification.

Grade	Myelin sheath	Axon	Endoneurium	Perineurium	Epineurium
I	Disrupted	Intact	Intact	Intact	Intact
II	Disrupted	Disrupted	Intact	Intact	Intact
III	Disrupted	Disrupted	Disrupted	Intact	Intact
IV	Disrupted	Disrupted	Disrupted	Disrupted	Intact
V	Disrupted	Disrupted	Disrupted	Disrupted	Disrupted

Peripheral Nerve Lesion

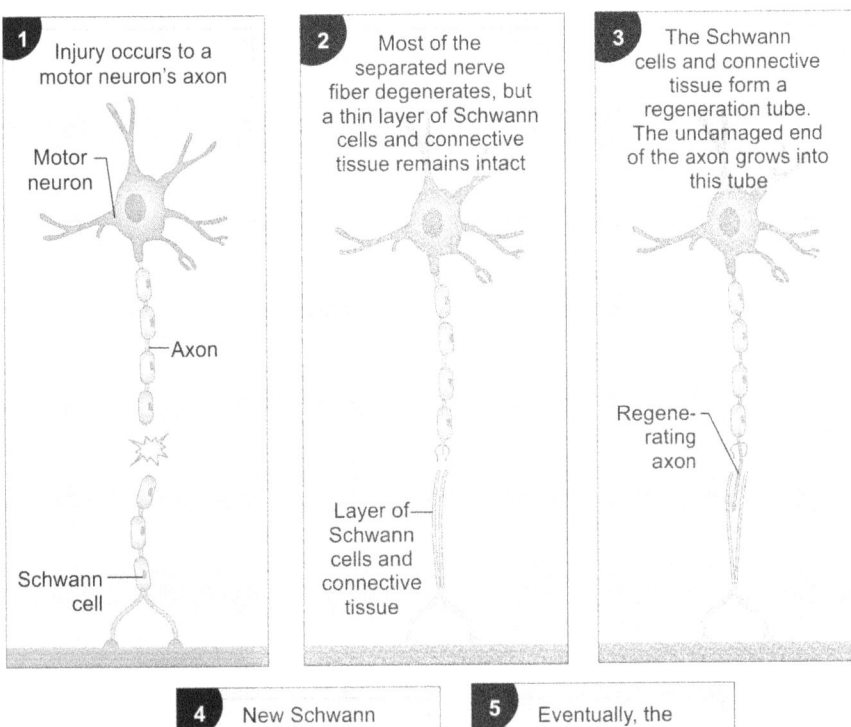
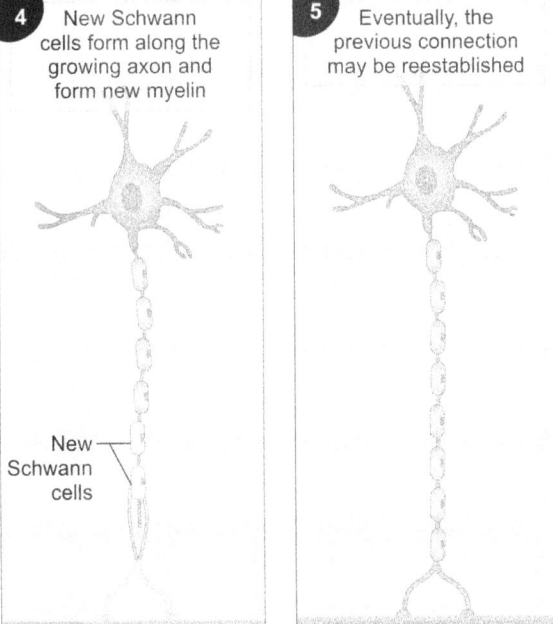

Fig. 3: Peripheral nerve regeneration.

and macrophages to the site of lesion to remove the damaged tissues by engulfing the degenerated axon and myelin. After complete removal of debris, the proximal segment which is still attached to cell body, swells and begins to sprout the axons.

These extensions are called fibrils. Some of these fibrils enter neurilemmal tube of distal end and forms an axis cylinder. Gradually the axis cylinder is fully formed inside neurilemmal tube. This process takes about 3 months after the injury to complete. At this stage the axon is quite fine but not myelinated. Progressively, the terminal axon increases in diameter due to the production of new neurofilaments. In later stages, the terminal axon becomes myelinated due to the formation of new Schwann cells along the axon. This myelination completes in around one year.

A nerve regenerates at the rate of 1 inch per month. Larger nerves regenerate comparatively faster than the smaller one, i.e. regeneration rate is 1 mm/day in small nerves and 5 mm/day in large.

Nerve Injury and Anticipated Recovery

Factors Affecting the Prognosis of Peripheral Nerve Injury

- **Age:** Prognosis of nerve injuries worsen with increasing age. Recovery is slow and partial in patients older than 50 years.
- **Type of injury:** Clean cut injuries gives better prognosis than crush or avulsion injuries.
- **Gap between the injured nerve ends:** The greater the gap, the poorer the recovery. With more gaps the fascicular pattern becomes more dissimilar between the ends, because the arrangement of fibers constantly changes as it progresses distally.
- **Time gap between the injury and repair:** The shorter the delay, the better the recovery. Motor recovery is good if repair occurs within 6 months of injury however sensory recovery have been reported following a delay of up to 48 months.
- **Level of injury:** Distal lesion have a better prognosis than proximal ones because distal lesion are located near the innervated muscles thus less time is needed to access to the endplates.
- **Type of nerve:** Although all the types of nerve have same spontaneous recovery rate but the surgical repair of pure motor or sensory nerve has better prognosis than mixed nerves due to similar fascicular pattern in pure nerves.
- **Associated vascular injury:** An associated vascular injury may delay the healing process.
- **Severity of injury:** The lesser the severity, the better the prognosis of injury (Table 3).

Diagnosis

Diagnostic Tests

After careful clinical assessment, neurophysiological testing may give additional information about nerve injury. Even when a nerve is divided, the axons in the distal segment continue to conduct for a few days. It may be nearly 2 weeks before conduction ceases completely and therefore reliable

Table 3: Nerve injury and anticipated recovery.

Grade of nerve injury	Spontaneous recovery	Recovery rate	Surgery
Grade I	Full	In days to 3 months after injury	None
Grade II	Full	1 inch/month	None
Grade III	Partial	1 inch/month	Neurolysis or none
Grade IV	None	1 inch/month after surgery	Nerve transfer, graft or repair
Grade V	None	1 inch/month after surgery	Nerve transfer, graft or repair

results can be obtained on testing. Therefore neurophysiology is not applicable in open injuries or other injuries requiring very early surgical exploration.
- **Electromyography (EMG):** It is useful to determine the extent and severity of nerve lesion and to demonstrate the neurological recovery. In EMG, muscle activity at rest and during electrical response is determined by placing a needle electrode through the skin into the specific muscle. In a normal resting muscle, there is complete silence. However in recently denervated muscle, spontaneous electrical activity known as spontaneous fibrillation can be recorded in resting phase. A period of 10-21 days may elapse after a nerve injury before spontaneous fibrillation can be recorded from denervated muscle.
- **Magnetic resonance neurography (MRN):** It is an advanced technique useful for diagnosing the disease of peripheral nerve.
- **Strength duration (SD) curve:** It is a graph of excitability of nerve, muscle or both. The purpose of SD curve plotting is to determine whether the stimulated muscle is innervated, denervated or partially denervated. It plots the graph between electrical stimuli of different intensities and the time needed by each stimulus to start the response. Optimal timing for SD curve is 10-14 days after the onset of lesion, when the motor end plate is no longer functioning and Wallerian degeneration would have occurred. The limitations of SD curve—it assess only the state of motor innervation of muscle but gives no indication of damage to sensory nerve and it does not localize the site of neuronal damage.
- **Nerve conduction velocity:** NCV test is used to measure the speed of conduction of an electrical impulse through nerve that may be slowed down following nerve injuries and neuropathies. It may help to determine the site of nerve damage and dysfunction.
- **Tinel's sign:** It refers to paresthesia elicited by lightly tapping along the course of a nerve. It is used to determine the irritation of nerve (compression or damage). Progressive distal advancement of Tinel's sign over time may be useful to follow the course of regenerating sensory axons. However the presence of Tinel's sign does not guarantee motor recovery.

Physical Examination
- **Motor function:**
  - **Observation:** Inspection of abnormalities such as clawing of fingers associated with ulnar nerve dysfunction.
  - **Muscle bulk** should be examined. Wasting of muscles indicates prolonged denervation.
  - **Manual muscle** testing to determine the muscle power.
- **Sensory function (Table 4):** There are different methods of sensory assessment of varying complexity. A simple assessment of touch sensation is—normal, altered, or absent sensation.

  More detailed tests of sensation include:
  - Localization
  - Two point discrimination (2PD)
  - Threshold

Table 4: MRC classification of sensory function.

Grade	Clinical features
S0	No sensation
S1	Deep pain sensation
S2	Skin touch, pain and thermal sensation, i.e. protective sensation
S3	S2 also with accurate localization but deficient stereognosis. Cold sensitivity and hypersensitivity are often present
S3+	Object and texture recognition but not normal sensation. Good but not normal, two point discrimination
S4	Normal sensation

- Temperature
- Vibration
- **Autonomic function:** It can be determined by assessing sweating. Loss of sweating occurs in complete interruption of nerve due to loss of autonomic function.
  - **Iodine starch test:** The test consists of dusting the area with quinizarine powder. In innervated area the powder becomes deep purple in color but in denervated area the powder remain dry and light gray in color due to absence of sweating.
  - **Ninhydrin print test:** Place hand (cleaned with soap and alcohol) under a lamp and obtain an imprint. Spray the imprint with ninhydrin. Purple pattern is obtained in normal sweating.
  - **Skin resistance test:** Innervated area offers the normal reistance whereas denervated area shows an increased resistance to the passage of electric current due to absence of sweating.

Management

Physiotherapy Treatment

- **For pain relief:** For neuropathic pain some therapies such as massage, TENS, cognitive exercises and yoga is given to reduce pain.
- **For edema:** Extremity elevation along with massage (effleurage) is given to dispel the edema.
  - When edema is severe (in case of nerve injury of hand) hand should be kept in sling with hand well up over the opposite shoulder.
- **Skin care:** In nerve lesion, skin of affected area is dry, scaly and anesthetic. Therefore, regular oil massage should be given to maintain the skin moisture.
- **Patient education:** Patients with absent or impaired protective sensation should be instructed with the various measures to protect skin integrity, such as:
  - Avoid holding cigarettes and cooking at stove in case of upper limb involvement.
  - Always wear shoes while walking in case of lower limb involvement.
  - Patient should be taught to use eyes to compensate for anesthesia. She/he should be vigilant while using sharp objects such as knife, nail cutters, etc.
  - Regularly inspect for any rashes and signs of maceration.
  - When trophic lesion does occur, saline soaks, eusol dressing should be applied until the lesion is healed.
- **Splinting/orthotics or assistive device:** After surgical technique of nerve the area is immobilized in splint for 2-3 weeks. Splints are used:
  - To protect insensate area and to reduce the amount of tension on repaired nerve.
  - To prevent contracture and deformity that occurs due to faulty positioning of limb, loss of muscle action, prolonged immobilization and unopposed pull of antagonistic muscles.
  - To improve functional ability by the assistance of dynamic splint.
- **Electrotherapy modalities:**
  - **Hot therapy:** Usually not recommended as it can increase the inflammation in recovery phase. Hot therapy can be given prior to muscle stretching in later stages.
  - **Cryotherapy:** To control edema and inflammation.
  - **Ultrasound:** Pulsed ultrasound below 1 W/cm^2 can be used in recovery phase to promote healing.
  - **LASER therapy:** Low level laser therapy is found to promote nerve recovery by enhancing energy production, reducing inflammation and promoting the formation of new blood vessels.
- **Sensory retraining:** This includes sensory desensitization and sensory reeducation

which are intended to reduce hyperesthesia and promote reorganization of cortical representation of involved limb.
- **Desensitization:** It reduces hypersensitivity that may occur with sensory nerve regeneration, new scar tissue, neuromas or other injuries. This consists of graded introduction of stimuli that produce the least painful response to the stimuli that produce the most painful response. Once the affected area begins to acclimate to initial stimulus, the next stimulus is incorporated, e.g. desensitization program may progress from a very soft material stimulus (i.e. silk) to a rougher material (i.e. wool) or textured fabric (i.e. velcro).
- **Sensory re-education:** It is a technique that therapists use in attempt to re-train sensory pathways or stimulate unused pathways. Therapists also teach adaptive technique to help compensate for sensory loss. Sensor re-education technique can include touching different textured objects, massage, vibration, pressure, determining joint position, identifying different temperature and electrical stimulation.
- **Joint mobilization:** Passive mobilization of the entire adjacent joint improves the circulation of synovial fluid and reduces the stiffness, adhesion formation, capsular tightness and joint deformity.
- **Nerve glide (also known as neural flossing or nerve stretching):** Sometimes inability of injured nerve to glide normally through the surrounding sheath may cause a sharp pain. Therefore, nerve gliding within the surrounding tissue is imperative for normal nerve function. For this, stretching of peripheral nerve should be performed with slow, steady movement not exceeding the nerve's allowable stretch limit.
- **Flexibility and ROM exercises:**
  - **Joint ROM and muscle stretching:** In nerve injury, ROM and flexibility can be seriously affected due to unopposed action of antagonistic muscles or after immobilization. Therefore, passive ROM and gentle muscle stretching should be given after the phase of immobilization i.e. 2-3 weeks to restore full ROM and flexibility. Static stretch are found to be more beneficial (withhold time of at least 30 seconds) as compared to dynamic stretching. Muscle stretching is also recommended in entrapment neuropathy to release the compression on the involved nerve.
  - **Proprioceptive neuromuscular Facilitation (PNF):** These are the exercise program used to facilitate recovery using neuromuscular pattern and sensory receptors.
- **Strengthening exercises:** This will not cause improvement in complete motor denervation but can be effective in partial innervation and during reinnervation. Strengthening exercise, after injury is important to maintain function in innervated muscles, to prevent atrophy of denervated muscles, to maintain muscle perfusion and to minimize scarring.
  - Initiate with concentric exercises, as it subject the injured noncontractile elements to less stress, then gradually progress to either isometric or eccentric programs.
  - Electrical stimulation (ES) may be used to stimulate contraction of denervated muscles, to facilitate contraction in weakened reinnervated muscles and for pain management. Although research on the use of ES in nerve injury is still controversial with mixed outcomes. So some therapist uses ES to maintain the strength of partially or completely denervated muscles and to reduce the rate of atrophy or fibrosis in these muscles.

Surgical Treatment

Indications
- Neuropraxia that failed to recover within first 3 months.
- Definite nerve injuries such as crushed injuries, open fracture, cut wounds, gunshot injuries, iatrogenic nerve injuries or animal bite injuries etc.
- Chronic nerve lesion with painful neuroma.
- Entrapment neuropathies.

Principles of nerve injury management: Although the classification of nerve injury provide the basis for prognosis and management but practically it is very difficult to diagnose the grade of injury to a nerve in early stages. Therefore it is useful to divide injuries into those which are open and closed.

Rule of three: Rule of three determines the surgical timing in a traumatic peripheral nerve injury.

1. **Immediate surgery**, i.e. within 3 days after injury is advised for clean and sharp open injuries.
2. **Early surgery**, i.e. within 3 weeks after injury is advised for blunt or contusion injuries.
3. **Delayed surgery**, i.e. within 3 months after injury is advised for closed injuries.

Surgical Techniques
- **Neurolysis:** It refers to the removal of scar from the nerve. It is used when scar tissue is blocking the nerve from regeneration.
- **Neurorrhaphy:** It is the surgical suturing of the divided nerve. It is usually possible in case of sharp cut of nerve.
- **Nerve grafting:** It is a surgical procedure in which a segment of donor nerve is used to bridge the gap between the two ends of nerve. It is usually performed in extensive damages where it may not be possible to suture the two ends of nerve directly together after the excision of the damaged portion of nerve. **Commonly used donor nerves for grafting** are sural nerve of leg and medial antebrachial cutaneous nerve of arm.
- **Nerve transfer:** It is a surgical technique that includes transfer of adjacent functional nerve to the area of injured nerve. It is used where nerve injury results in complete loss of muscle function or sensation.
- **Nerve transplant:** In this surgical technique in which the donor nerve from cadaver or a family member is used for nerve graft. It is used where adequate nerve graft material cannot be taken from the same patient without causing a substantial deficit.
- **Tendon transplant:** It is performed by releasing one end of a tendon from bone or soft tissue and reattaching it to another bone or tendon to restore the muscle function. It is used when the nerve gap is more than 4 cm or associated with extensive scarring or soft tissue damage over the nerve.

UPPER LIMB NERVE LESIONS

■ RADIAL NERVE INJURY

Anatomical course (Fig. 4): Radial nerve is a continuation of the posterior cord of brachial plexus. It arises in axillary region behind axillary artery and exits the axilla inferiorly where it gives branches to supply long and lateral heads of triceps brachii.

The nerve descends down the arm through the radial groove of humerus and then wraps around the humerus laterally and gives a branch to supply the medial head of triceps. The radial nerve moves anteriorly over the lateral epicondyle through the cubital fossa and terminates by dividing in two main branches.

1. **Superficial radial nerve (sensory):** It contributes to the cutaneous innervation of hand and fingers.
2. **Deep radial nerve (motor):** It supplies most of the muscles of posterior compartment of the forearm.

Peripheral Nerve Lesion

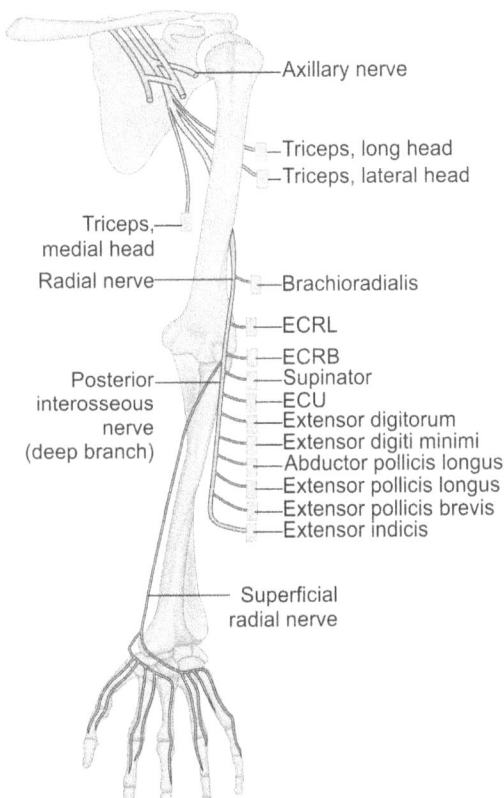

Fig. 4: Anatomical course of radial nerve.
(ECRL: extensor carpi radialis longus; ECRB: extensor carpi radialis brevis; ECU: extensor carpi ulnaris)

Nerve roots: C5-T1.
Sensory supply: It supplies most of the skin of posterior side of forearm and the dorsal surface of the lateral side of hand and three and a half fingers.
Motor supply: It supplies the triceps brachii and most of the extensors muscles in forearm that extends the wrist and fingers and supinates the forearm.

Clinical Presentation
Clinical presentation depends on the site of nerve injury (Table 5).

Special Test for Examination of Radial Nerve
- **Test for triceps:** Patient is asked to extend elbow against the resistance applied by the therapist. A positive test is determined by the inability of patient to extend the elbow.
- **Test for supinator:** Patient is asked to supinate forearm with the arm by the side of trunk against the resistance applied by therapist. A positive test is determined by the inability of patient to supinate the forearm.
- **Test for brachioradialis:** The forearm is positioned in midprone position with 90º elbow flexion. Patient is asked to flex elbow against the resistance applied by the therapist at wrist. A positive test is determined by the inability of patient to flex the elbow.
- **Test for wrist extensor:** Positive test is determined by the inability of patient to extend the wrist, thumb and fingers.
- **Test for extensor digitorum:** Positive test is determined by the inability of patient to extend the fingers at MCP joint.
- **Thumbs up test (Fig. 5):** It is used to examine extensor pollicis longus muscle: Inability to extend the thumb determines muscle paralysis.

Attitude and Deformity
Wrist drop: Inability to extend the wrist due to the paralysis of wrist extensors along with the unopposed action of wrist flexors.
Splint used: Unlike in median and ulnar nerve injury where sensory loss impairs the hand function, patient with radial nerve palsy can perform normal function with hand. Therefore, splint is used to facilitate normal function of the hand.
- Static volar wrist cock up splint (Fig. 6)
- Dorsal wrist cock up with dynamic finger extension splint.
- Dynamic tenodesis suspension splint: It allows partial wrist movement along with full finger movements (Fig. 7).

MEDIAN NERVE INJURY

Anatomical course (Fig. 8): Median nerve is derived from the medial and the lateral

Table 5: Clinical presentation of radial nerve injury.

Site of injury	Causes	Clinical presentation	
		Motor paralysis	Sensory loss
In axilla	• Dislocation of shoulder • Fracture of proximal humerus • Crutch palsy	• Triceps and muscles in posterior compartment are paralyzed • Inability to extend forearm, wrist and fingers	Over the lateral and posterior aspect of arm and posterior aspect of forearm, dorsal and lateral aspect of hand and three and a half fingers
In radial groove	• Prolonged application of tourniquet • Fracture shaft humerus • Intramuscular injection • Saturday night palsy	• Triceps and anconeus spared • Muscle of posterior compartment of forearm are paralyzed • Inability to extend wrist and fingers	Over dorsal and lateral aspect of hand and three and a half fingers
At elbow joint and in forearm. • Deep branch: Posterior interosseous nerve (PIN) is injured	• Fracture of neck of radius • Dislocation of radius • Excision of head of radius	• Extensors of wrist and fingers.	No sensory loss because PIN is pure motor nerve
At elbow joint and in forearm. • Superficial branch	• Stabbing/laceration of forearm	None	Over dorsal and lateral aspect of hand and three and a half fingers with associated area of palm

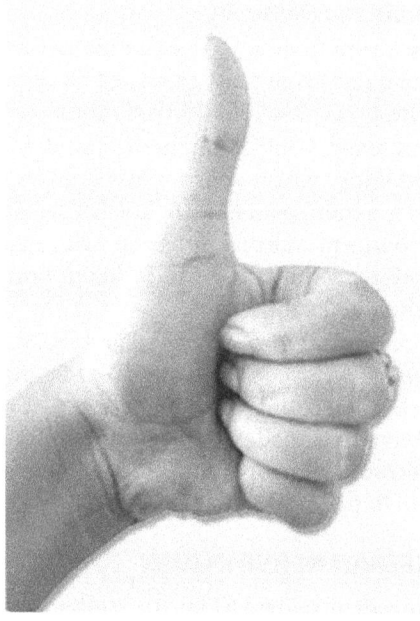

Fig. 5: Thumbs up test.

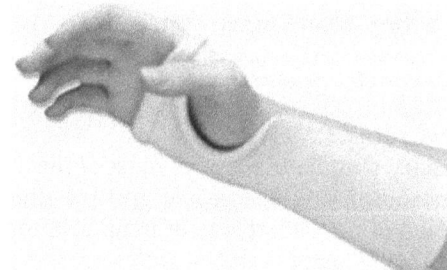

Fig. 6: Static wrist cock up splint.

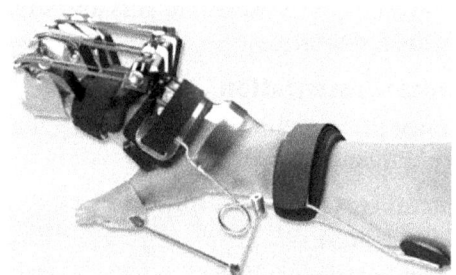

Fig. 7: Dynamic wrist and finger extension splint.

Peripheral Nerve Lesion

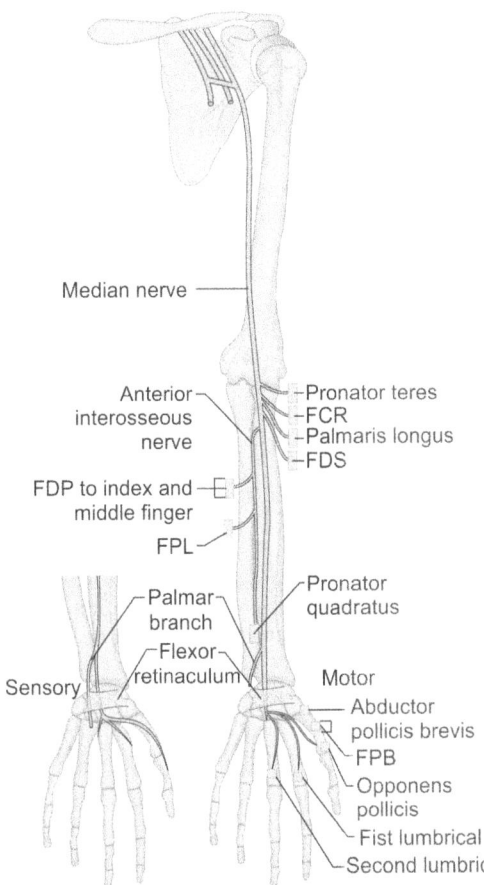

Fig. 8: Anatomical course of median nerve.
(FDP: flexor digitorum profundus; FPL: flexor pollicis longus; FCR: flexor carpi radialis; FDS: flexor digitorum superficialis; FPB: flexor policis brevis)

cords of brachial plexus. It arises in axilla and descends down the arm initially lateral to the brachial artery. Subsequently the nerve crosses over the artery from lateral to medial. Then the nerve enters the anterior compartment of forearm via the cubital fossa.

In forearm, the nerve travels between the flexor digitorum profundus (FDP) and flexor digitorum syperficialis (FDS) muscles and gives rise to two major branches in forearm:
1. **Anterior interosseous nerve:** It supplies the deep muscles of anterior forearm.
2. **Palmar cutaneous nerve:** It supplies the skin of the lateral aspect of palm.

Median nerve then enters the hand via the carpal tunnel and terminates by dividing into two branches:
1. **Recurrent branch:** It supplies the thenar muscles.
2. **Palmar digital branch:** It supplies the palmar surface and the fingertips of lateral three and half digits along with lateral two lumbrical muscles.

Nerve Roots: C6-T1

Sensory supply: It supplies the palmar surface of thumb and lateral two and half fingers.

Motor supply: It supplies the flexor muscles in the anterior compartment of forearm (except flexor carpi ulnaris [FCU] and part of flexor digitorum profundus [FDP] that are supplied by ulnar nerve). It also supplies the thenar muscles and lateral two lumbricals in hand.

Clinical Presentation

Clinical presentation depends on the site of nerve injury (Table 6).

Special Test for Examination of the Median Nerve (Individual Muscles)

- **Pen touching test (Fig. 9):** It is used to test abductor pollicis brevis: Hand is placed flat on a table with palm facing upwards. Patient is asked to abduct the thumb to touch the pen held above it. Inability to do so is considered to be positive.
- **Okay test (Fig. 10):** It is used to examine opponens pollicis. Positive test is determined by the inability to touch the tips of index finger and thumb.
- **Test for flexor pollicis longus (Fig. 11):** The positive test is determined by the inability of patient to flex the distal phalanx of thumb when the proximal phalanx is stabilized by the therapist to prevent the action of the short flexors.

Table 6: Clinical presentation of median nerve.

Site of injury	Causes	Clinical presentation	
		Motor paralysis	Sensory loss
At elbow	• Supracondylar fracture of humerus • Elbow dislocation • Application of tourniquet for prolonged period	• Flexors of wrist and fingers and pronators are paralyzed Except FCU and medial part of FDP • FCR paralysis leads to ulnar deviation of hand particularly when hand is flexed. • FDP (lateral part) paralysis • FPL and FPB paralysis leads to inability of flexion of thumb at DIP joint. • Thenar muscle paralysis—paralysis of first dorsal interosseous and 2 lateral lumbricals	Lateral half of palmar surface of thumb and radial 2 and half fingers
In wrist	• Carpal tunnel syndrome • Cut injury • Fracture of lower radius • Lunate dislocation	• Only thenar muscles are paralyzed • Paralysis of first dorsal interosseous and 2 lateral lumbricals	Lateral half of palmar surface of thumb and radial 2 and half fingers

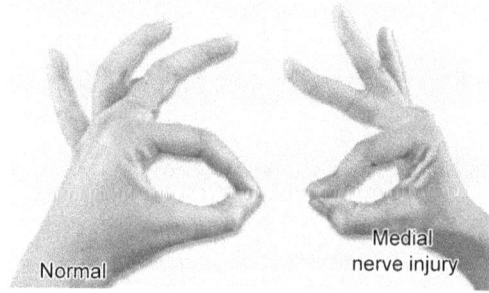

Fig. 10: Okay test.

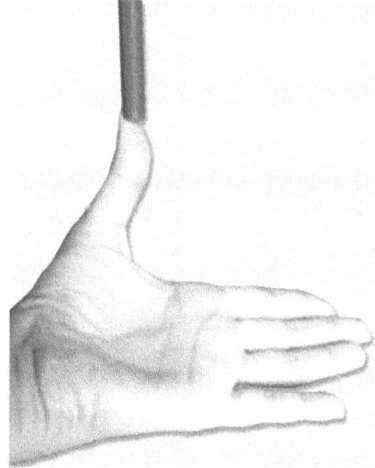

Fig. 9: Pen touching test.

- **Pointing index/Oschner's clasping test (Fig. 12):** Inability to flex index finger while clasping hands that looks like a pointing finger. This test is used to examine the flexor digitorum superficial and profundus muscles. It is the inability to flex the index finger while clasping the hands that looks like a pointing finger.

Attitude and Deformity

- **Ape thumb deformity or Simian hand (Fig. 13):** It occurs due to the paralysis of opponens palsy. In this deformity the thumb being in the line with the other metacarpals.
- **Hand of benediction or pope's blessing (Fig. 14):** Inability to flex the MCP joint

Peripheral Nerve Lesion

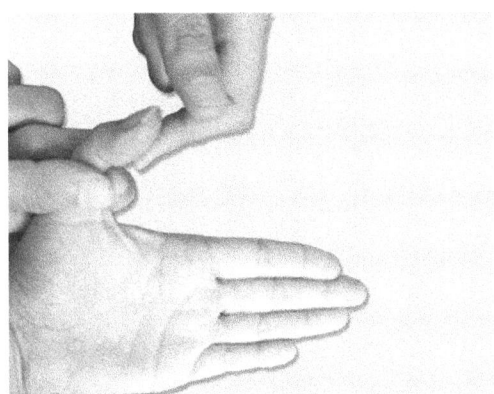

Fig. 11: Flexor pollicis longus test.

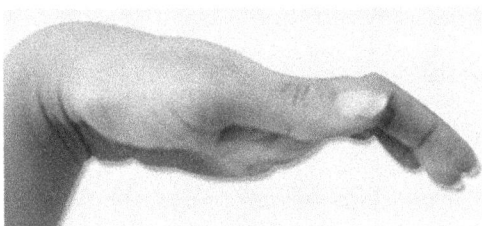

Fig. 13: Simian hand.

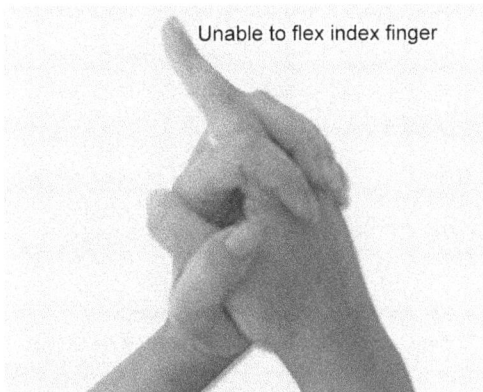

Fig. 12: Oschner's clasping test.

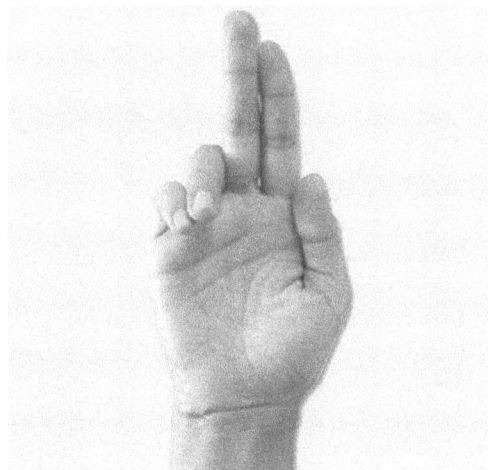

Fig. 14: Hand of benediction.

of middle and index finger due to the paralysis of lateral two lumbricals.

Splint used (Figs. 15 and 16): It is used to maintain the web space between the thumb and index finger and to place the thumb in palmar abduction or in opposition, e.g. C bar splint, opponens splint.

■ ULNAR NERVE INJURY

Anatomy course (Fig. 17): Ulnar nerve is the continuation of the medial cord of brachial plexus. After originating from brachial plexus, it descends down on the medial side of arm and then passes posterior to the medial epicondyle at the elbow and enters the forearm.

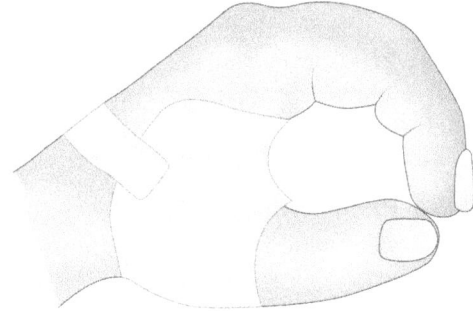

Fig. 15: C bar splint.

In forearm, it penetrates between the two heads of FCU and gives three branches:
1. **Muscular branch:** It supplies some of the muscles of anterior compartment of forearm.

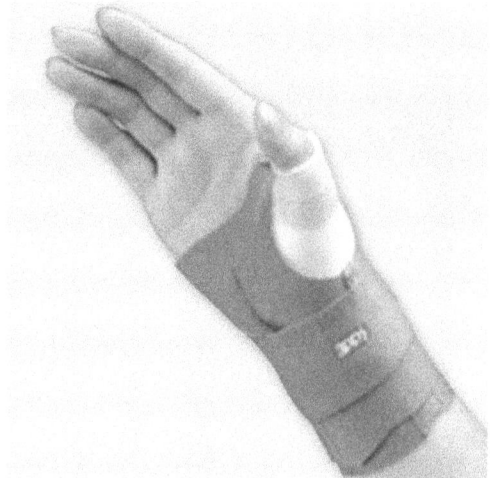

Fig. 16: Opponens splint.

2. **Palmar cutaneous branch:** It supplies the skin on the medial half of palm.
3. **Dorsal cutaneous branch:** It supplies the skin of medial one and half fingers and associated area of hand.

At wrist, it passes superficial to the flexor retinaculum and enters the hand through Guyon's canal and terminates by giving superficial and deep branches.

Spinal roots: C8-T1

Sensory supply: It supplies anterior and posterior surfaces of medial one and half fingers with associated area of hand.

Motor supply: It supplies the muscles of hand (except thenar muscles and laterals two lumbricals), FCU and medial half of FDP.

Clinical Presentation

Clinical presentation depends on the site of nerve injury (Table 7).

Special Test for Examination of Ulnar Nerve

- **Froment test (Fig. 18):** It is used to test adductor pollicis muscle. Patient is asked to hold paper between the thumb and index finger. A positive test is determined by flexion at DIP joint using flexor pollicis longus to maintain the grip.

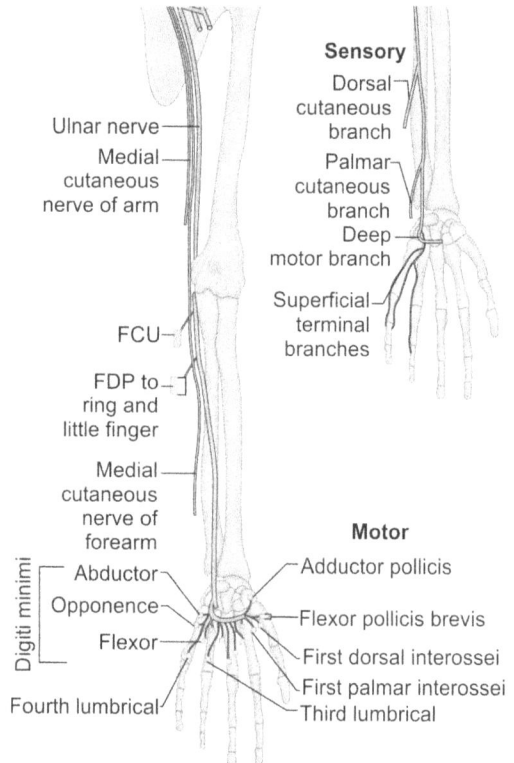

Fig. 17: Anatomical course of ulnar nerve.
(FCU: flexor carpi ulnaris; FDP: flexor digitorum profundus)

- **Card test (Fig. 19):** It is used to test the function of palmar interossei muscles of hand. Patient is asked to hold card between the adjacent fingers while the therapist tried to pull the card from the grip. A positive test is determined by inability to maintain the grip.
- **Egawa test (Fig. 20):** It is used to test the function of dorsal interossei muscles of hand. Patient is asked to move the middle finger sideways. A positive test is determined by the inability of middle finger to move on either side.
- **Test for abductor digiti minimi (Fig. 21):** Patient is asked to abduct the little finger against the resistance applied by therapist by placing the hand flat on table. A positive test is determined by inability to abduct the little finger.

Table 7: Clinical presentation of ulnar nerve injury.

Site of injury	Causes	Clinical presentation	
		Motor paralysis	Sensory loss
At elbow	• Fracture of medial epicondyle • Supracondylar fracture of humerus • Elbow dislocation • Cubitus valgus	• FCU and medial half of FDP are paralyzed leads to radial deviation of hand when wrist is flexed • Hypothenar muscles paralysis • All interossei except first dorsal interossei are paralyzed leads to inability of adduction and abduction of fingers. • Paralysis of third and fourth lumbricals lead to "partial claw hand"/main en griffe deformity/ulnar claw hand	Medial border of hand along with palmar and dorsal surface of one and half fingers
In wrist	Cut injury	• Only the hand muscles are paralyzed and forearm muscles are spared. • Hypothenar muscles paralysis. • All interossei except first dorsal interossei are paralyzed leads to inability of adduction and abduction of fingers. • Paralysis of third and fourth lumbricals leads to "partial claw hand"/main en griffe deformity	Palmar aspect of medial one and a half fingers due to the involvement of palmar branch whereas the dorsal branch is spared

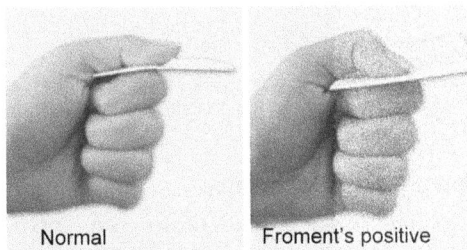

Fig. 18: Froment test.

- **Test for flexor carpi ulnaris:** Patient is asked to perform palmar flexion at wrist joint against the gravity. A positive test is determined by the radial deviation of affected hand along with palmar flexion.
- **Cross finger test (Fig. 22):** It is used to test palmar interossei muscles of hand. A positive test is determined by inability to cross index finger over middle finger or vice versa.

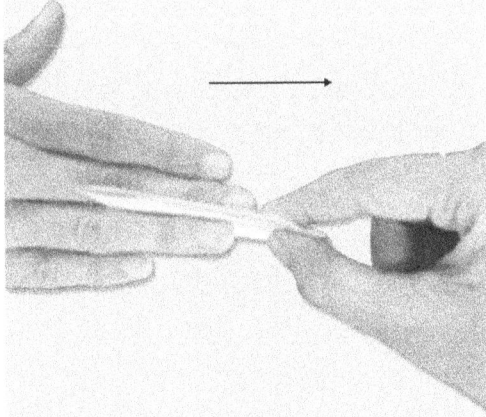

Fig. 19: Card test.

- **Peace sign (Fig. 23):** It is used to test dorsal interossei muscles. A positive test is determined by inability to spread index and middle finger.

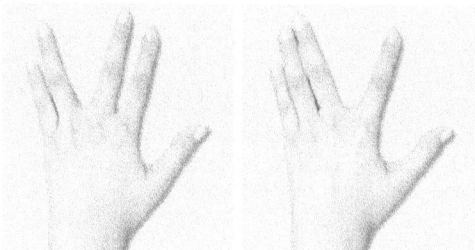

Fig. 20: Egawa test.

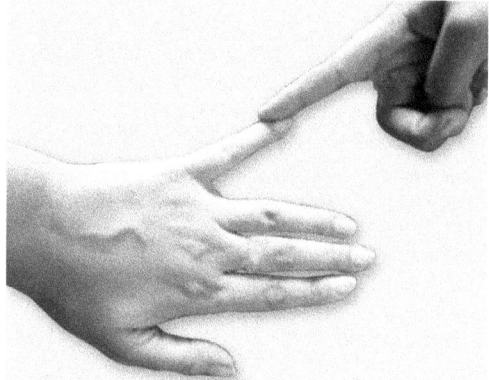

Fig. 21: Test for abduction digiti minimis.

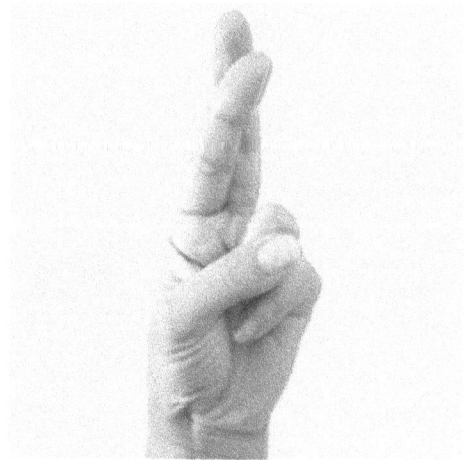

Fig. 22: Cross finger test.

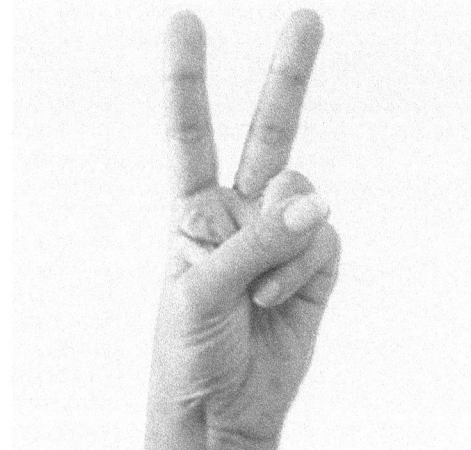

Fig. 23: Peace sign.

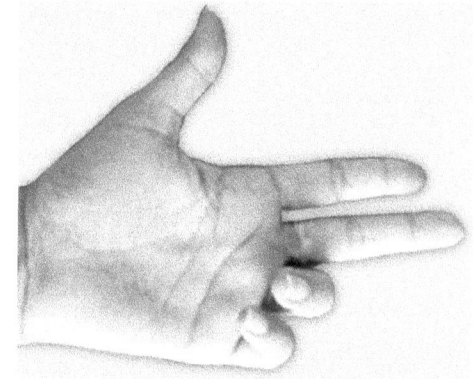

Fig. 24: Duchenne sign.

Attitude and Deformity

- **Partial claw hand/main en griffe deformity/Duchenne sign (Fig. 24):** It is a deformity of little and ring finger in which there is extension at the MCP joint and flexion at IP joints of the affected fingers.
- **Masse's sign (Fig. 25):** Flattened palmar metacarpal arch and loss of hypothenar elevation.

Splint used: Goal of low lesion of ulnar nerve is to prevent the overstretching of denervated intrinsic muscles of little and ring finger. Splint is designed to maintain the MCP joints in slight flexion to prevent the clawing of fingers.

- **Pollock's sign:** It is used to test the flexor digitorum profundus muscle. A positive test is determined by inability to perform flexion at DIP joints of ring and little finger.

Peripheral Nerve Lesion

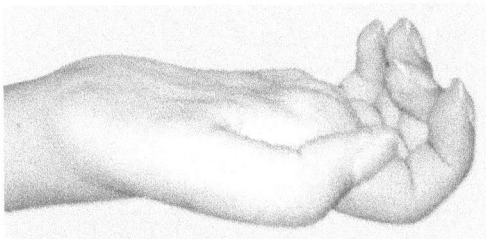

Fig. 25: Masse's sign.

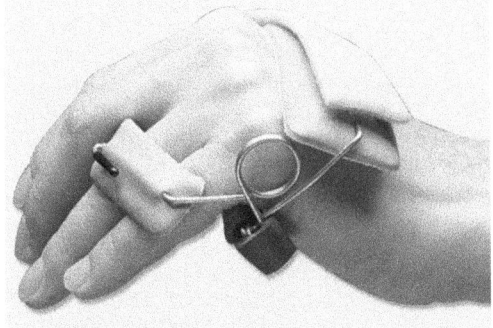

Fig. 26: Knuckle bender splint.

- **Knuckle bender splint (Fig. 26):** It blocks the hyperextension of MCP joints and allow full flexion of all the joints of fingers.

LOWER LIMB NERVE LESIONS

■ SCIATIC NERVE

Anatomy course (Fig. 27): Sciatic nerve is derived from lumbosacral plexus. It exits the pelvis and enters the gluteal region via greater sciatic foramen. It emerges inferiorly to piriformis muscle and descends downwards in inferolateral direction.

As the nerve passes through the gluteal region, it crosses the posterior surface of superior gemellus, obturator internus, inferior gemellus. Then it enters the posterior aspect of thigh by passing deep to the long head of biceps femoris. In posterior thigh, the nerve gives branches to hamstring and adductor magnus muscles. On reaching the apex of popliteal fossa it terminates by bifurcating into two branches:

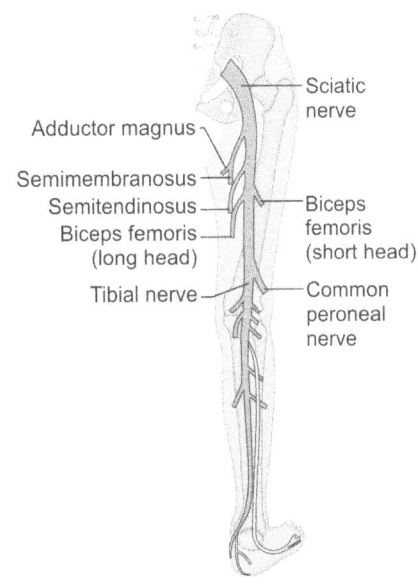

Fig. 27: Anatomical course of sciatic nerve.

1. Tibial nerve
2. Common peroneal nerve.

Nerve roots: L4-S3

Sensory supply: No direct sensory innervation. Indirectly supplies the skin of the lateral aspect of leg, heel and both plantar and dorsal surfaces of foot via its terminal branches.

Motor supply: It supplies the muscles of posterior thigh and hamstring portion of adductor magnus. Indirectly supplies the muscles of leg and foot via the terminal branches.

■ TIBIAL NERVE

Anatomy course (Fig. 28): Tibial nerve is a branch of sciatic nerve that arises at the apex of popliteal fossa. It passes the popliteal fossa and gives off branches to superficial muscles of the posterior compartment of leg and a branch that contributes towards the sural nerve that supply the posterolateral aspect of leg.

Tibial nerve descends down the leg over the posterior surface of tibia and supplies

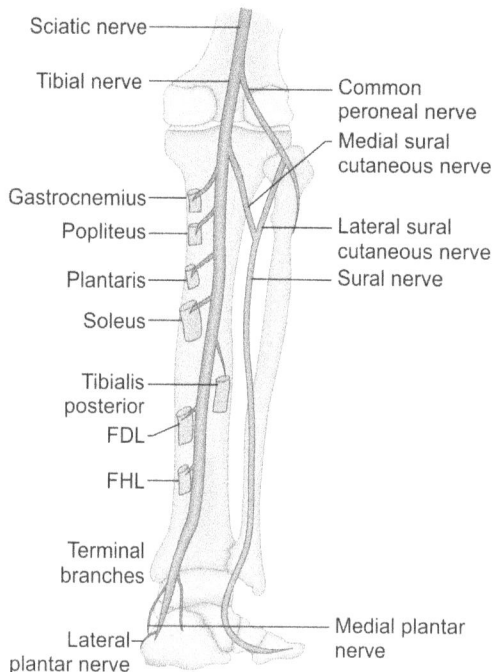

Fig. 28: Anatomical course of tibial nerve.
(FDL: flexor digitorum longus; FHL: flexor hallucis longus)

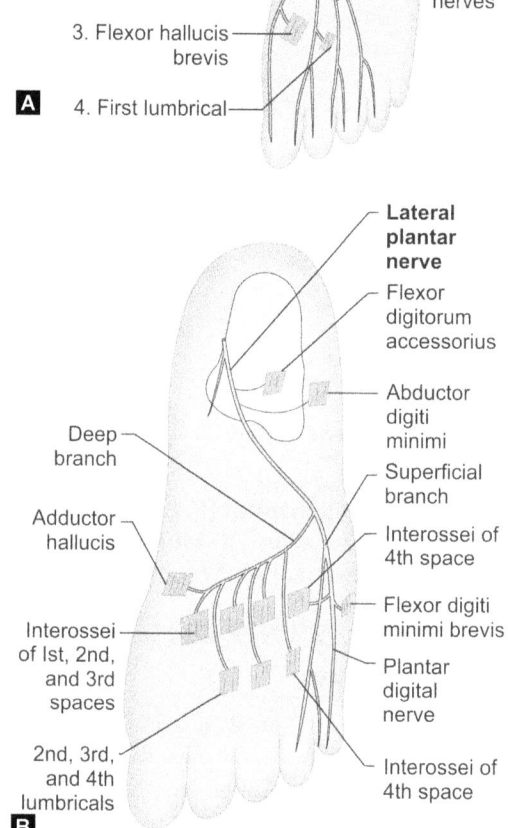

Figs. 29A and B: Medial and lateral plantar nerve.

the deep muscles of the posterior compartment of leg. At ankle, it passes posteriorly and inferiorly to the medial malleolus through the tarsal tunnel. Within the tunnel, tibial nerve gives a branch for cutaneous innervation to heel. Immediately distal to the tarsal tunnel, tibial nerve terminates by dividing into lateral and medial plantar nerves that innervates the sole of foot (Figs. 29A and B).

Nerve roots: L4-S3

Sensory supply: It supplies the posterolateral aspect of leg, lateral aspect and sole of foot.

Motor supply: It supplies the muscles of posterior compartment of leg.

■ COMMON PERONEAL NERVE

Anatomy course (Fig. 30): It is a branch of sciatic nerve that arises at the apex of popliteal fossa.

It lies on the medial border of biceps femoris and descends downward in inferolateral direction over the lateral head of gastronemius and gives off two cutaneous branches that innervates the skin of leg. The nerve wraps around the neck of fibula to enter the lateral compartment of leg. Common peroneal nerve terminates by dividing into superficial and deep peroneal nerves.

Nerve roots: L4-S3

Sensory supply: It supplies the skin of upper lateral and lower posterolateral aspect of

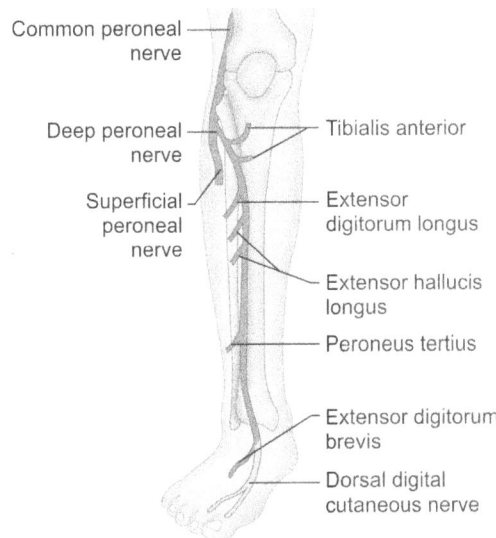

Fig. 30: Anatomical course of common peroneal nerve.

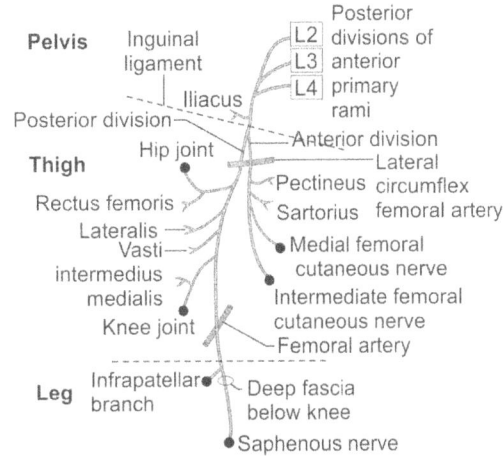

Fig. 31: Anatomical course of femoral nerve.

leg. It also supplies the skin of anterolateral aspect of leg and dorsum of foot via its terminal branches.

Motor supply: It supplies the short head of biceps femoris and also indirectly supplies the muscles of anterior and lateral compartment of leg via its branches.

■ FEMORAL NERVE

Anatomy course (Fig. 31): It is the largest branch of lumbar plexus. After its origination from lumbar plexus, it passes through the psoas major muscle then travels through the pelvis till the midpoint of inguinal ligament where it transverses behind the inguinal ligament into the thigh and divides into an anterior and posterior division. Its posterior division passes through femoral triangle lateral to the femoral vessels and gives off articular branches to hip and knee joint. The terminal branch of femoral nerve is the saphenous nerve that continues with the femoral vessels through the adductor canal.

Nerve roots: L2–L4

Sensory supply: It supplies the anteromedial aspect of thigh through the anterior cutaneous branch and medial aspect of leg and foot through the saphenous nerve.

Motor supply: It supplies the muscle of anterior compartment of thigh.

Clinical Presentation of Lower Limb Nerve Lesions

Clinical presentation depends on the site of nerve injury (Table 8).

ENTRAPMENT NEUROPATHY

It refers to the pressure induced injury to a segment of peripheral nerve. It is also known as nerve compression syndrome (Tables 9 and 10).

■ PATHOGENESIS

Gradual compression of nerve over a prolonged period leads to ischemia of nerve characterized by a variety of symptoms that depends on the nerve injured, site of compression and the duration of injury. Progressive compression leads to the demyelination of nerve that may compromise the function of normal nerve and may result in distal axonal degeneration if left untreated.

Table 8: Clinical presentation of lower limb nerve lesions.

Nerve	Causes	Clinical presentation	
		Motor paralysis	Sensory loss
Sciatic nerve	• IVDP • Hip joint dislocation • Piriformis syndrome • Intramuscular injection • Penetrating wound • Fracture of pelvis	**Muscles** • Hamstrings • All muscles below knee **Motor loss** • Loss of knee flexion. • Loss of all foot movements **Deformity:** Foot drop due to the paralysis of dorsiflexors and pull of gravity on foot	All sensation below knee except on the medial side of leg and foot up to the 1st MTP joint.
Common peroneal nerve	• Fibular neck fracture • Entrapment by leg splint or cast	**Muscles:** Anterior and lateral leg muscles **Motor loss:** Loss of eversion and DF of foot **Deformity:** • Equinovarus: PF and inversion of foot. • Foot drop due to the paralysis of dorsiflexors and pull of gravity on foot	• Anterior and lateral side of leg. • Dorsum of foot and digits. • Medial side of big toe.
Tibial nerve	• Fracture of proximal end of tibia. • Penetrating wound	**Muscles:** All the posterior muscles of leg and sole. **Motor loss:** Loss of inversion and PF of foot. **Deformity:** Calcaneovalgus: DF and eversion of foot.	Sole of foot.
Femoral nerve	Stab or gunshot injuries.	**Muscles:** Quadriceps muscles. **Motor loss:** Loss of knee extension	• Anterior and medial aspect of thigh • Medial aspect of leg • Medial border of foot up to 1st MTP joint.

Clinical Presentation

Sensory dysfunction, paresthesia, pain, muscle weakness and muscle wasting on the progression of the injury.

■ THORACIC OUTLET SYNDROME

It refers to the compression of neurovascular structures as they exit through the thoracic outlet (cervicothoracobrachial region), the area between the base of the neck and the armpit, including the front of shoulder and chest (Fig. 32).

It is also known as costoclavicular compression syndrome, hyperabduction syndrome, scalenus anticus syndrome, anterior scalene syndrome, Droopy shoulder syndrome, Paget-Schroetter syndrome, cervical rib syndrome and thoracic outlet syndrome (TOS).

Potential Sites of Compression (Fig. 33)

■ **Scalene triangle:** It is also called scalene groove that transmits C5- T1 nerve roots of brachial plexus and subclavian artery.

Table 9: Common upper extremity entrapment neuropathy.

Entrapment syndrome (Name of nerve)	Causes	Site of entrapment	Symptoms
Quadrilateral space syndrome (axillary nerve)	Shoulder dislocation; upward pressure (e.g. from improper crutch use); repetitive overload activities (e.g. pitching a ball, swimming); and arthroscopy or rotator cuff repair	As it passes through the quadrilateral (bounded by the teres minor, teres major, long head of the triceps, and the neck of the humerus)	• Fatigue with overhead activity, i.e. weak lateral abduction and ER. • Paresthesia of the lateral and posterior upper arm.
Suprascapular nerve syndrome (suprascapular nerve)	Prolonged wearing of heavy backpacks and direct blows to the nerve	Mostly as it pass through suprascapular notch and rarely more distal entrapment at the spinoglenoid notch	• Severe, deep, aching pain that radiates from the top of the scapula to the ipsilateral shoulder. • Tenderness over suprascapular notch is usually present. • Painful shoulder movements especially reaching across the chest • Weakness and atrophy of the supraspinatus and infraspinatus muscles.

Saturday night palsy (radial nerve)	• Falling asleep with the arm over the back of a chair
	• Falling asleep with your arm tucked underneath you
		In armpit or arm	• Pins and needles or sharp burning pain or numbness of the area supplied by radial nerve.
			• Muscle weakness
			  – Inability to extend elbow
			  – Wrist drop
			  – Decreased grip strength

Radial tunnel syndrome/ supinator syndrome (posterior interosseous nerve)	• Bone fractures • Soft tissue injuries surrounding the nerve • Repetitive motion resulting in inflammation of the muscle	In radial tunnel/at the arcade of Frohse	• Fatigue or a dull, aching pain at the top of the forearm with use • Weakness of the extensor muscle group of forearm and wrist
Wartenberg's syndrome/ Cheiralgia paresthetica (superficial branch of the radial nerve)	• Constriction of the wrist, as with a bracelet or watchband • Iatrogenic injury related to vein cannulation	At the level of distal wrist where it crosses over the first dorsal wrist compartment	• Numbness, tingling, or burning pain on the posterior aspect of the thumb • No motor impairment

Contd...

Contd...

Entrapment syndrome (Name of nerve)	Causes	Site of entrapment	Symptoms
Cubital tunnel syndrome (ulnar nerve)	• Cubitus valgus • Subluxation of the ulnar nerve over the medial epicondyle • Trauma/direct compression by soft tissue mass or bony spurs	In cubital tunnel at elbow	Pain, loss of sensation, tingling and/or weakness. "Pins and needles" usually are felt in the ring and small fingers. These symptoms are often felt when the elbow is bent for a long period of time
Guyon's canal syndrome (ulnar nerve)	• Space occupying lesions • Trauma • Anomalous muscles • Ulnar artery aneurysms	In Guyon's canal in wrist	Associated with either motor or sensory findings, depending on whether the nerve compression involves the ulnar nerve prior to its bifurcation to the superficial (sensory) and deep (motor) branches or if the compression is limited to one of the branches
Handlebar palsy/ cyclist palsy (ulnar nerve)	Long periods of direct pressure on the nerve when the weight of the upper body is resting on hand rest on handlebars during prolonged cycling	In wrist/palmar aspect of hand	Numbness, tingling, weakness, clumsiness, cramping, pain and possibly motor limitation. The condition can impact both sensory and motor functions of the hand, depending on the branch of the ulnar nerve that is affected
Pronator syndrome (median nerve)	• Trauma • Congenital abnormalities • Pronator teres hypertrophy	Compression or entrapment of the median nerve between the ulnar and humeral heads of the pronator teres muscle	Pain, tingling, numbness and paresthesia over volar aspect of the elbow, forearm, and wrist without muscle weakness
Anterior interosseous nerve syndrome/ Kilo-Nevin syndrome (anterior interosseous nerve)	• Direct nerve trauma • Enlarged bicipital bursa • Compression from a thrombosed radial or ulnar artery	In proximal forearm	• Anterior elbow and forearm pain • Motor weakness and paralysis in the FPL, FDP, and pronator quadratus muscles • Pure motor neuropathy with no sensory deficit
Carpal tunnel syndrome (median nerve)	• Idiopathic • Repetitive trauma • Conditions related to metabolic and hormonal changes • Ganglion cysts	In carpal tunnel at wrist	• Numbness, tingling and pain in thumb and the first three fingers of your hand. • Weakness in the muscles of the hand

Table 10: Common lower extremity entrapment neuropathy.

Entrapment syndrome (Name of nerve)	Causes	Site of entrapment	Symptoms
Piriformis syndrome (sciatic nerve)	• Anatomical variation of piriformis muscle • Piriformis muscle spasm or tightness • Prolonged sitting	Entrapment of the sciatic nerve at the level of the greater sciatic notch by the piriformis muscle	Pain, tingling and numbness in the hip/buttocks and along the path of the sciatic nerve descending the lower thigh and into the leg
Meralgia paresthetica or Bernhardt-Roth syndrome (lateral femoral cutaneous nerve)	• Tight clothing • Obesity • Pregnancy • Local trauma • Disease such as diabetes • Seat belt injury after a motor vehicle accident	Often compressed as it pass under the inguinal ligament	• Tingling, numbness and burning pain in your outer thigh
Superficial peroneal tunnel syndrome (common peroneal nerve)	• Space occupying lesions such as tumor • Exostosis • Chondromatosis • Associated with Baker's cyst	In superior peroneal tunnel/ fibular tunnel	• Pain, numbness and paresthesia over lateral aspect of leg and dorsum of foot • Weakness of dorsiflexion or foot drop
Tarsal tunnel syndrome (posterior tibial nerve)	Post-traumatic fibrosis due to fracture • Tenosynovitis • Ganglion cysts space occupying lesions • Dilated or tortuous veins	In tarsal tunnel at ankle	Pain, numbness, tingling and burning sensation on the sole of the foot • Weakness of the foot muscles
Soleal sling syndrome (proximal tibial nerve)	• Local trauma • Prolonged compression • Peripheral neuropathy by diabetes	Entrapment of the tibial nerve in the proximal leg by a fibrous sling at the origin of the soleus muscle	Numbness, paresthesia in the sole of the foot, and posterior calf pain
Morton neuroma (Interdigital nerve)	Repetitive mechanical stress with subsequent perineural fibrosis due to high heeled or narrow shoes, high impact athletic activity or foot deformities.	Entrapment of the interdigital nerve near the distal edge of the intermetatarsal ligament, most commonly occurs in the second and third intermetatarsal spaces	• Burning pain, numbness and tingling sensation in ball of foot radiating to the affected toes • Burning pain and paresthesia in the affected web space • May report the sensation of walking on a lump/ pebble

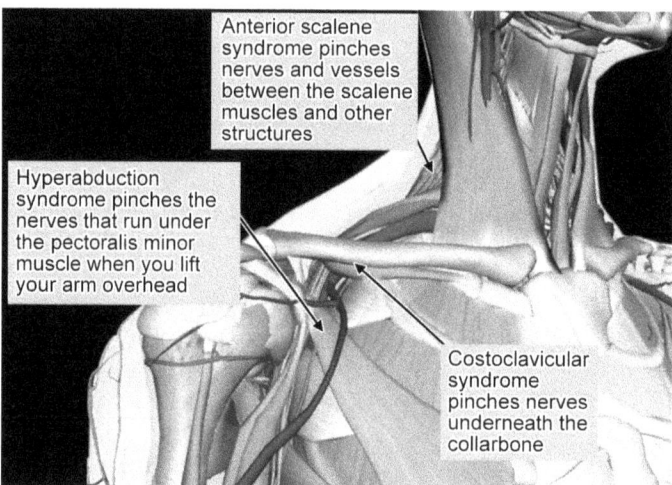

Fig. 32: Thoracic outlet syndrome.

- **Costoclavicular space:** Costoclavicular interval between the clavicle and first rib that transmits subclavian vessels.
- **Subcoracoid space:** Inferior to coracoid process posterior to the insertion of pectoralis minor muscle that transmits the trunk and divisions of brachial plexus and subclavian vessels.

Epidemiology

- **Age:** Neurogenic TOS commonly affects the middle aged women.
- **Gender:** TOS is more common in females than males with 2:1 ratio because of poor posture i.e. drooped shoulders, additional breast tissue, narrow thoracic outlet, poor muscular development and a lower sternum which changes the angle between the scalene muscles and consequently causes a higher prevalence in females.

Etiology

It is caused by the compression of neurovascular structures in the narrow passageway of thoracic outlet. So any factor that reduces the space in thoracic outlet may result in the symptoms.

- **Congenital abnormalities:** Cervical rib, prolonged transverse process, congenital unilateral or bilateral elevated scapula, fibrous muscular band, etc.
- **Repetitive activities of arm and shoulder:**
  - **Occupation related activities:** Assembly line work, keyboard typing, overhead reaching, carrying heavy shoulder loads, etc.
  - **Athletic activities:** Baseball, golf, weight lifting, volleyball, etc.
- **Post-traumatic:** Injury to neck e.g. whiplash injury, hyperextension injuries, fracture of cervical spine or ribs.
- **Poor posture:** Drooped shoulder, cervicodorsal scoliosis, forward head posture.
- Tumor or large lymph nodes in pectoral or axillary region.
- Heavy mammaries
- **Psychological disorder:** Sleep disorder, depression or stress, etc.
- Muscular causes:
  - Hypertrophy of scalene, pectoralis minor muscles
  - Hypotonus muscles—trapezius, levator scapulae, rhomboids
  - Muscle tightness—scalene muscles, trapezius, levator scapulae, pectoralis minor muscles, subscapularis (Fig. 34).

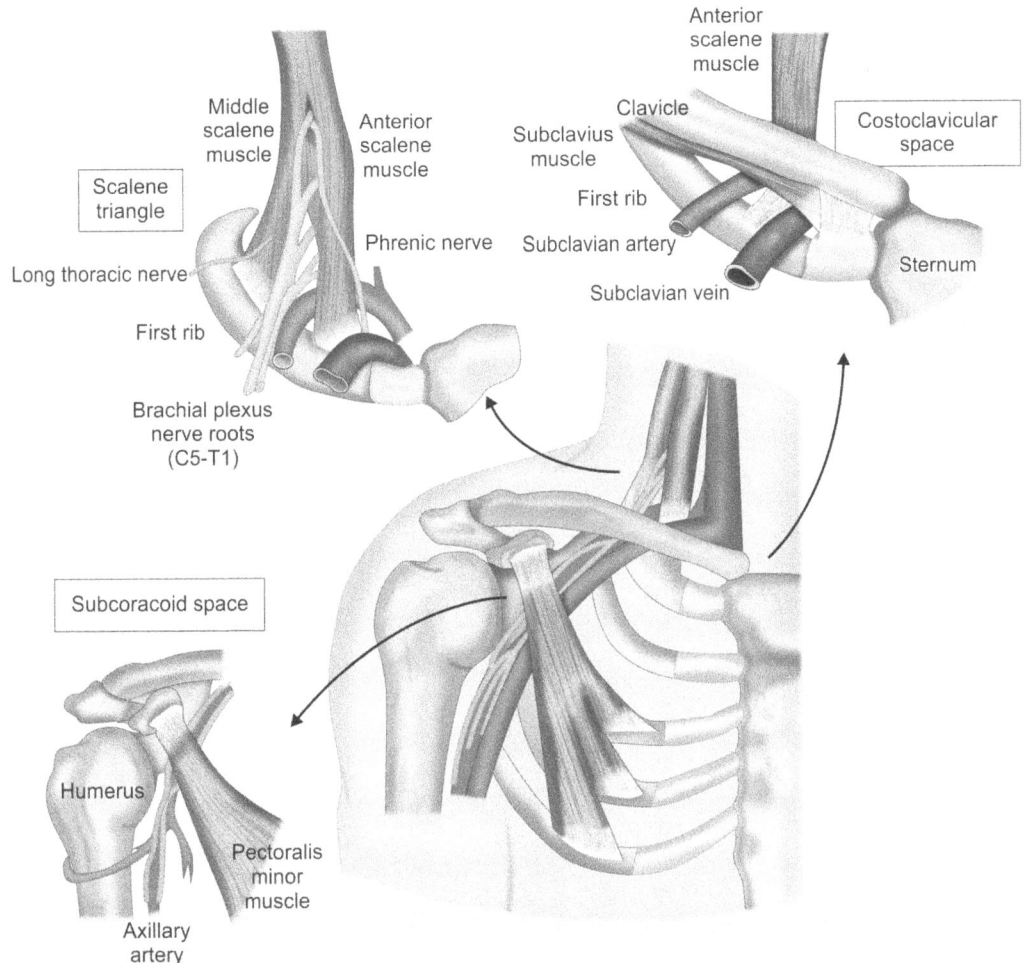

Fig. 33: Potential sites of compression.

Types of Thoracic Outlet Syndrome

- **Neurogenic TOS**: About 80% of TOS are neurological. It is caused by the compression of brachial plexus nerves due to some bony or soft tissue abnormalities in the lower region of neck.
- **Venous TOS**: About 15% of TOS are of venous type. It is caused by the compression of subclavian vein that progressively results in the injury of vein, its scarring, narrowing and eventual clot formation and occlusion of vein. It is also named as "Paget-Schroetter syndrome". It is characterized by sudden swelling and bluish discoloration of arm.
- **Arterial TOS**: Only 5% of TOS are diagnosed with arterial type. It is caused by the occlusion or aneurysm of subclavian artery in the neck that is usually associated with cervical rib anomaly. It is characterized by feeling of coldness, pain and numbness in hand.

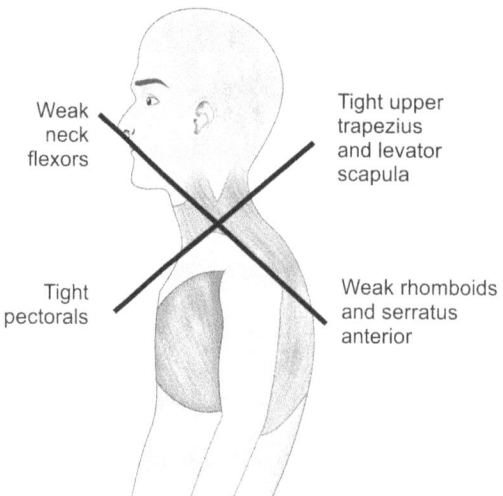

Fig. 34: Muscular imbalance due to poor posture.

Clinical Presentation (Table 11)
Worsens with repetitive overhead activities.
- **Neurogenic TOS:**
  - Occipital headache, neck pain or shoulder pain.
  - Burning pain, numbness and tingling sensation in upper extremity.
  - Muscle spasms in scapular or upper back region.
  - Muscle wasting of thenar muscles (Gilliatt-Sumner hand).
  - Muscle weakness of arm and hand.
- **Venous TOS:**
  - Cyanotic discoloration and heaviness of upper extremity.
  - Abrupt spontaneous swelling and pain in upper extremity.
- **Arterial TOS:**
  - Pain, numbness and tingling sensation in fingers or whole hand.
  - Coldness and paleness of fingers.
  - Cramping/claudication of forearm and hand with activity.
  - Non-healing wounds in the fingers.
  - Absence of neck and shoulder pain.

Chest pain (mimicking a heart condition that does not improves with rest) often relieved with the elevation of arm.

Table 11: Clinical presentation of TOS.

Upper extremity	Arterial	Numbness of arms and hands
		Tingling of arms and hands
		Positional weakness of arms and hands
	Venous	Swelling of fingers and hands
		Heaviness of upper extremity
	Nerves	Pain in upper extremity
		Paresthesia of C8-T1 distribution
		Weakness of hands
		Coldness of hands
		Clumsiness of hands
		Tiredness, heaviness and paresthesia on elevation of arms
Neck and shoulder	-	Pain and tightness
Chest	-	Anginal chest pain
		Interscapular pain
Head	-	Headache
		Funny feeling in face and ear
Vertebral artery	-	Dizziness, light headedness
		Vertigo, syncope
		Diplopia, dysarthria, dysphagia, dysphonia
		Tinnitus, ear pain

Diagnosis
Investigations
- **Chest roentgenography:** To determine the presence of cervical cysts or thoracic masses.
- **X-ray:** To rule out the presence of cervical rib, malunited fracture of clavicle, elongated transverse process of cervical spine
- **Angiography:** Transfemoral subclavian angiography to check the vascular compression.

- **EMG and NCV studies:** To evaluate the electrical activity of muscle or nerve to check the nerve compression.
- **MRI or CT scan:** To determine the cause and location of compression.

Physical Examination
- **Observation:** Skin discoloration, swelling, muscle atrophy, any wound or ulcer in hand.
- **Palpation:** Skin temperature, swelling, tenderness, muscle spasm.
- **Muscle strength and tightness** of scalene, trapezius, levator scapulae, serratus anterior, sternocleidomastoid and pectoralis muscles.

Special Tests
Neurologic Signs
- **Roos test (Fig. 35):** Patient is asked to hold the arm at 90° abduction with elbow in flexion and open and close the fingers repeatedly. Positive test is determined by reproduction of the symptoms of TOS within 90 seconds.
- **Supraclavicular pressure (Fig. 36):** Patient lies in high sitting position with both the arms at side. Therapist squeezes the area by placing the fingers on upper trapezius and thumb on anterior scalene muscle near the first rib for around 30 seconds. Reproduction of TOS symptoms determines the possible compression of brachial plexus through scalene triangles.
- **Cyriax release:** Patient is in seating position and therapist stands behind the patient and grasp both the wrist of patient under the forearm with elbow at 90° flexion. Therapist then passively elevates the shoulder girdles by raising the forearm and hold for 90 seconds. Test is considered to be positive if the symptoms subside gradually.
- **Supraclavicular Tinel's sign (Fig. 37):** Elicited by direct palpation or percussion of brachial plexus in supraclavicular area.

Vascular Signs
- **Adson test (Fig. 38):** Therapist extends, abducts and externally rotates the arm of patient. Patient is asked to take a deep breath and hold it and then extend the neck and rotate it towards the side being tested. A positive test is determined by weak or absent radial pulse.
- **Wright test (Fig. 39):** Therapist hyperabduct and extend the arm of patient and ask the patient to take deep breath and

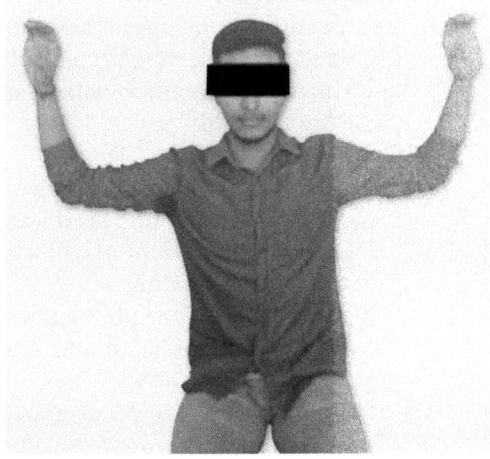

Fig. 35: Roos test.

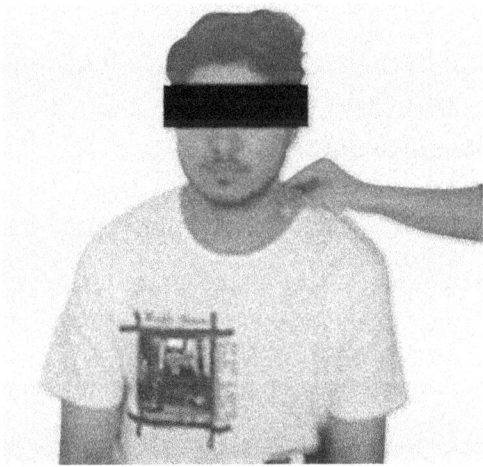

Fig. 36: Supraclavicular pressure.

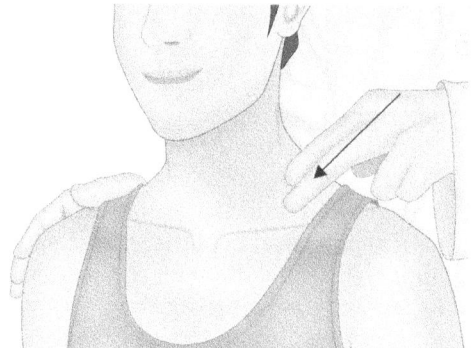

Fig. 37: Supraclavicular Tinel's sign.

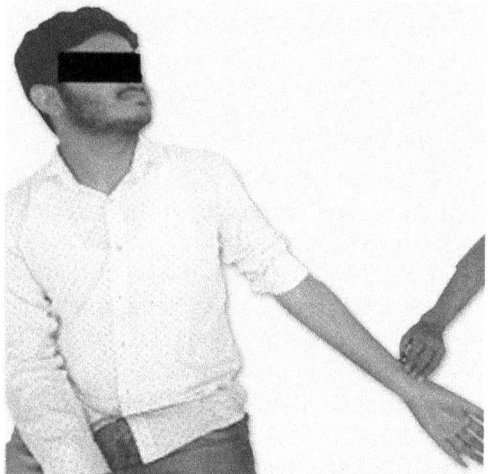

Fig. 38: Adson test.

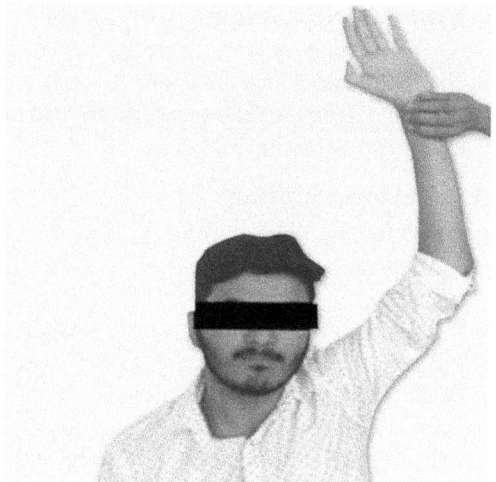

Fig. 39: Wright test.

hold, i.e. positive test is determined by weak or absent radial pulse.

Management

Conservative Treatment

- NSAIDS are used to reduce pain and inflammation.
- Botulinum injections: Given to anterior and middle scalene to decrease pain and associated muscle spasm.
- In venous or arterial TOS, medication such as
  - Thrombolytic medicines are given to dissolve blood clots.
- Anticoagulant medicines (warfarin, heparin) decrease the blood ability for clot formation.

Physiotherapy Treatment

In neurogenic TOS
- **Postural awareness:** Patient should be taught about bad posture such as forward head posture or drooped shoulder or increased thoracic kyphosis accompanied with increased compensatory lumbar lordosis that result in forward head posture.
- **Sleeping posture:**
  - **Bad posture:** Bringing the arms up overhead, lying on the affected side and lying on the stomach with head turned to one side.
  - **Good posture:**
    - Side lying on unaffected side with one pillow under the head and another pillow in front of trunk to support the upper arm.
    - Supine lying with one pillow under the head and shoulder and one pillow under each arm.
- **Working posture:** Avoid overhead activities because this compresses the neurovascular bundle in costoclavi-

cular space and beneath the coracoids insertion of pectoralis minor muscle.
- **Good posture:** Using a step stool to reach high objects. One must prevent traction of the plexus over glenohumeral joint which is produced by carrying items with affected arm.
- **Sitting posture:** Use forearm supporting surface that do not cause excessive elevation or depression of shoulders.
- **Driving posture:** Keep the hands low and relaxed on the steering wheel. A small pillow should be used to support the affected arm.

- **To control pain:** Hot fomentation, pain relieving modalities like TENS, IFT, micro currents, HVPGS, phonophoresis and gentle ROM exercises may be used to reduce pain.
- **To control edema:** AROM exercises, retrograde massage, phonophoresis, tendon and nerve gliding exercises of neck and upper extremity helps to minimize the edema, improves the tissue nutrition and alleviate traction neuropathy by minimizing the scarring.
- **Diaphragmatic breathing exercise:** Relaxed diaphragmatic breathing helps to reduce the dependency on accessory respiratory muscle such as scalene and decrease the potential elevation of first rib. As these two factors, i.e. overactivity of scalene muscle and elevation of first ribs are the contributory factors in causing TOS.
- **Cyriax release technique (Fig. 40):** This maneuver is used to unload neurovascular structures in thoracic outlet. In this technique, patient sits on the chair with well supported spine and head in neutral position. Elbow 90° flexed and forearm placed on the arm rests which is elevated by placing the towels/pillow to cause passive elevation of shoulder girdle.

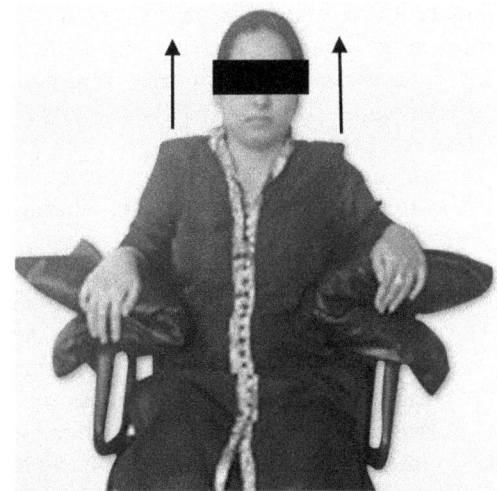

Fig. 40: Cyriax release technique.

- **Cervical traction:** Cervical traction helps to reduce the associated symptoms of TOS by stretching the scalene muscle and decreasing the compression on brachial plexus. Regular application of cervical traction additionally found to increase the patient's awareness of muscular tension and postural imbalance.
- **Therapeutic exercises:** To correct muscular imbalance in cervicoscapular region.
  - **Strengthening exercises:** Strengthening of levator scapulae, sternocleidomastoid and upper trapezius muscle helps to open the thoracic outlet by raising the shoulder girdle and opening the costoclavicular space also.
  - **Stretching exercises:** Stretching of pectorals, scalene and lower trapezius muscles as tightness of these muscle causes the narrowing of thoracic outlet.
- **Joint mobilization:** Mobilization of cervicothoracic, sternoclavicular, acromioclavicular and costotransverse joints is used to decompress neurovascular structures by increasing costoclavicular space.
- **Nerve gliding exercises:** Gliding exercises of ulnar, median and radial nerve. Nerve gliding exercises helps to maintain the

mobility of nerves in a tight concised space, to minimize scarring and to milk out the excessive fluid if present around the nerve.
- **General precautions:**
  - Stressful situations lead to tension of cervical muscles. Therefore, sharing of tension with other and relaxation techniques should be used.
  - Large mammaries contribute to poor posture by pulling the chest down and protracting the shoulder. Thick bra straps, strapless or bralessness will assist in direct pressure on thoracic outlet. Therefore custom measured supporting bra with wide and crossed back strap should be used.
  - Cold climate or decreased temperature often leads to shivering and hyper tonicity of muscles including upper cervical muscles. Therefore wearing several layers of light clothing is advised.
  - Avoid strenuous breathing—as strenuous breathing requires the action of secondary musculature that causes the elevation of ribs which may provoke these symptoms.
  - Avoid carrying heavy purse or bag over the affected shoulder as it may cause the sustained scapular depression and puts tractional force on brachial plexus.
  - Avoid prolonged slouched postures and neck flexion that aggravates the symptoms.

Surgical Management
Indications
- Persistence of symptoms inspite of regular conservative treatment.
- In limb-threatening complications of vascular TOS
- 90% cases are of arterial or venous TOS.

Surgical Interventions
Decompression surgery: Goal of surgery is to repair the compressed structures and remove the source of compression on neurovascular structures which is usually accomplished by removing first rib, abnormal muscle or fibrous band (scalenotomy).

It may perform using several approaches:
- **Transaxillary approach:** Through an incision on the chest to remove the first rib to relieve the compression on neurovascular structures.
- **Supraclavicular approach:** Through an incision under the neck to expose brachial plexus region. In this procedure, muscles causing compression are removed and compressed blood vessels are also repaired.
- **Infraclavicular approach:** Through incision under clavicle and across chest to treat compressed vein with extensive repair.

CARPAL TUNNEL SYNDROME

This condition refers to the entrapment neuropathy of median nerve characterized by numbness, pain, tingling and weakness in the hand. It occurs due to the compression of median nerve as it passes through carpal tunnel in the wrist (Figs. 41A and B).

Epidemiology
- Females are more affected than males with ratio of 3:1.
- Usually occurs between 40 to 70 years of age.

Predisposing Factors
Any condition that increases the pressure in the carpal tunnel.
- Medical condition: High BP and endocrinal disorders such as diabetes and hypothyroidism.
- Fluid retention from pregnancy or menopause
- Obesity: Being obese is a significant risk factor for CTS.
- Any form of arthritis such as OA, RA in the wrist joint that cause swelling of wrist joint or the tendon that passes through the tunnel.

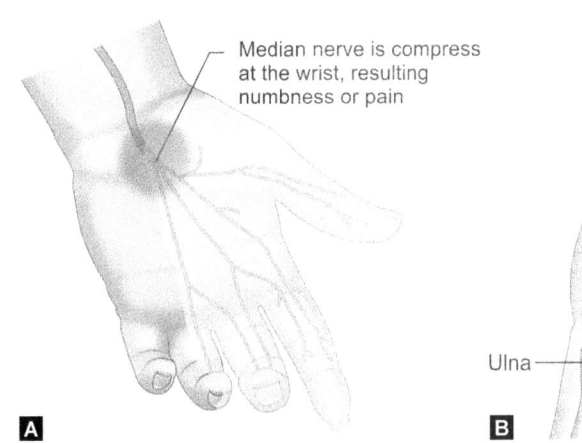
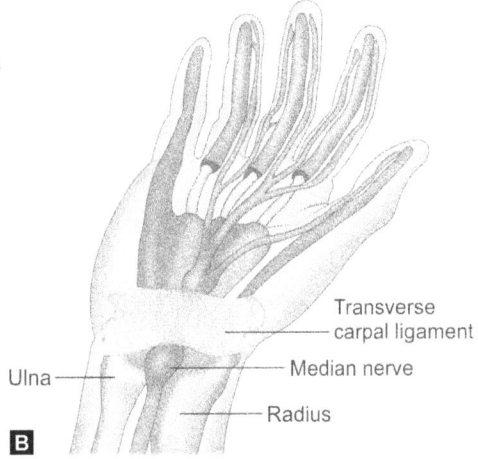

Figs. 41A and B: Carpal tunnel syndrome.

- Repeated use of vibrating hand tools
- Development of space occupying lesions such as cyst, ganglion or tumor in the tunnel.
- Inflammation of the tendons that passes through carpal tunnel such as tendons of FDP, FDS, FPL.
- Fracture, dislocation or trauma to the wrist.
- Occupations that require repetitive movement that overextends the wrist such as playing the piano, typing.

Clinical Presentation

- Burning pain, numbness, pins and needle sensation in thumb and radial two and a half fingers (Fig. 42).
- Nocturnal pain: Symptoms are more pronounced at night that may be due to excessive flexion at wrist during sleeping or due to the accumulation of fluid around wrist during prolonged inactivity.
- Cramping and weakness of hand.
- Dropping of objects from hand due to decreased grip strength.
- Difficulty doing tasks such as brushing, blow drying or washing hair, writing, doing up buttons, grasping small objects, driving or typing on keyboard.
- Occasionally, sharp shooting pain in forearm.
- Stiffness of hand and wrist.

Diagnosis

Imaging Studies

- **X-ray:** Carpal tunnel view: To demonstrate the osseous structure of carpal tunnel including the hook of hamate and to rule out other possible causes like wrist fracture or arthritis.
- **MRI/US:** To identify any soft tissue abnormality or any space-occupying lesion in and around the median nerve that causes CTS.

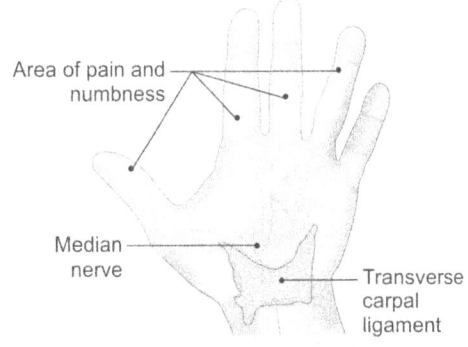

Fig. 42: Pain pattern in carpal tunnel syndrome.

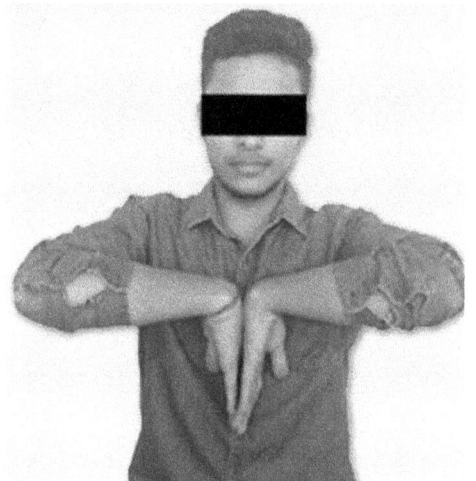

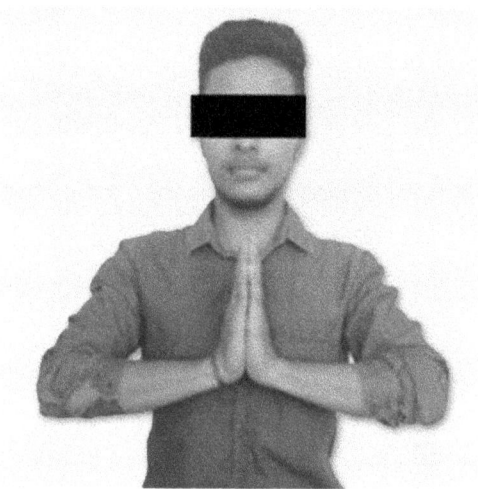

Fig. 43: Phalen test.

Fig. 44: Reverse phalen test.

- **NCV:** To identify the extent of involvement of median nerve by measuring the speed of electrical impulse travel in median nerve.
- **EMG:** This test used to determine any muscle damage and can rule out other conditions that mimics CTS.

Physical Examination

- ROM of wrist joint.
- Sensory evaluation of hand.
- Muscle strength: Muscle weakness and wasting of median nerve innervated hand muscle, i.e. LOAF muscles.
  L: 1st and 2nd lumbricals
  O: Opponens pollicis
  A: Abductor pollicis brevis
  F: Flexor pollicis brevis.

Special Test

- **Phalen test (Fig. 43):** Patient is asked to push the dorsal surface of both the hands and hold the wrist in complete flexion for 30-60 seconds. A positive test is determined by the onset of symptoms of carpal tunnel syndrome (CTS).
- **Reverse phalen test (Fig. 44):** Patient is asked to place the palm of both hands

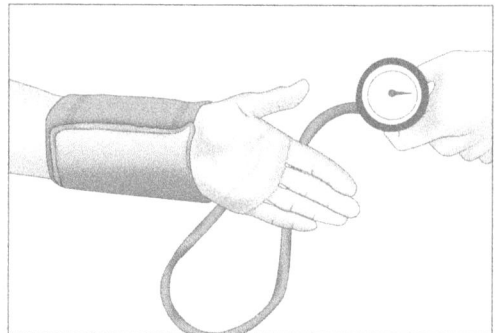

Fig. 45: Carpal compression test.

together in front of the body and raising both the elbows superiorly in a position resembling prayer position and hold this position for 30-60 seconds. A positive test is determined by the onset of symptoms of CTS.

- **Tourniquet test/Carpal compression test (Fig. 45):** Apply a blood pressure cuff to upper arm and inflate it between the systolic and diastolic pressure. This results in the onset of symptoms i n CTS due to increased pressure in carpal tunnel as a result of obstruction of venous return from arm.

CTS Preventive Measures
- Don't smoke: It interferes with blood flow and may worsen the condition.
- Avoid repetitive and strong grasping with wrist in flexed position and activities that overextends the wrist.
- Perform stretching exercises of wrist and fingers before and after activities.
- Keeping the wrist straight while sleeping or using tools.
- Appropriate treatment of conditions such as diabetes, high BP, arthritis, etc. to reduce the risk factors for developing it.

Management
Conservative Treatment
- **NSAIDs:** Helps to reduce pain and inflammation.
- **Corticosteroid:** Orally or intra-articular injection if not responding to anti-inflammatory drugs, to reduce pain and inflammation.
- **Vitamin B6 (Pyridoxine):** Helps to decrease the symptoms.
- **Diuretics** are used to remove excess amount of fluid.

Physiotherapy Treatment
- **Rest:** Avoid aggravating positions and activities.
- **Night splint:** Mueller carpal tunnel wrist brace helps to decrease pressure in carpal tunnel by maintain the wrist in neutral position.
- **To reduce pain:** Therapeutic pain relieving modalities such as TENS, IFT, Heat therapy or Cryotherapy.
- **To reduce edema:** Elevation of hand, crape bandaging or therapeutic Ultrasound.
- **Carpal bones mobilization:** It helps in improving the circulation and nerve function by relieving the pressure in carpal tunnel, increase the ROM, removing the excess fluid, break down the adhesions or scar tissue and stretching the soft tissues.
- **Nerve gliding exercises:** Nerve gliding helps to maintain the mobility of the nerves in carpal tunnel and to minimize the scarring (Figs. 46A to F).
- **Tendon gliding exercises:** Tendon glides helps to minimize the edema, improves the tissue nutrition and alleviates the chances of nerve entrapment by minimizing the nearby scarring (Fig. 47).
- **Myofascial release of flexor retinaculum of wrist:** It is used to stretch soft tissues, release tissue adhesions, eliminate the restricted motion of carpal bones, increase the length of transverse carpal ligament (TCL) to enlarge carpal tunnel space and

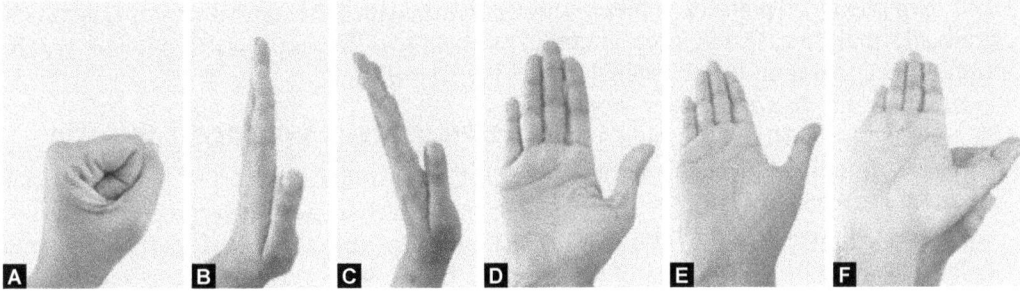

Figs. 46A to F: Median nerve gliding technique. A. Wrist in neutral with fingers and thumb in flexion; B. Wrist in neutral with thumb in neutral and fingers extended; C. Wrist and fingers are extended with thumb in neutral; D. Wrist, fingers and thumb in neutral; E. Wrist, fingers and thumb in neutral with forearm in supination; F. Opposite hand applies a gentle stretch to the thumb.

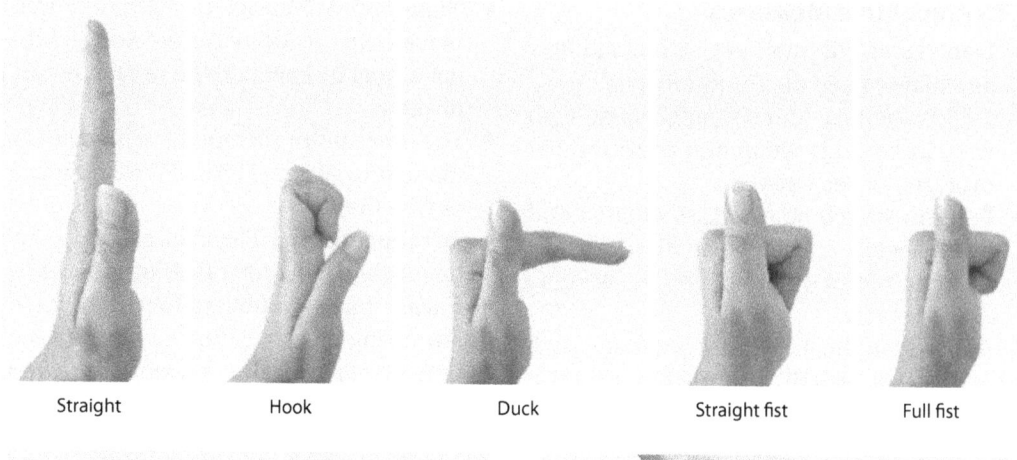
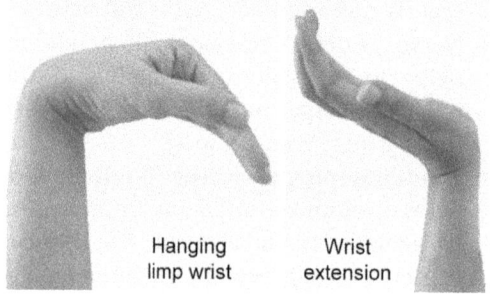
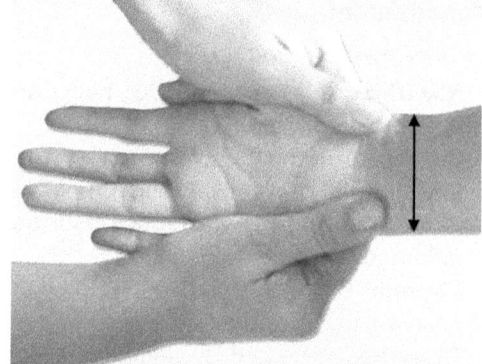

Fig. 47: Tendon gliding exercises.

Fig. 48: Myofascial release of flexor retinaculum.

lower intratunnel pressure, increase ROM, and reduce edema. In this transverse distraction is applied to retinaculum until release of restriction is attained (Fig. 48).
- **Thenar and carpal ligament release (Figs. 49A and B):** Opponens roll maneuver: Therapist holds the thenar and hypothenar region of patient and gradually pulls the thenar area laterally with moving the thumb into extension to create traction. This maneuver stretches the opponens pollicis muscle and TCL to decrease intratunnel pressure and unload the median nerve pressure.
- **Stretching exercises:** Stretching of wrist, fingers and thumb to improve the flexibility of wrist, hand, fingers and thumb.
- **Strengthening exercises:** Strengthening of hand, fingers and forearm muscles to improve the grip strength.
- **Maintain ROM:** AROM of wrist and fingers to reduce stiffness and restore mobility.

Surgical Treatment
Carpal tunnel release: It is a surgical technique in which the transverse carpal ligament is divided to decompress the median nerve in carpal tunnel.

■ PIRIFORMIS SYNDROME (FIG. 50)

Piriformis syndrome is a neuromuscular condition characterized by pain, tingling and numbness in buttock that may radiate into the hip, posterior aspect of thigh and up to the proximal portion of the leg. It is caused by the compression of sciatic nerve as it passes through the shortened, inflamed or tender piriformis muscles.

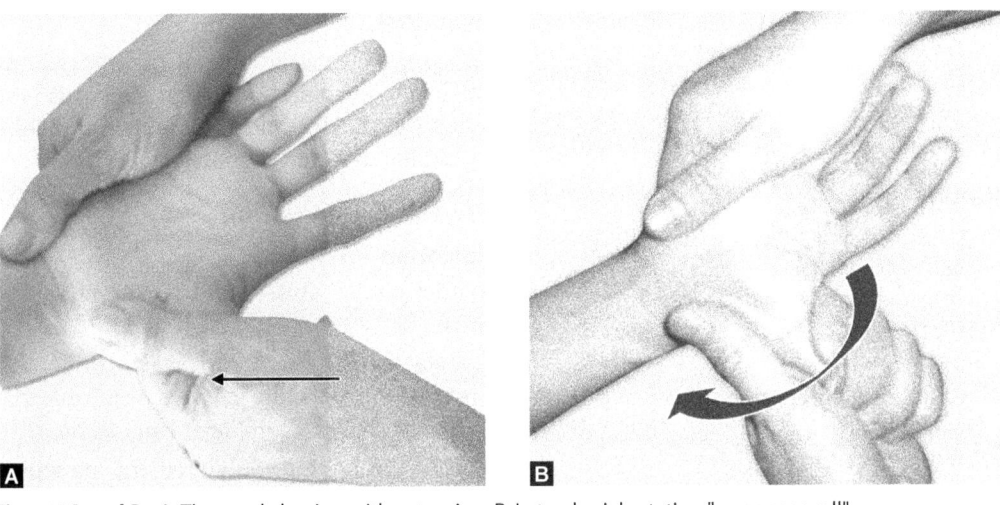

Figs. 49A and B: A. Thenar abduction with extension; B. Lateral axial rotation "opponens roll".

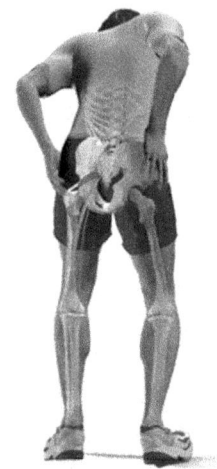

Fig. 50: Piriformis syndrome.

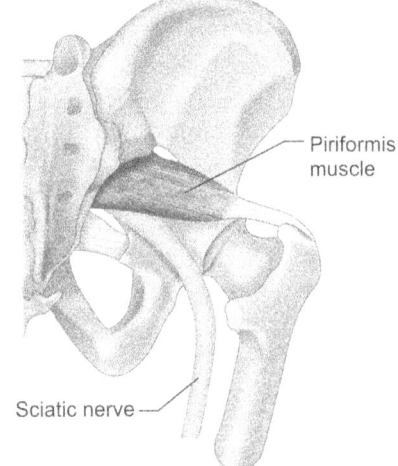

Fig. 51: Anatomy of piriformis muscle.

Anatomy

Piriformis muscle is a small muscle located deep in the buttock behind the gluteus maximus. It attaches to the anterior surface of sacrum and the greater trochanter of femur and helps in the external rotation of leg (Fig. 51).

In majority of population the sciatic nerve passing vertically beneath the piriformis muscle and therefore it is easily affected by this muscle.

Two common theories that explains the possible causes of piriformis syndrome:
1. **Tightness or spasm of piriformis muscle:** Tight piriformis muscle causes compression of sciatic nerve that is passing beneath it.
2. **Weakness of agonist muscle:** Excessive adduction and internal rotation of hip occurs during weight bearing activities due to the weakness of the agonist muscles of piriformis, i.e. gluteus maximus and/

or medius that causes the elongation and increased eccentric load on piriformis muscle. The over lengthening and high eccentric loading on piriformis may result in sciatic nerve compression or irritation.

Etiology
Exact cause is still unknown but the predisposing factors are:
- Piriformis muscle spasm
- Piriformis muscle tightness in response to injury or spasm
- Swelling or inflammation of piriformis muscle
- Prolonged sitting
- Pregnancy
- Weakness of hip adductor and external rotator.

Clinical Presentation
- Acute pain and tenderness in gluteal region
- Burning pain, numbness and tingling sensation radiating down the leg along the course of sciatic nerve
- Pain aggravates on stairs climbing, prolonged sitting or running.
- Pain decreases on lying down, walking or bending the knee
- Reduced ROM of hip joint.

Diagnosis
Imaging studies is needed to rule out the other possible conditions that may cause the symptoms, such as sacroiliac joint dysfunction or lumbar disc herniation, etc.

Physical Examination
Palpation

Tenderness in gluteal and retrotrochanteric area.

Special test: These are provocative test which are used to stretch the irritated piriformis that in turn compresses the sciatic nerve.

Freiberg test (Fig. 52): Freiberg maneuver reproduces pain when the therapist performs passive internal rotation of extended hip.

FAIR (flexion, adduction, internal rotation): FAIR maneuver reproduces pain in buttock when the therapist passively flex, adduct and internally rotate the hip joint (Fig. 53).

Management
Conservative Treatment
- **NSAIDs:** Used to reduce pain and inflammation.
- **Muscle relaxants:** Used to reduce pain and muscle spasm.

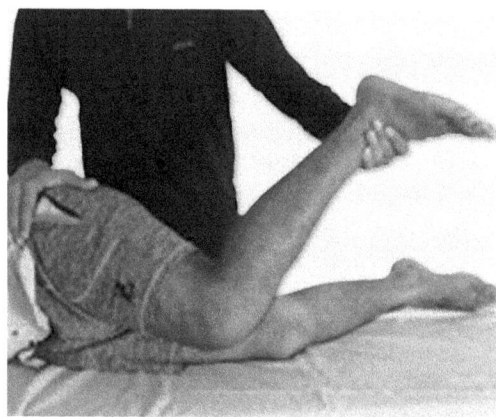

Fig. 52: Freiberg test.

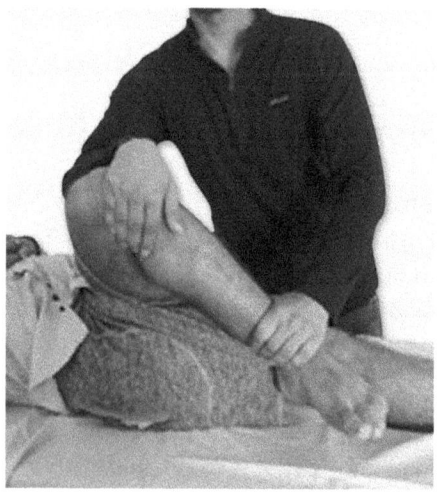

Fig. 53: FAIR test.

Physiotherapy Treatment

- **Therapeutic electrical modalities:** Helps to decrease pain and inflammation.
  - Ultrasound: 2-2 w/cm² for 10-15 minutes. US is applied in FAIR position of hip.
  - Cold application for acute cases and hot pack for chronic conditions to decrease pain and muscle spasm.
  - Laser therapy/TENS/IFT/EMS to reduce pain, inflammation and muscle spasm.
- **Massage:** It helps to decrease pain, muscle spasm and improve the extensibility of soft tissues.
- **Stretching exercises:** Piriformis muscle stretching along with stretching of hamstrings, groin, hip abductors and lower back.
- **Myofascial release at lumbosacral paraspinal muscles and trigger point release therapy:** These are used for the decompression of nerve by breaking the connective tissue adhesion in the affected area.
- **Muscle energy technique (MET) of piriformis muscle:** It helps to stretch the muscle and decompress the nerve.
- **Strengthening exercise:** Strengthening of piriformis and other hip muscles as weakness of piriformis and its agonistic muscles may be the contributing factor of causing the problem.

Surgical Management

Indications
- Not responding to conservative treatment.
- Functional disability because of progressive symptoms.
- Any underlying pathological cause e.g. hematoma, abscess, neoplasm etc.

Surgical Technique
Surgical release is done to decompress the sciatic nerve. It may be performed by tenotomy of piriformis tendon at its attachment to greater trochanter or by cutting the piriformis muscle.

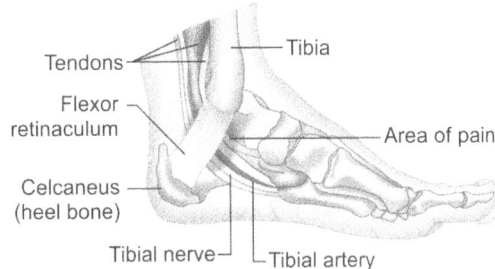

Fig. 54: Tarsal tunnel syndrome.

■ TARSAL TUNNEL SYNDROME

This condition refers to the entrapment neuropathy of posterior tibial nerve as it passes through tarsal tunnel in the foot (Fig. 54).

Anatomy of Tarsal Tunnel
Tarsal tunnel is found on the medial aspect of foot behind the medial malleolus. It is floored by posterior talus and calcaneus bone and covered with a thick fibrous band called flexor retinaculum. Inside the tunnel, the posterior tibial nerve splits into 2 branches:
1. Medial plantar nerve
2. Lateral plantar nerve.

Etiology
Any condition that increases the pressure in tarsal tunnel.
- Inflammation and swelling in or around the tunnel due to soft tissue or bony injury.
- Space occupying lesion, e.g. ganglion cyst, varicose vein, bone spur, etc.
- Repetitive activities like running, walking or jumping
- Systemic disease like diabetes or arthritis.

Types of Tarsal Tunnel Syndrome
- **Proximal tarsal tunnel syndrome:** Compression of posterior tibial nerve in tarsal tunnel.
- **Distal tarsal tunnel syndrome**
  - **Medial plantar nerve entrapment:** It is also known as jogger foot. In this the

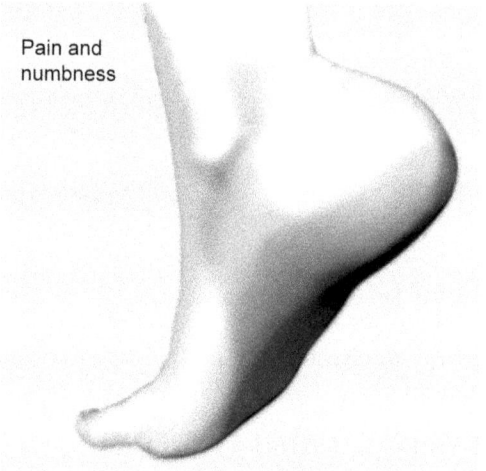

Fig. 55: Pain and numbness pattern in tarsal tunnel syndrome.

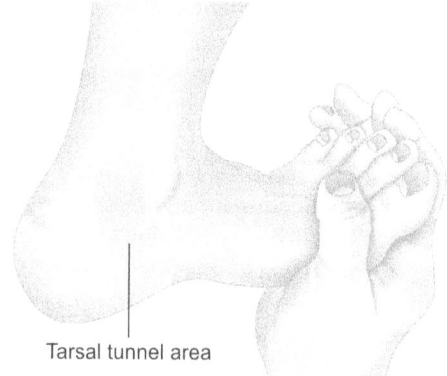

Fig. 56: Dorsiflexion-eversion test.

medial plantar nerve is compressed as it passes through the intermuscular septum of abductor hallucis muscle.
- **Lateral plantar nerve entrapment:** It is also known as Baxter neuropathy. In this lateral plantar nerve is compressed between the abductor hallucis and quadratus plantae muscle or between the flexor digitorum muscle and calcaneus.

Clinical Presentation (Fig. 55)
- Burning pain and tingling sensation in foot.
- Numbness on the plantar surface of foot.
- Radiation of paresthesia along the course of nerve.
- Pain on forced eversion and dorsiflexion of foot.
- Pain aggravates on weight bearing and relieves by rest.
- Tenderness behind the medial malleolus.

Diagnosis
- Imaging studies (X-ray, CT, MRI scan) or Ultrasonography: To determine the presence of the causative factors like ganglion, synovitis, arthritis or any soft tissue or bony injury.

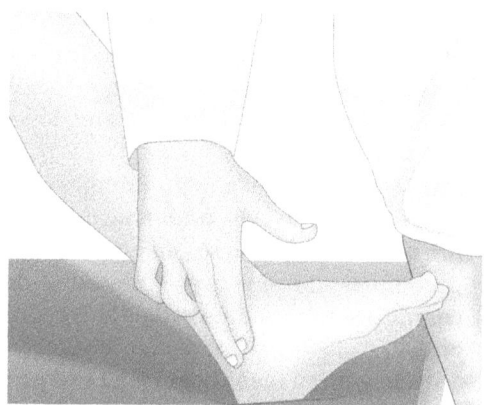

Fig. 57: Ankle Tinel's sign.

Physical Examination
Special Test
- **Dorsiflexion-eversion test (Fig. 56):** Patient is sitting with ankle in neural position. Therapist passively dorsiflex and evert the patient's ankle onset of symptoms indicates a positive test.
- **Positive Tinel's sign (Fig. 57):** Tapping over the affected nerve between the medial malleolus and Achilles tendon produces a tingling sensation that travels along the course of nerve.

Management
Conservative Treatment
- **Medication:** NSAIDs to decrease pain and inflammation.

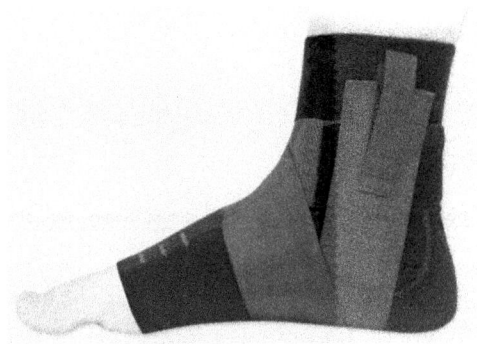

Fig. 58: Ankle brace.

- **Cryotherapy:** It is used to decrease the swelling.
- **Brace:** Immobilizing the ankle in brace is required for healing of nerve and surrounding tissue and improving the hind foot alignment (Fig. 58).

Physiotherapy Treatment
- **Pain relieving modalities:** TENS, IFT, ultrasound, neuromuscular electric stimulation or iontophoresis used to reduce pain and inflammation.
- **Plantar arch taping:** Taping is used to reduce the amount of stress on tissues.
- **Shoe modifications:** Medial heel wedge may be useful in reducing the stretch over the tibial nerve by limiting the eversion and supporting the longitudinal arch of foot.
- **Neural glide:** Tibial nerve glide is required to maintain the mobility of nerve and to break done any nearby adhesion or scar tissue. Tibial nerve glide is performed by ankle dorsiflexion with hip flexion and knee extension; it can be further sensitized by everting the ankle, extending the toes and stretching the plantar fascia.
- **Soft tissue mobilization:** Soft tissue mobilization over the area helps to break down any adhesion in the surrounding tissues and to encourage the movement of accumulated fluid in the tunnel.
- **Immobilization:** Restricting movements of foot by wearing a brace is required to heal the nerve and surrounding tissues and to maintain ideal foot biomechanics.
- **Stretching of calf muscles:** It is essential to stretch calf muscle as tight calf muscle may further cause traction of nerve due to increase pronation of foot.

Surgical Treatment

Tarsal tunnel release: It is the surgical release of tight flexor retinaculum from its attachment in foot to decompress the posterior tibial nerve.

CHAPTER 5

Spinal Disorders

■ SPONDYLOSIS

It refers to degenerative condition affecting the bones, discs and joints of spine. Therefore it is also known as *Spinal Osteoarthritis*.

Commonest Sites
- Cervical spine: C4–T1
- Lumbar spine: L2–L4
- Thoracic spine: T4–T6

Etiology
- Primary cause is age. Although it can occur at any age, however, older people are more susceptible.
- Females are more affected than males.

Predisposing Factors
- Occupations require repeated bending and lifting activities can hasten the progress of spondylosis.
- Any direct or indirect injury that causes undue physical stress and loading on disc.
- Diseases such as vertebral tumor, Pott's spine, spondylolisthesis, osteoporosis, etc.
- Congenital vertebral anomalies and disc or vertebral infection may lead to early spondylosis.

Pathophysiology
- **Degeneration of intervertebral disc (IVD):** Disc becomes hard, stiff and shrinked due to progressive decrease in water content. The shrinked disc loses its shock absorbing qualities and cause increased strain on surrounding joints and soft tissues.
- **Degeneration of facet joint:** Loss of disc height gradually causes degeneration of the facet joint due to increased mechanical stress.
- **Osteophyte formation:** Abnormal excessive bone growth known as osteophytes (Bony spur) forms on the vertebral body in an effort to repair itself.
- **Narrowing of intervertebral space:** Degeneration of IVD and bony spur formation progressively reduces the IVD space that leads to the compression of the nerve emerging from the spinal cord causing pain, paresthesia, numbness and loss of function of the areas supplied by the nerve.
- **Degeneration of spinal ligaments:** In degenerative spondylosis, ligament attached to vertebrae becomes hypertrophied, calcified and lost their strength also.
- **Fusion of intervertebral joints:** Degeneration of facet joints, fusion of bony spur and calcification of spinal ligament gradually leads to the fusion of interverbral joints.

Clinical Presentations
Depends on the stage of disc degeneration and the part of vertebral column involved.

Cervical Spondylosis
- Neck pain that worsen over time.
- Neck pain increases with movement.
- Radiating pain in arm.
- Neck stiffness particularly after night rest.

- Numbness, tingling sensation and weakness may appear in arm, hands and fingers.
- Cervical muscles spasm.
- Suboccipital headache.
- Patient may experience fatigue, disturbed sleep and impaired functional ability.
- Cervical movement restrictions in all directions.
- Loss of balance and control over bladder and bowel may occur due to significant compression of spinal cord.

Lumbar Spondylosis
- Mild and intermittent low backache.
- Pain gradual in onset, worsen on exertion and eased by rest.
- Morning low back stiffness.
- Referred pain in buttock, hip, groin and thigh.
- Paravertebral muscle spasm.
- Radiating pain in legs.
- Numbness, tingling sensation and weakness in legs and feet.
- Significant impingement of spinal cord may cause poor bowel and bladder control, unsteady gait and severe neurological problems.

Diagnosis
X-ray Findings (Fig. 1)
- Presence of osteophytes.
- Intervertebral disc space narrowing.
- Loss of cervical or lumbar lordosis.
- Uncovertebral joint hypertrophy.
- Apophyseal joint arthritis.
- Decreased vertebral canal diameter.
- Irregular articular margins.

CT scan and MRI: These are used to evaluate the soft tissue changes along with degenerative changes in bone.

Physical Examination
Palpation
- Areas of tenderness
- Assess the spinal deformities
- Paravertebral muscle spasm.

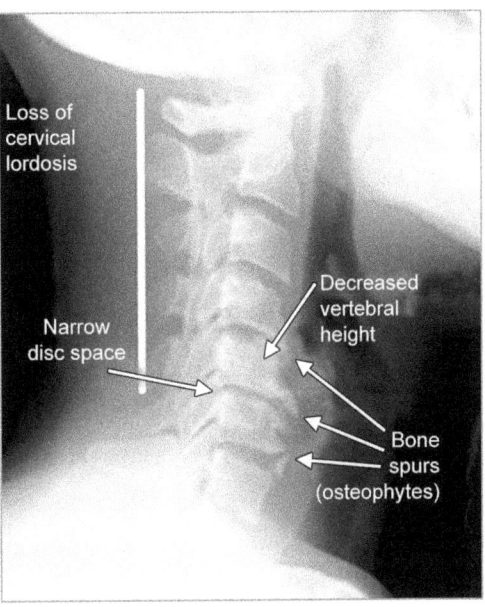

Fig. 1: X-ray findings of cervical spondylosis.

Range of Motion (ROM)
- Spinal movements, i.e. flexion, extension, lateral flexion and rotation.

Neurological Examination
- Sensory examination
- Reflexes
- Bladder/bowel changes
- Motor function.

Management
Conservative Treatment
- **Rest:** Used to relieve stress on spine and to subside the symptoms.
- **Medications:**
  - Non-steroidal anti-inflammatory drugs (NSAIDs) used to decrease pain and inflammation.
  - Muscle relaxants and analgesics are used to decrease pain and relax the paravertebral muscles.
  - Epidural steroid injection are used to decrease pain and inflammation.
- **Activity modification:**
  - Avoid repetitive bending movements and repetitive flexion and extension of spine.

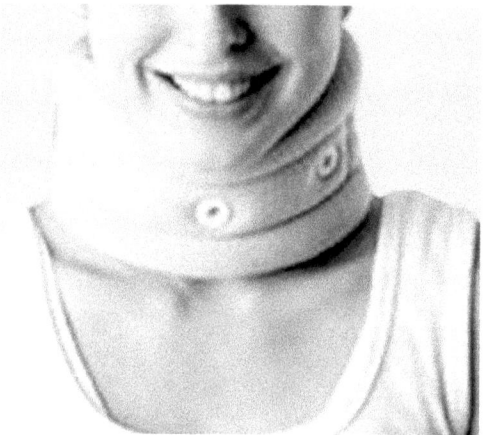

Fig. 2: Cervical collar.

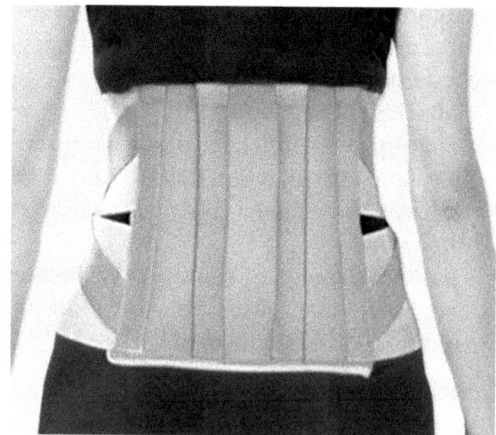

Fig. 3: Lumbar corset.

- **Corset (Figs. 2 and 3): Cervical or lumbar corset are used:**
  - To reduce excessive mechanical forces
  - To restrict spinal movements
  - To stabilize the spine in neutral position.

Physiotherapy Treatment

- **Pain relieving modalities:** Hot pack, shortwave diathermy (SWD), cold pack, ultrasound, TENS, IFT and NMES are used to reduce pain and inflammation.
- **Traction:** Gentle intermittent traction is used
  - To inhibit painful muscle response.
  - To facilitate the movement of synovial fluid within the joint that aids in the healing process and movement of the stiff joint.
  - To open the IVD space and decrease the lordosis of spine. This temporary spinal realignment relieves the mechanical stress and nerve compression.
- **Static contraction:**
  - Isometric exercises of cervical muscles for cervical spondylosis
  - Core stability exercises for lumbar spondylosis to support the spine, reduce the pain and to strengthen the abdominals and spinal extensors.
- **Mobilization:** Restoration of intersegmental mobility by accessory pressure helps to regain full functional painfree movement.
- **Gentle ROM within the limits of pain:** To maintain the mobility of spine.
- **Soft tissue techniques:** Massage is used to relieve paravertebral muscle spasm and tightness.
- **Strengthening and stretching exercises of surrounding muscles:** Used to increase the stability and flexibility of spine.
- **Relaxation:** Hydrotherapy, deep breathing exercises and physiological relaxation techniques are used to reduce discomfort and uneasiness caused by pain and muscle spasm.
- **Postural awareness:**
  - Good posture for cervical spondylosis: Straight neck with chin tucked in position.
  - For lumbar spine: While sitting, low back should be well supported by a small cushion, legs should be placed over small stool. And while sleeping, side lying is most preferred position.

SPONDYLOLISTHESIS

Greek word *"Spondylos"* means spine and *"Olisthanein"* means to slip. It is a condition of spine in which one of the vertebra slips forward or backward compared to adjacent vertebra.

Anterolisthesis is forward slippage of one vertebra on another vertebra (Fig. 4).

Retrolisthesis is backward slippage of vertebra.

Epidemiology

Most common site is between L_4-L_5 and L_5-S_1
Females are more commonly affected than males.

Etiology

- **Dysplastic/Congenital spondylolisthesis:** Includes developmental abnormalities in posterior element of vertebra, e.g. neural arch defect in upper sacrum or L5.
- **Isthmic spondylolisthesis:** Due to the defect in the portion of vertebra called pars interarticularis (PIA). The pars may be congenitally defective or undergone repeated stress under hyperextension and rotation, resulting in microfractures.
Isthmic spondylolisthesis has following subtypes:
  - Type IIA: Secondary to stress fracture of PIA.
  - Type IIB: Denotes an intact but elongated PIA.
  - Type IIC: Acute fracture of PIA.
- **Degenerative spondylolisthesis:** In this, intersegmental instability is present because of degenerative disc disease or facet arthropathy. It commonly occurs in elderly females.
- **Traumatic spondylolisthesis:** Unstable vertebral subluxation may occur due to direct trauma or injury to vertebrae.
- **Pathological spondylolisthesis:** It results from generalized or localized bone disease which causes abnormal mineralization, remodeling and attenuation of the posterior elements leading to the skip.
- **Post-surgical/iatrogenic:** Due to the loss of posterior element secondary to some surgical procedures.

Predisposing Factors

- Genetic predisposition
- Repetitive trauma or hyperextension of lower back.
- Athletic activities, e.g. gymnasts, weight lifters, etc.

Meyerding classification (Fig. 5): Meyerding grades the slippage on the basis of the degree of displacement of vertebra.

Meyerding classification divides the superior endplate of the caudal vertebra into four quarter and measures the percentage of slippage.

- **Grade I:** Slippage of 0–25%, i.e. up to ¼ length of vertebra.
- **Grade II:** Slippage of 25–50%, i.e. up to ½ length of vertebra.
- **Grade III:** Slippage of 50–75%, i.e. up to ¾ length of vertebra.
- **Grade IV:** Slippage of 75–100%.
- **Grade V:** More than 100%, i.e. when the vertebra completely dislocates from the supporting vertebra. It is also known as *spondyloptosis*.

Clinical Presentation

- Low back pain which may feel like muscle strain.

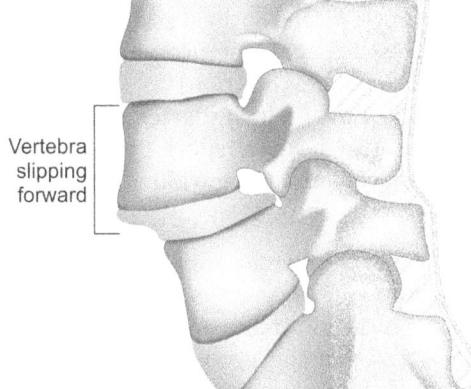

Fig. 4: Anterolisthesis.

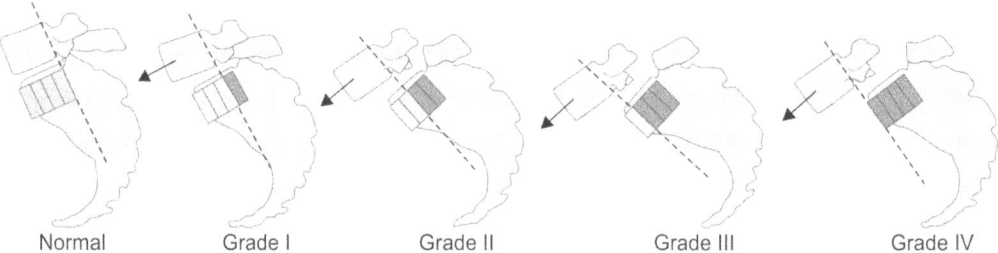
Fig. 5: Meyerding classification.

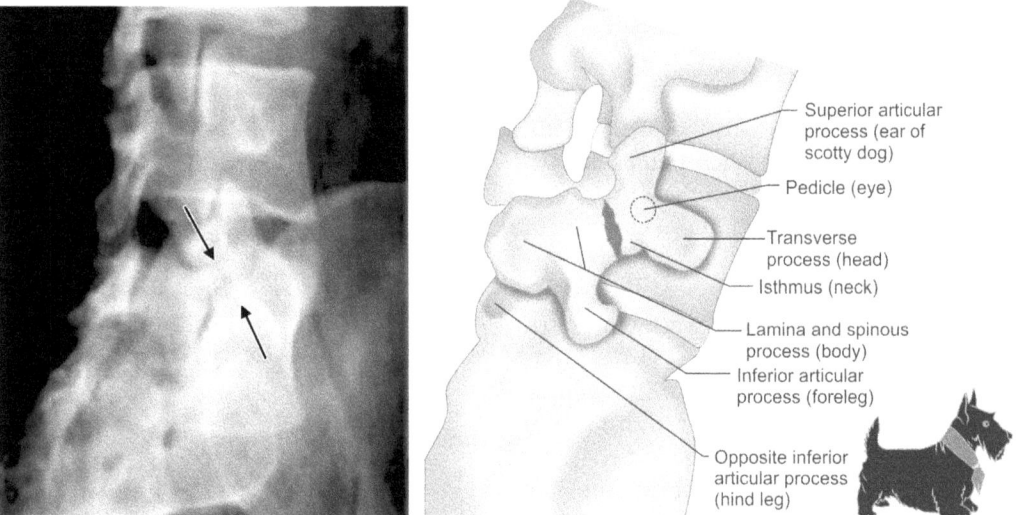
Fig. 6: X-ray finding: Scotty dog appearance.

- Pain worsens with standing and walking and relieved by sitting and lying down.
- Patient can bend forward only by the support of his hands kept on his knees and feels a sudden jerk while returning back from bending position.
- Stiffness in the back.
- Nerve compression may cause radiating pain, numbness or weakness in the leg.
- Significant spinal cord compression may cause the loss of bowel and bladder function or cauda equine syndrome.

Diagnosis

X-ray findings: Pars interarticularis identified by break or collar in neck of "**Scotty dog appearance**" on oblique view (Fig. 6).

Physical Examination

Palpation

- Tenderness over lumbosacral region (easier to palpate in fetal position as the paraspinal muscles becomes thinned and the defect opens up in this position)
- "**STEP**" can be felt on affected region when fingers run down the spine.
- Spasm of hamstring and glutei muscles.

Observation

- Increased lumbar lordosis.
- Sacrum appears to extend to the waist and transverse loin crease is seen.
- Sometimes associated with scoliosis.

Range of motion: Commonly associated with reduced spinal ROM and lumbopelvic rhythm.

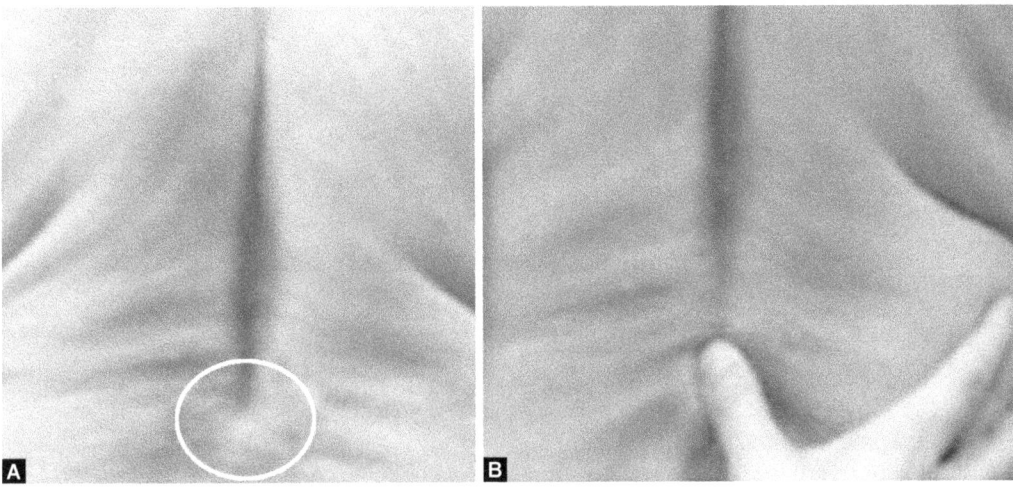

Figs. 7A and B: Low midline sill sign test.

Muscle tightness: Hamstring tightness is usually present.

Special Tests

- **Low midline sill sign test:** Therapist inspect the midline of patient's low back and notice for any increased lumbar lordosis and sill like capital "L" on the midline. If the sill is present then the therapist palpate the interspinous space in the area of the sill and evaluates the upper spinous position in relation to the lower spinous position. The test is considered to be positive if sill like capital "L" and the displacement of anterior spinous process in relation to the lower spinous process is palpated (Figs. 7A and B).
- **Interspinous gap change test for lumbar instability:** Patient stands with feet shoulder width apart in front of the examine table. Ask the patient to flex his back with both the hands on the edge of table. Therapist inspect the midline of lower back of the patient for any change in interspinous space. If interspinous space is wide or bent than adjacent interspinous space, the therapist then palpates and evaluate the width of the individual interspinous space and the position of upper spinous process in relation to the lower spinous process.

Thereafter the patient is asked to extend or to hollow the lower back, the therapist evaluates the change in interspinous gap during the motion. The test is considered to be positive if the width of interspinous space abruptly becomes narrow as compare to adjacent space or when the position of upper spinous process changes in relation to lower spinous process during the flexion and extension movements (Fig. 8).

Management

According to grades of slippage.
- Grade I and II can be managed conservatively.
- Grade III and IV require surgical intervention.

Conservative Treatment

- **NSAIDs:** To reduce pain and inflammation.
- **Analgesics:** To reduce pain.
- **Steroid:** It may be used to get immediate pain relieving effect. It also reduces the swelling and inflammation.
- **Epidural steroid injection:** It involves the injection of steroid and an analgesic numbing agent in epidural space of spine

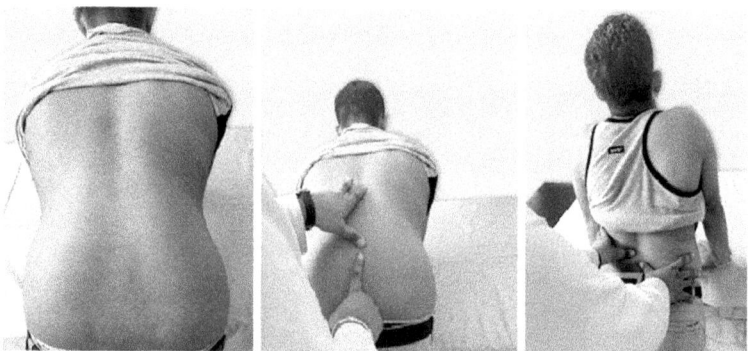

Fig. 8: Interspinous gap change test.

to reduce pain, swelling and inflammation. Results observed in 50% cases but are temporary. If injections prove to be helpful then they can be done up to 3 times a year.

Physiotherapy Treatment

Aims
- To control pain.
- Restoration of normal function.
- To maintain maximum correction of exaggerated lordosis.

Treatment
- **Bracing:** Brace may help to decrease pain and muscle spasm by immobilizing the spine and facilitating the healing process. Thoracolumbosacral orthosis (modified Boston overlap brace) (Fig. 9) is used to prevent lordosis. The orthosis should wear for 23 hrs/day up to 6 months to 1 year.
- **Activity modification:** Avoid pain aggravating activities, e.g. Spinal extension for around one to two months.
- **Electrotherapeutic modalities:** These modalities are used to control pain and muscle spasm
  - SWD, Hot pack, TENS, IFT or US
- **Stretching exercises:** Stretching of hip flexors, hamstring, rectus femoris, tensor fascia lata, lumbar erector spine muscle and paraspinal muscles helps to reduce the undue strain on unstable vertebrae by restoring the normal alignment of pelvis

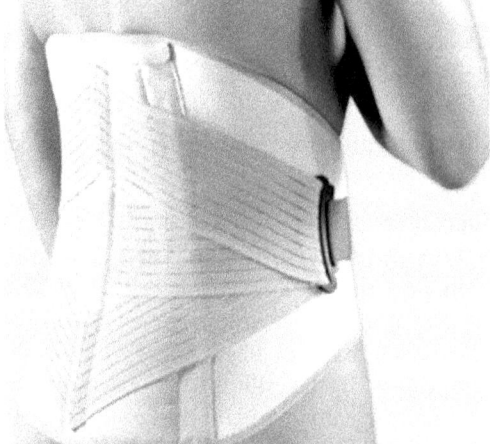

Fig. 9: Modified Boston overlap brace.

and maintaining the neutral position of spine.
  - Initially hamstring stretching should be given in spinal flexion position and then in neutral spine position to decrease the abrupt stress on the posterior elements during the stretch.
- **Strengthening exercises:** It helps to maintain the segmental spinal mechanism and to increase the stability of the spine. Strengthening of core muscle of spine, i.e. deep abdominal muscle, multifidus and paraspinal muscle. These muscles help to support the spine and maintain the neutral alignment of pelvis and thereby reduce the stress on the unstable vertebrae.

- Deep abdominal muscle (transverse abdominus, rectus abdominus, internal and external oblique) strengthening exercises.
- Active posterior tilting: To compensate the exaggerated lumbar lordosis.
- Strengthening multifidus muscle has the ability to pull the vertebra backward and to stabilize the condition directly.
* **Guidelines for postural correction and its maintenance.**
  - Prone lying is advised to control advancement of lordosis.
* **Muscle relaxation training by using biofeedback** helps to reduce pain and paravertebral muscle spasm.
* **Spinal flexion exercise program**, for e.g. sitting on a chair with back resting, then gradually bending the trunk forward from the lumbar region. Spinal flexion exercise helps to decrease stress on posterior element.

Surgical Treatment

Indication
* Slip is progressing
* Persistence of symptoms despite of aggressive conservative treatment
* Intense pain
* Slippage of Grade III and IV
* High slip angle.

Surgical Interventions

Spinal fusion is performed with or without the reduction of the slippage to prevent the further progression of slippage.

■ ANKYLOSING SPONDYLITIS (FIG. 10)

It is a chronic inflammatory disease characterized by progressive stiffness of joints of axial skeletal especially sacroiliac joint.

Epidemiology
* It may occur at any age but usually the age of onset is between 18–30 years.
* Males are more commonly affected than females with the ratio of 3:1.

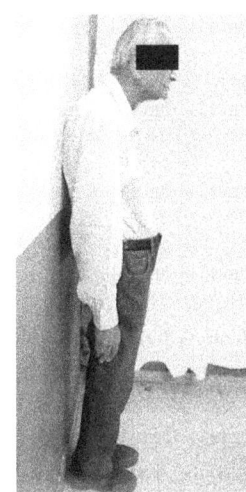

Fig. 10: Ankylosing spondylitis.

* Genetic predisposition: First degree relatives are at major risk of developing this condition.

Etiology

Although the exact cause of ankylosing spondylitis is not known, genetics plays a key role in the disease.
* People having genetic factor "HLA B27" are at greatly increased risk of developing ankylosing spondylitis.

Pathogenesis (Fig. 11)
* **Synovitis:** Initially the inflammation of the synovial membrane occurs. Synovitis most commonly starts from SI joint followed by other region of the spine.
* **Enthesopathy:** This is an inflammatory reaction at the Enthesis, i.e. zone of ligamentous attachment to the bone. It occurs commonly in spine and near the pelvis.
* **Capsular inflammation:** Capsular inflammation occurs after the inflammation of the synovium and ligament.
* **Cartilage destruction and bony erosion:** Cartilage of the involved joint gets destroyed and bone becomes eroded. This occurs due to the inflammation of periarticular structures.

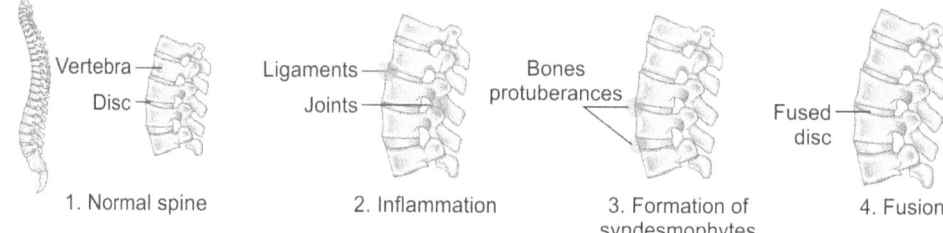

Fig. 11: Pathogenesis of ankylosing spondylitis.

- **Ossification:** All the above factors leads to the formation of new bones at the edges of the bones and bridging takes place between the vertebral bodies along the outer layer of the disc. This is known as *"Marginal syndesmophyte formation"*. The formation of syndesmophyte usually starts at dorsolumbar region. Ossification also occurs in the anterior and posterior longitudinal ligament along with other ligaments of the spine.
- **Bony ankylosis:** Gradually fusion of all the vertebrae of the spine occurs and this condition is known as *"Bamboo spine"*. After the fusion of the bone the pain may subside but the spine becomes permanently stiff.

Clinical Presentation

- Pain at the site of tendon insertion like heel and pelvic girdle.
- Pain and stiffness of lower back, sacroiliac joint that may radiate down the legs.
- Pain worsens at night.
- Stiffness is worse in the morning or after the period of rest.
- Pain and stiffness in other joint might also present, e.g. neck, upper back, shoulder, ribs, knee and feet (Fig. 12A).
- Chest pain due to the ossification of costovertebral joints or involvement of heart or lung.
- Eye pain, visual changes and increased watering.
- Fatigue, weight loss, loss of appetite and fever are the less common symptoms.

Extra-articular Manifestations (Fig. 12B)

- **A**ortic valve problems.
- **N**eurologic: Myelopathy secondary to atlanto-axial subluxation.
- **K**idney: Renal amyloidosis.
- **S**pine: Vertebral fracture, osteoporosis
- **P**ulmonary: Apical pulmonary fibrosis.
- **O**cular: Anterior uveitis, conjunctivitis (20–30%, pain and redness of the eyes).
- **N**ephropathy
- **D**iscitis

Complications

- Cauda equina syndrome
- Spinal cord compression
- Reduced chest expansion and vital capacity
- Risk for chest infection.

Diagnosis

- ESR: It is commonly raised in proportion to the inflammation activity.
- HLA B27: This is positive in about 90% of patients.
- Pulmonary function test: Diminished vital and total lung capacity and increased residual volume.

X-ray Findings

- **Sacroiliac joint (Fig. 13):**
  - Periarticular sclerosis of ilium and sacrum
  - Narrowing of joint space
  - Haziness of joint margins.

Spinal Disorders

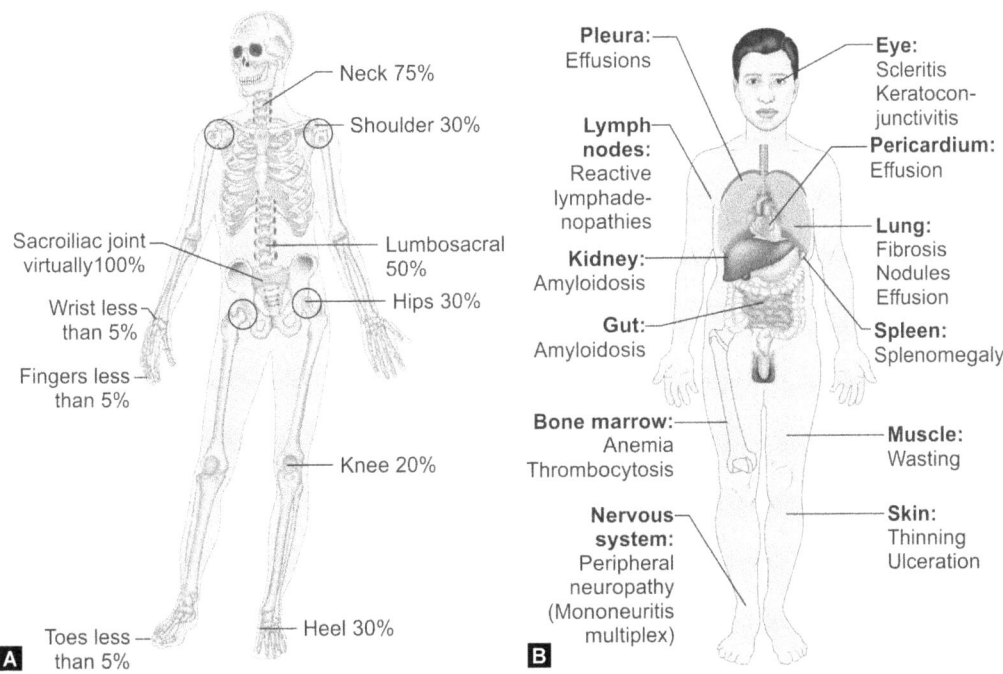

Figs. 12A and B: A. Articular manifestations; B. Extra-articular manifestations.

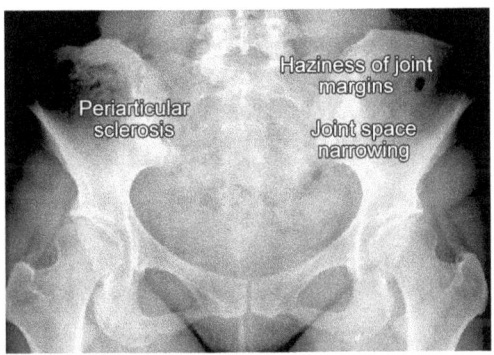

Fig. 13: X-ray finding of sacroiliac joint in AS.

- **Spine (Fig. 14):**
  - Squaring of vertebral body, i.e. loss of anterior concavity of vertebral body.
  - Romanus sign: It is erosion surrounded by the sclerosis at the margins of vertebral body.
  - Syndesmophyte formation.
  - Arthritic changes.
  - Atlantoaxial subluxation.
  - Calcification of paraspinal ligaments.
  - Fusion of apophyseal joints.

Diagnostic criterion: Presence of criterion B with any one clinical criterion OR Presence of any 4 clinical criterions in the absence of radiological findings.

A. Clinical criterion:
- Low back pain (LBP) and stiffness for more than 3 months not relieved by rest.
- Pain and stiffness in thoracic region.
- Limited motion in lumbar spine.
- Limited chest expansion.
- History of evidence of iritis or its sequel.

B. Radiological criterion:
Bilateral S-I changes of ankylosing spondylitis.

Physical Examination

Test for Sacroiliac Joint

- **Lateral compression test:** Patient is placed in side-lying position. Lateral compression of pelvis will reproduce the pain in SI joint (Fig. 15).
- **Gaenslens test:** Patient is placed in supine lying position with buttock of the affected side over the edge of the couch to allow the hyperextension at hip. Therapist passively

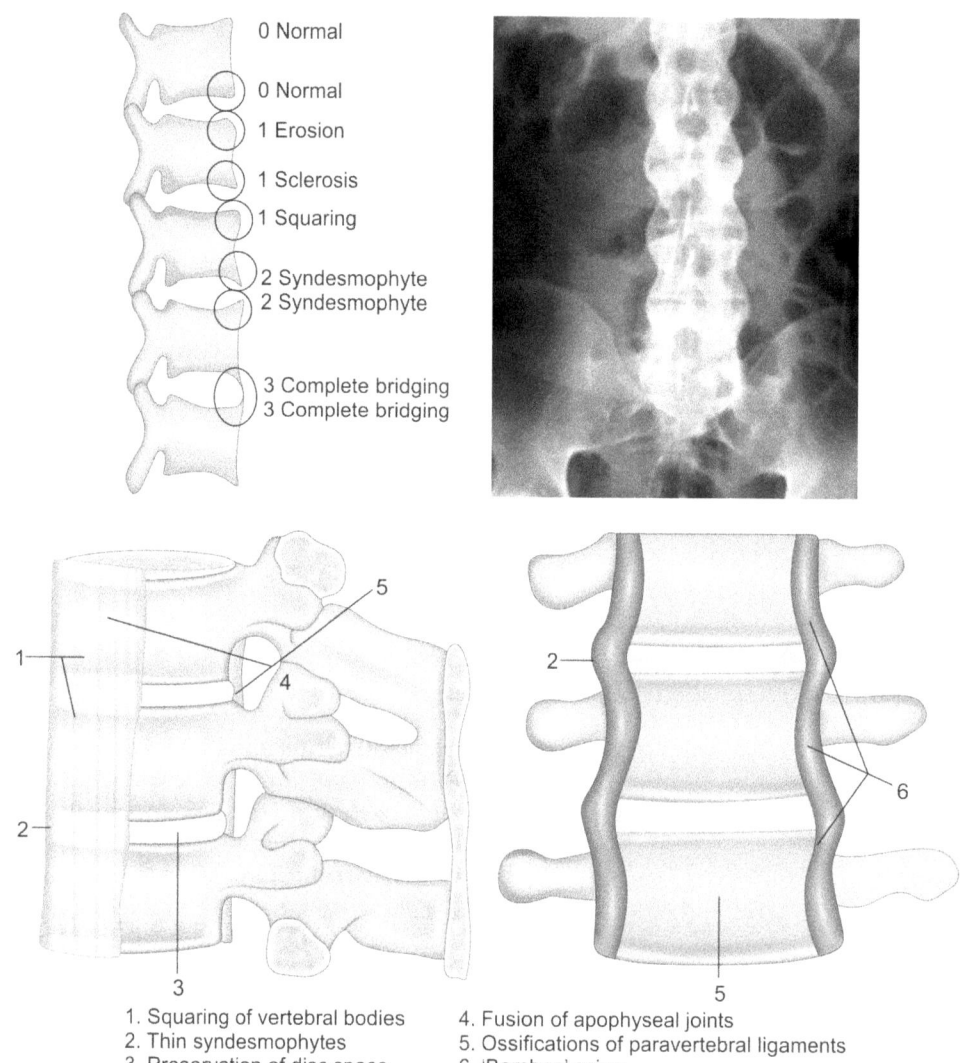

Fig. 14: X-ray findings of spine.

flexes the hip and knee of the unaffected side towards the chest of the patient. The test is considered to be positive if this reproduces the pain in the SI joint in the hyperextended side (Fig. 16).

- **Pump handle test:** Patient is placed in supine position. Therapist flexes the hip and knee of affected joint and tries to push the flexed knee towards the shoulder of opposite side. The test is considered to be positive if pain is felt in SI joint of the affected side (Fig. 17).

Cervical spine: ROM of the spine is restricted and flexion deformity develops at cervical spine.

- **Tragus to wall test:** It is used to evaluate the flexion deformity of cervical spine. Patient is asked to stand against the flat surface and the therapist measures the distance between the tragus of ear and the

Spinal Disorders

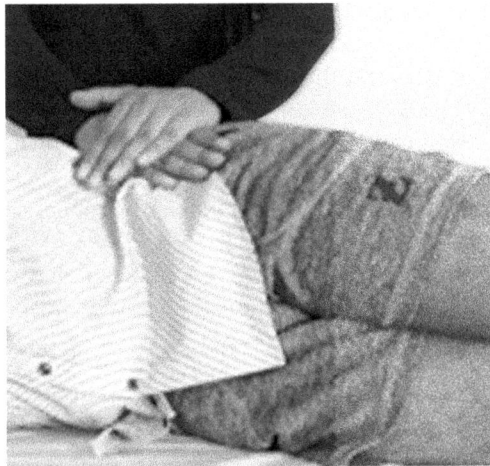

Fig. 15: Lateral compression test.

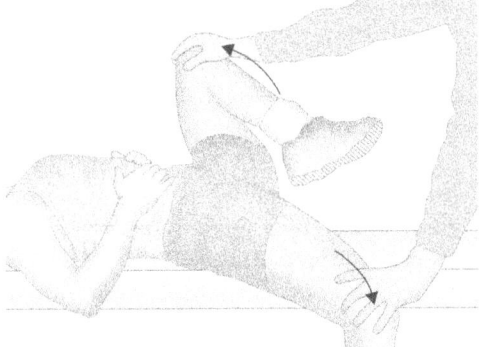

Fig. 16: Gaenslens test.

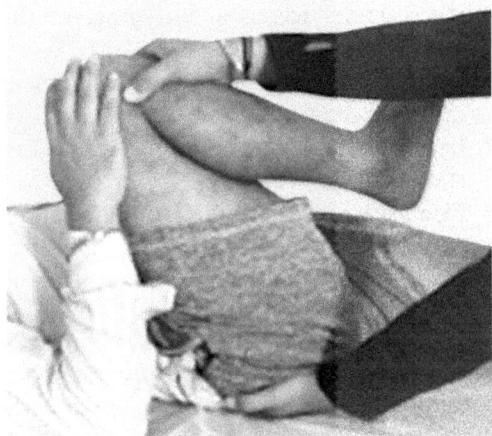

Fig. 17: Pump handle test.

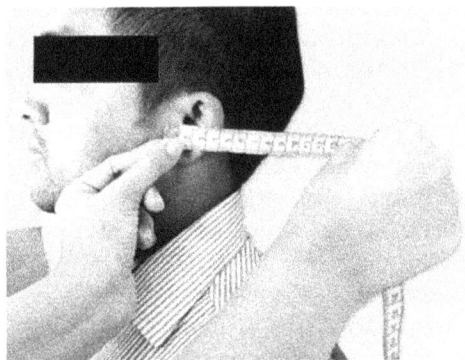

Fig. 18: Tragus to wall test.

wall. Normal tragus to wall distance is less than 15 cm. More than 15 cm is considered to be flexion deformity (Fig. 18).

- **Flesche test or occiput to wall distance:** Patient stands against the wall and asked to touch the back of head to the wall without the upward movement of chin, i.e. to maintain the neutral position of spine. The test is considered to be positive if the patient is not able to touch the occiput to the wall. Normal occiput to wall distance should be Zero (Fig. 19).

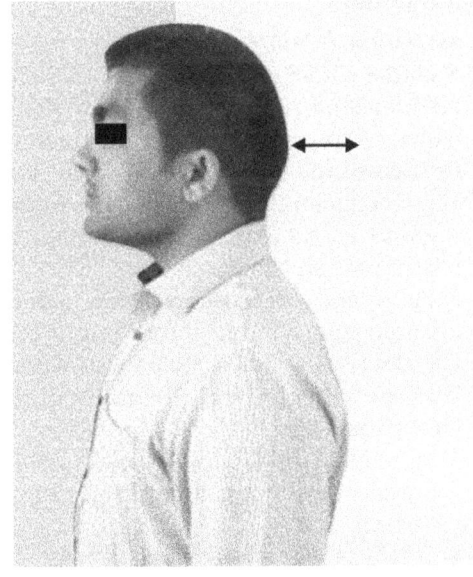

Fig. 19: Flesche test.

- **Thoracolumbar, lumbar and lumbosacral ROM:** Active and passive ROM of flexion, extension, lateral bending and rotation are measured using Goniometer.
- **Peripheral joint movements:** Active and passive ROM of all the joints should be examined especially hip, knee, shoulder and temporomandibular joints.
- **Lung function test:**
  - Involvement of costovertebral joints are examined using spirometer that measures the volume of air inspired and expired by lungs.
  - Rib cage movement is examined by measuring chest expansion using measuring tape. In adult the normal chest expansion around the level of nipple at the end of deep inspiration and expiration is 2–5 inches.
- **Postural deformity:** Spondylometer is used for the measurement of postural deformity. Usually "**QUESTION MARK deformity**" is present, i.e. the loss of secondary curve of lumbar and cervical lordosis and increase of thoracic kyphotic curve.

Management

Conservative Treatment

- **NSAIDs:** NSAIDs reduces pain and inflammation but do not prevent tissue damage or progressive joint deterioration.
- **Corticosteroid drugs:** Steroids are usually recommended for those who do not respond to NSAIDs. These are used to reduce pain and inflammation.
  NSAIDs and corticosteroid can reduce inflammation but are not disease modifying and do not prevent joint destruction.
- **Disease modifying anti-rheumatic drugs (DMARDs):**
  - It reduces inflammation e.g. methotrexate, hydroxychloroquine, sulfasalazine.
  - It reduces or prevents joint damage.
  - It preserves joint structure and function.
- **Biologic DMARDs:**
  - It reduces the pain and stiffness.
  - It blocks the immune system messenger called cytokines.
  - A cytokine TNFα is known to be involved in causing AS.
  - Anti-TNFα agent block the effect of cytokines
  - These agents can be injected in the skin or intravenously, e.g. etanercept, infliximab.

Physiotherapy Treatment

General instruction to patients:
- Exercise on regular and daily basis.
- Heat and cold application prior to the exercises.
- Start gentle exercises and progress the exercises gradually.
- Pay attention to the postures and alignment during exercise.
- Exercise should be performed on a firm surface.
- Exercise gently without causing any jerk.
- Avoid holding the breath while exercising.
- Exercise should not increase pain.

Treatment

- **To reduce pain:** Electrotherapeutic modalities are used to reduce pain and muscle spasm.
  - Superficial heating modalities like Infrared, hot packs and steam bath.
  - Cryotherapy.
  - IFT/TENS/US.
- **Mobility exercises:** Mobility exercises are used for maintaining the range of motion.
  - AROM exercises for upper and lower extremity (especially of the joints that are more involved like shoulder joint, hip joint and knee joint).
  - Thoracic mobility exercises.
  - Spinal mobility exercises (extension exercises are advisable to counteract flexion deformity).

- **Flexibility exercises:** Flexibility exercises helps to:
  - Correct and maintain an erect posture.
  - Prevent tightness and contracture of soft tissue.
  - Maintain and improve the mobility of joint.
  - Reduce the risk of injury during exercise.
  - Reduce soreness after exercise.

  Gentle static stretching of calf muscles, hamstring, hip flexors, lumbar erector spinae, pectoralis, latissimus dorsi, upper trapezius and levator scapulae muscle should be incorporated in the treatment to prevent any postural deformity.

- **Joint mobilization:** Joint mobilization helps in mitigating capsular restrictions, breaking adhesions, distracting impacted tissues and provides lubrication of normal articular cartilage. It also decreases the pain and muscle tension through the stimulation of fast conducting fibers to block fast conducting fibers and through the activation of dynamic mechanoreceptors to produce reflexive relaxation. Mobilization of facet joint, SI joint and costovertebral joints helps to improve the chest expansion, posture and spinal mobility.

- **Hydrotherapy:** It helps to
  - To reduce pain and muscle spasm: Warm water provide relaxation effect to the tight and spasmodic muscles.
  - To maintain or improve the joint mobility without loading the joint.
  - To strengthen weak muscles.
  - To improve the circulation.
  - To improve the functional abilities.
  - To improve the balance and coordination.

- **Prevent and correct deformity by postural awareness:**
  - Maintain erect posture during sitting, standing or walking.
  - Sleeping posture: Patient should sleep on a firm mattress using a thin or no pillow to maintain the spine in extended position.
  - Sitting posture:
    – Patient should use an upright chair with some cushioning to support the lower lumbar spine.
    – Avoid low arm chair.
    – Table height should be adjusted according to the height of chair so that the patient does not stoop on the table.
  - Avoid prolonged immobilization or bed rest that could lead to weakness of spinal extensors.

- **Breathing exercises:** It helps to increase chest expansion and vital capacity.
  - Apical breathing exercises.
  - Diaphragmatic breathing exercises
  - Lateral coastal breathing exercises
  - Deep breathing exercises
  - Resisted exercises for inspiratory muscles
  - Ballooning exercises.

- **Massage:** Massage helps to reduce pain, stress, stiffness and improves the flexibility.

- **Aerobic exercises:** Aerobic exercises help to improve and maintain the cardiorespiratory fitness by improving the capacity and efficacy of lung and heart. Additionally, it also increases the feeling of wellbeing by facilitating the release of endorphins and decreasing the level of stress hormone in the body. Aerobic exercises such as swimming, walking, jogging and cycling are used in ankylosing spondylitis for cardiorespiratory conditioning.

- **Yoga:** Yoga incorporates exercises and postures aimed at maintaining balance in body through strength and flexibility. It uses the combinations of stretches, postures and poses with deep breathing which also promotes relaxation. The roles

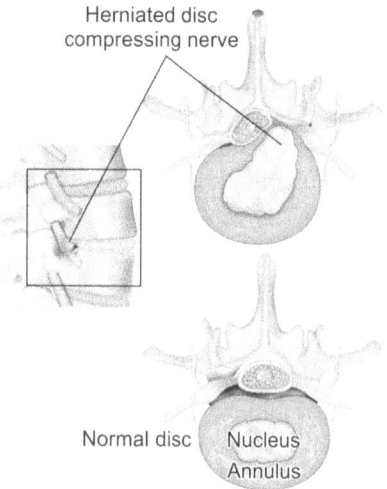

Fig. 20: Intervertebral disc herniation.

to Yoga in Ankylosing spondylitis are to maintain an erect posture, balance and improving strength and flexibility along with whole body relaxation.

■ PROLAPSED INTERVERTEBRAL DISEASE (PIVD)

PIVD refers to the herniation of nucleus pulposus through a rent in annulus fibrosus of intervertebral disc into the spinal canal (Fig. 20).

Causes
- Sudden strenuous activity like lifting heavy weight, twisting violently, etc.
- Occupation require repetitive bending, lifting and prolonged sitting.
- Poor and inadequate strength of the trunk muscles.
- Being overweight.
- Through traumatic injury such as Road traffic accident (RTA) or fall.
- Recurrent episodes of back strain.
- Advance age.

Types of Disc Herniation (Fig. 21)
- **Central bulge:** The bulge pushes the center of spinal canal and spinal cord that impinge the dura.
  - In lower lumbar segment, central herniation may result in S1 radiculopathy.
  - Less frequently a protruded disc above L2 may result in cauda equina syndrome.
- **Paramedial/Posterolateral bulge:** The bulge pushes towards the posterior and left side or posterior and right side which can impinge the nerve roots.
  - Posterolateral herniation does not affect the nerve corresponding in number to that of intervertebral disc.
  - Protruded disc usually compress the next lower nerve as that nerve crosses the level of disc in its path to its foramen.
  - For example: L4–L5 herniation will impinge L5 nerve root (Fig. 22).
- **Lateral bulge:** The bulge pushes towards the left or right side of the spinal canal where it may impinge the nerve roots that branches off the spinal cord in intervertebral foramen.
  - It compresses the nerve above the level of herniation.

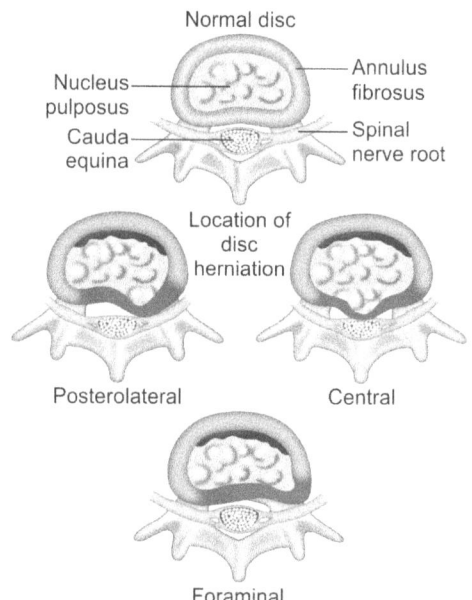

Fig. 21: Types of herniation.

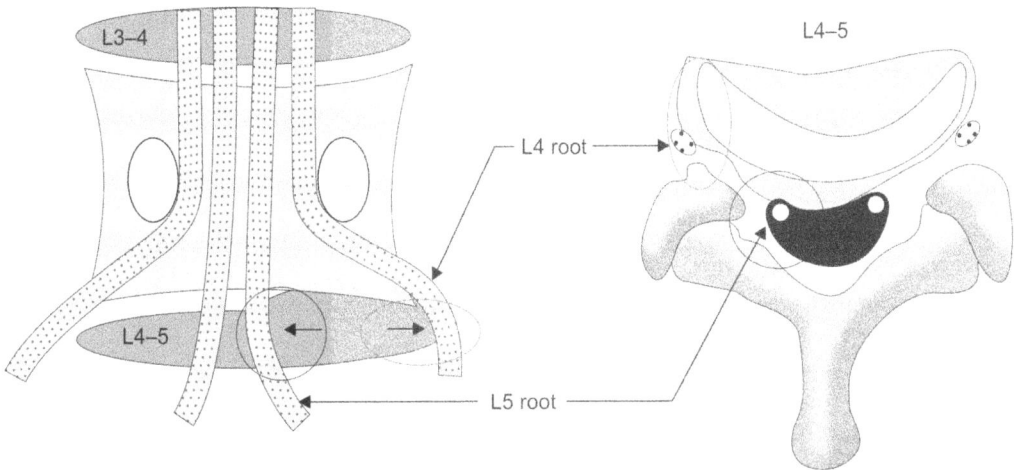

Fig. 22: Anatomy of lumbar disc herniation and nerve root impingement.

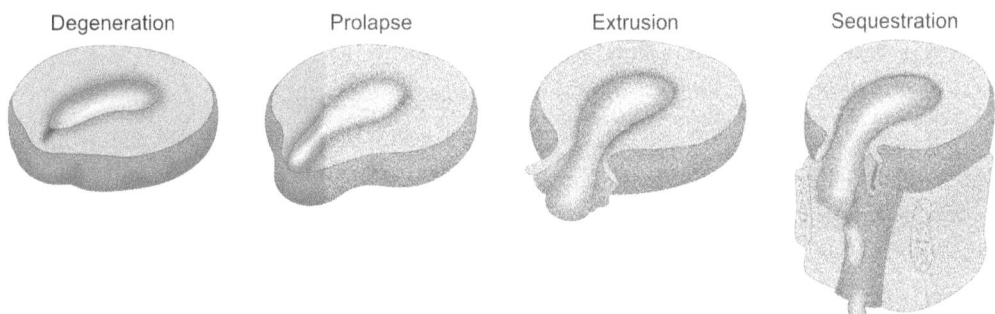

Fig. 23: Four stages to a disc herniation.

- For example: L4–L5 herniation will impinge L4 nerve root (Fig. 22).

Site

- Lumbosacral region (L4-5 and L5-S1): 80%
- Lower cervical region (C5-6 and C6-7): 19%
- Dorsal region: 1%

Pathogenesis

It has four stages (Fig. 23):
1. **Nucleus degeneration:** Degenerative changes gradually causing fragmentation of nucleus pulposus (NP) and softening of annulus fibrosis (AF) results in weakening and disintegration of posterior part of annulus.
2. **Nucleus prolapsed:**
    - **Nucleus protrusion:** When annulus becomes weak, the nucleus bulges into annulus posterolaterally or laterally and causes a bulge.
    - **Nucleus extrusion:** Finally, the NP comes out of AF and lies under posterior longitudinal ligament (PLL) though it has not lost contact with the parent disc. Once extruded, the disc does not go back. PLL is not strong enough to prevent the further protrusion of nucleus pulposus.
3. **Stage of sequestration:** The extruded disc may lose its contact with parent disc then it is known as sequestrated disc.

4. **Stage of fibrosis:** Extruded NP becomes flattened, fibrosed and finally undergoes calcification. At the same time new bone formation occurs at points where PLL has been stripped from vertebral body.

Clinical Presentation

Lumbar Disc Herniation
- Severe low back pain (LBP).
- Radiating pain in legs, buttocks and feet.
- Pain worsens with coughing, straining or laughing.
- Paravertebral muscle spasm.
- Tingling or numbness in legs or feet.
- In later stages, muscle weakness or atrophy of the posterior compartment of lower extremity may occur.
- Loss of bladder and bowel control may occur in case of significant impingement.
- Postural scoliosis (contralateral protective scoliosis with disc prolapsed occurs on the lateral side of involved nerve root and ipsilateral scoliosis with the disc prolapsed occurs on the medial side of involved nerve root) (Fig. 24).

Cervical Disc Herniation
- Deep pain near or over the shoulder blades on the affected side.
- Radiating pain in the shoulder, upper arm, forearm and rarely in the hand, fingers or chest (less common because of the comparative smaller size of cervical disc).
- Pain worsens with coughing, straining or laughing.
- Neck pain on the posterior and lateral aspect along with the spasm of neck muscles.
- Pain increases on flexion and rotation of neck.
- Tingling and numbness sensation in one arm
- Arm muscle weakness.

Diagnosis

Imaging Studies
- **X-ray findings** show decreased disc space, facet hypertrophy and bone spur (osteophytes)
- **CT scan, MRI and myelography** will determine the stage and location of herniated disc.

Physical Examination

Palpation: Tenderness of cervical or lumbar spine. Paravertebral muscle spasm present.

Special Tests for Lumbar Disc Herniation
- **Straight leg raising test:** Patient lies in supine position. Therapist passively flexes the hip while keeping the hip in medial rotation, adduction and knee in fully extended position. Test is considered positive if the pain reproduces at back or leg (Fig. 25).

Different degree of hip flexion and their possible causes:
- **Between 0–30° of hip flexion:** Pain at less than 30° hip flexion might be due to spondylolisthesis, gluteal abscess, disc protrusion or extrusion, tumor of buttock, acute dural inflammation or a malingering patient.
- **Between 30–70°:** Leg and low back pain between 30–70° of hip flexion may be due to the disc herniation at L4–S1 nerve roots.
- **Above 70°:** Pain at more than 70° of hip flexion may be due to tightness of

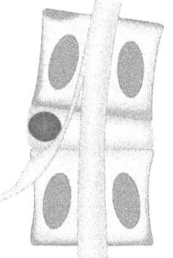
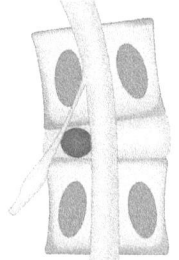

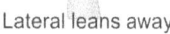
Lateral leans away   Medial leans towards

Fig. 24: Protective scoliosis in relation to the disc herniation.

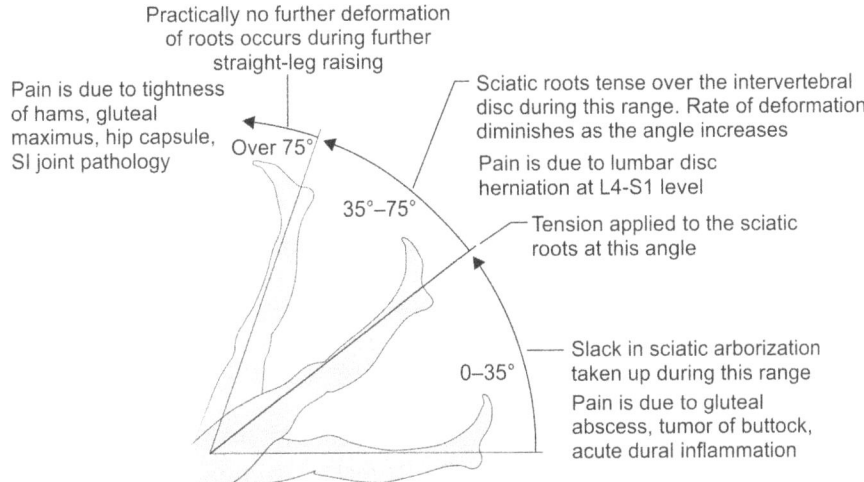

Fig. 25: Straight leg raising test.

hamstring muscles, gluteus maximus muscle, hip capsule or pathology of hip or sacroiliac joints.
- Inclusion of neck flexion in SLR is known as **Hyndman sign, Brudzinski sign, Linder sign or Soto-Hall test**.
- Inclusion of ankle dorsiflexion in SLR is known as **Lasegue test or Bragard test**.
- Inclusion of great toe extension in SLR is known as **Sicard test**.
- **Bowstring test:** Patient lies in supine position. Therapist performs passive SLR on the affected side. If this will elicit the pain then therapist flexes the knee until the disappearance of pain and then applies pressure with the thumbs on the popliteal fossa that will reproduce the pain again. This reproduction of pain indicates the sciatic nerve pathology (Figs. 26A and B).
- **Femoral stretch test/Nachlas test:** Patient lies in prone position. Therapist passively flexes the knee to the thigh. Anterior thigh pain indicates the protrusion at levels of L2-L3 and L3-L4 (Fig. 27).
- **Gait pattern in PIVD:** Excessive hip flexion or Trendelenburg gait (due to weakness of hip abductor as in L5 radiculopathy).

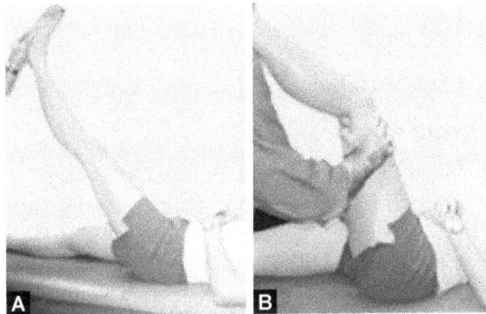

Figs. 26A and B: Bowstring test.

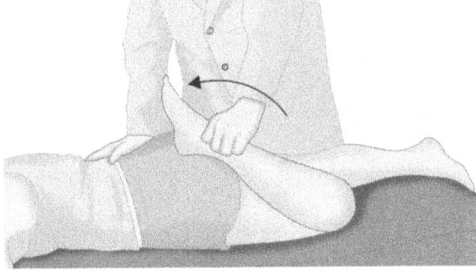

Fig. 27: Femoral stretch test.

Preventive Measures

- **Do not lift by bending the trunk:** Lift an object by bending the knees and squatting to pick up object while keeping the back

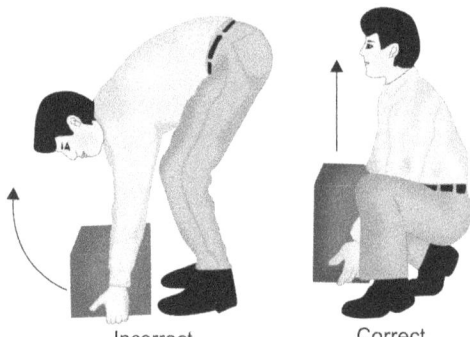

Fig. 28: Correct method for lifting an object.

straight and hold the object close to the body (Fig. 28).
- Avoid twisting body while lifting.
- Push rather than pull heavy object.
- Break up times with stops to stretch during long travelling.
- Wear flat shoes with heel less than 1 inch.
- Exercise regularly.

Sitting Posture
- Sit in upright chair with low back support. Keep the knees little higher than the hips by placing a low stool below the feet (Fig. 29).

Standing Posture
- Rest one foot on low stool to relieve pressure on the low back (Fig. 29).

Sleeping Posture
- Side lying with knees bent.
- Supine lying by keeping the pillows under the knees and a small pillow under the lower back (Fig. 29).

Management

Conservative Treatment
- **Rest:** Optimal amount of bed rest during acute phase founds to be helpful. During first two days, when the symptoms are intense, bed rest is required to aid early healing, but it should be mingled with short intervals of standing, walking and properly controled movements. Resting on a hard bed promotes lumbar extension and stimulates fluid mechanics to help reduce swelling in the discs or connective tissue.
- **Medication:** NSAIDs or analgesics are used to reduce pain and inflammation.
- Usually continuous bed rest and spinal traction for 2-3 weeks helps in reducing the herniation in over 90% cases.
- **Postural awareness and activity modification:** Avoid flexion, bending or lifting activities, prolonged sitting and combine movements or asymmetric movements, e.g. flexion or extension with rotation.
- **Epidural steroid injection:** Used to decrease pain and inflammation.

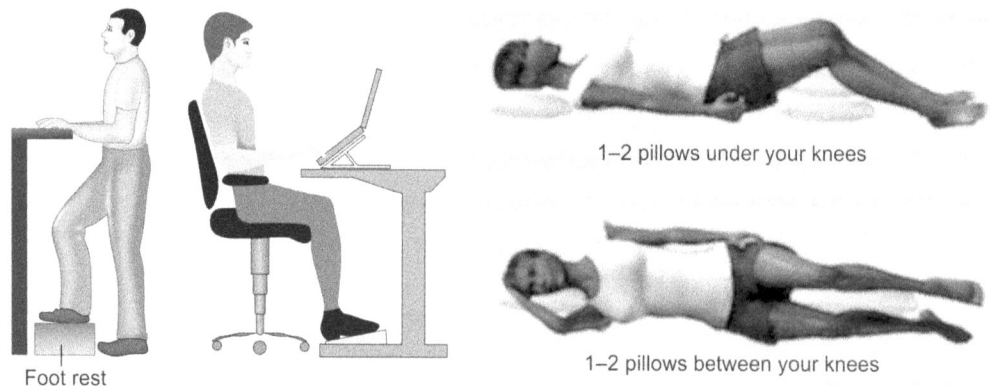

Fig. 29: Correct standing, sitting and sleeping postures.

Spinal Disorders

- **Chymopapain injection:** It is an injection of enzyme material into the nucleus of disc that helps to shrink the herniated disc which further relieves the pressure on the affected nerve root. This technique is known as *Chemonucleolysis*. Although it is proved to be less effective and contains the potential risk of anaphylaxis following intradiscal injection.

Physiotherapy Treatment

Acute Phase
- Modalities to reduce pain and spasm:
  - Cryotherapy: It is used in acute phase to reduce muscle spasm and inflammation.
  - Moist heat and SWD: In chronic conditions it is used to reduce pain and spasm by relaxing the muscles and promoting the blood flow.
  - Ultrasound: It reduces the muscle spasm, stiffness, cramping, swelling and pain by facilitating the healing process and improving the blood circulation.
  - IFT and TENS: It is used to reduce muscle spasm and relieves pain.
  - LASER: It is also used to reduce pain and inflammation.
- **Traction:**
  - May reduce nuclear protrusion by decreasing intradiscal pressure by 20%–30% or by placing tension on PLL.
  - Causes vertebral body separation
  - Decreases the compressive force on nerve root by increasing the neuroforaminal size.
  - Improves the blood flow to nerve roots.
  - Causes the stretching of spinal muscles.

In acute phase, the time of traction should be short. Long duration of traction may increase the intradiscal pressure due to imbibition of fluid and result in the aggravation of pain. So, less than 15 minutes of intermittent traction and less than 10 minutes of sustained traction are advisable.

Traction is contraindicated when the disc protrusion is medial to nerve root.

- **Corset:**
  - It maintains the normal physiological lumbar curvature.
  - It provides support and reassurance to the patient, especially in acute phase.
  - It facilitates the neutral splintage provided by abdominal and spinal musculature.
  - It uplifts and supports the abdomen and therefore unloads the effects of gravity on the intervertebral discs.
  - It provides partial immobilization that helps to protect the lumbar spine from abnormal stress of movement.

  Disadvantage: Prolonged use of corset may cause the muscle to become weaker and deconditioned through disuse.

- **Therapeutic exercises:**
  - Exercise plays an important role in the treatment of PIVD. Initial exercise position is determined by the movement which lessen the radicular or extremity pain (Centralize the pain).
  - Acute discogenic pain usually decreases or centralizes by extension-based exercise.
  - Pain cause by large central, paracentral, foraminal herniation may increase with extension-based exercise because central canal and foraminal diameter are decreased with extension. Therefore neutral or slightly flexion-based training may be least painful.

- **Joint mobilization:** Spinal mobilization of the proximal segment to the affected segmental level helps to reduce pain.

- **Nerve mobilization:** It uses specific postures that can tension neural tissues and gently stretch the nerve.

  Nerve mobilization of sciatic nerve is performed:
  - To maintain and improve the mobility of the nerve.
  - To reduce the tightness in the nerve and break down its adhesions to the surrounding tissues.

- It also helps to relieve pain associated with tight nerve.
- **Active ROM exercise:** Active ROM exercise of alternative lower limb, e.g. Hip flexion, extension, abduction, adduction, heel drag, and ankle toe movements.
- **Muscle stretching:** Piriformis muscle stretch may be given to reduce the stress over the sciatic nerve and to maintain the flexibility of muscle.

Subacute Stage (After 5–7 Days)
- Carry on with the acute phase exercises.
- **Strengthening exercises:** Initiate with isometric exercises, i.e. spinal stabilization exercise in supine position.
- **Pelvic tilt exercises:** Anterior pelvic tilt should be emphasized to promote the spinal extension and to stretch the tight lower back muscles. Pelvic tilt in different positions like supine, sitting, side lying, prone, quadruped and standing position.
- **Cardiovascular conditioning exercises:** Low impact aerobic exercises like walking, cycling and swimming. Low impact aerobic exercise improves the cardiovascular fitness along with the strengthening of abdominal and low back muscles without over straining the back.

Chronic Phase (After 3 Weeks)
- **Spinal mobility exercise:** Initiate with gentle pain free movement of spine, e.g. flexion, extension, side flexion.
- **Stretching exercise:** To restore the tissue flexibility and segmental movement of spine.
  - **Hamstring and hip flexors:** Healthy hamstring and hip flexors are responsible for the mobility and stability of the spine. Iliopsoas muscle is attached to T12–L5 vertebrae and has the strongest pull on the spine. Therefore a tight psoas can pull on the spine that compress the discs and vertebral joints and may lead to anterior pelvic tilt. This constant anterior tilt of pelvis causes an increased pull on the hamstring which also causes tightness. Therefore tight hamstring and hip flexors often occurs together. So hamstring and hip flexors stretches are necessary to maintain the neutral position of pelvis and evenly distribute the pressure on the vertebral discs.
  - **Lumbar erector spinae and quadratus lumborum:** Muscles that are more prone to tightness are erector spinae, quadratus lumborum, etc. which may further lead to muscle imbalance, decreased spinal stability and postural alteration. Therefore, it is very important to stretch these muscles.
- **Strengthening exercises:** The goals of strengthening exercises are to correct muscle weakness and imbalances, to improve postures, to enhance the cardiovascular fitness, flexibility and strength of patient.
  - **Core strengthening exercises,** e.g. bridging, plank, side planks, wall squat and basic crunches. The CORE is described as a box with abdominals in the front, paraspinal and gluteals in the back, diaphragm on the roof and pelvic floor and hip girdle musculature at the roof. They together serve as a muscular corset that works as a unit to stabilize the body and spine. Weakness of any of the core muscles can affect the stability and leave the back vulnerable to injury. Therefore strengthening training of these muscles are necessary to maintain the spinal stability and pelvic balance.
- **Balance and coordination exercises of core muscles:** It helps to stabilize and maintain the normal posture of spine which in turn reduces undue stress on the spine.
- **Hydrotherapy exercises:** Hydrotherapy helps to improve the muscle strength, circulation and mobility without the strain or potential for injury.
  - Benefits of hydrotherapy:
    – Warm water helps to reduce pain, muscle spasm, enhance muscle relaxation and improves circulation.

- Buoyancy of water counters the effects of gravity which helps to reduce the loading on the joints.
- Increased muscle strength benefits may be achieved by exercising in water due to greater resistance to movement in water.

Surgical Treatment

Indications for the surgical removal of disc:
- Cauda equina compression syndrome that does not resolve with six hours of bed rest and traction.
- Neurological deterioration in spite of regular conservative treatment.
- Presence of constant pain and symptoms of sciatic nerve compression even after 30 days of conservative treatment.
- Major postural alterations that impair the functional abilities of the patient who are not responding to conservative treatment are absolute indication of surgery.

Surgical interventions are: Aim to relieve compression on spinal cord and emerging nerve roots. Disc is excised by following techniques:
- **Hemilaminectomy:** Part of lamina and ligamentum flavum on one side is removed.
- **Laminectomy:** Lamina on both sides with spinous process is removed. It is performed when central disc bulge is causing cauda equine syndrome.
- **Microdiscectomy:** The prolapsed portion of disc is removed.
- **Fenestration:** In this procedure the ligamentum flavum bridging the two adjacent laminae is excised and spinal canal at affected level is exposed.
- **Laminotomy:** In laminotomy, along with fenestration, a hole is made in lamina for wider exposer of spinal canal.

■ TB SPINE (POTT'S SPINE)

It refers to the tubercular infection of the spine characterized by bone destruction, fracture and collapse of the affected vertebra resulting in kyphotic deformity.

Pott's spine is the presentation of extra-pulmonary tuberculous arthritis of the intervertebral joints. The causative agent is **Mycobacterium Tubercule**.

It is also known as:
- Tuberculosis spondylitis
- Tuberculous spondyloarthropathy
- Spinal TB
- Musculoskeletal tuberculosis
- Caries spine.

Epidemiology

Vertebral TB is always the secondary TB that comprises around 50% cases of bone and joint TB. It most commonly occurs during first 3 decades of life and equally distributed in both the genders. Dorsal region is the most commonly affected region in Pott's spine.

Predisposing Factors
- Malnutrition
- Poor sanitation
- Over crowding
- Immunocompromised patients
- Close contact with TB patients
- Multiple pregnancy.

Regional Distribution
- Cervical: 12%
- Cervicodorsal: 5%
- Dorsal: 42% (most commonly affected site)
- Dorsolumbar: 12%
- Lumbar: 26%
- Lumbosacral: 3%.

Pathophysiology

Like TB of bone and joint elsewhere in the body, TB of spine is always secondary. Bacteria reach the spine through the hematogenous route from the lungs or lymph nodes. It may reach from viscera via paravertebral plexus of veins, i.e. Baston plexus, which has free communication with the visceral plexus of the abdomen (a common site of TB). Anterior aspect of vertebral body adjacent to the subchondral plate is usually affected which may spread to intervertebral disc. In adult, the involvement of disc is secondary to the infection of vertebral body whereas in children the disc can be the primary site because of its proficient vascularization. Progressive bone destruction leads to anterior vertebral collapse resulting in kyphotic deformity. Spinal canal can be narrowed by abscesses, granulation tissue or direct dural invasion leading to spinal cord compression and neurological deficits. Abscess in the lumbar region may descend down the sheath of the psoas to femoral trigone and eventually erode the skin (Flowchart 1).

Cold abscess (Fig. 30): Collection of pus of tubercular debris in diseased vertebra is called cold abscess. It is called so because it is not associated with the usual sign of inflammation found with a pyogenic abscess. Tubercular pus can tract in any direction from the affected vertebra. If it travels backward, it may press upon the spinal cord. Pus may come out anteriorly or on the side of vertebral body. Once outside the vertebra, the pus may travel along the musculofascial plexus to appear superficially at places far away from the site of lesion.

An abscess from cervical or dorsal regions may present far from vertebral column along the fascial planes or course of neurovascular bundle. Commonly present at the back in posterior/anterior cervical triangles, along the intercostal spaces on chest wall.

An abscess from dorsolumbar and lumbar spine follows the psoas sheath. It may be palpable in iliac fossa, lumbar triangle, upper part of thigh below inguinal ligament or even downwards up to the knee.

Types of Vertebral Lesions (Fig. 31)
- **Paradiscal lesion:** This is the commonest type, in this contiguous area of two adjacent vertebra along with the intervening disc is affected.

Flowchart 1: Pathophysiology of Pott's spine.

Focus of infection: possible from any sites M/C pulmonary, abdomen
↓
Route of infection: 1. Hematogenous (Batson plexus), 2. Lymph node spread 3. Direct spread
↓
Infection begins in cancellous area of vertebral body (central/anterior/ epiphyseal in location)
↓
Advances and destroys the cortex, intervertebral disc and adjacent vertebrae
↓
Infectious exudate may spread anteriorly beneath anterior longitudinal ligament and neighboring vertebrae

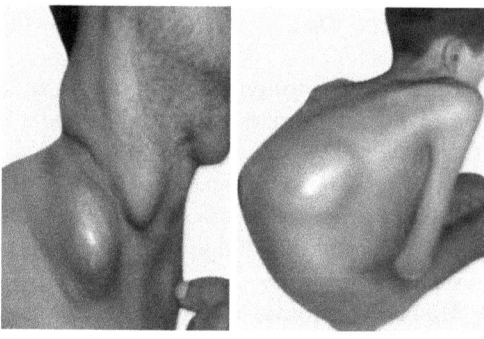

Fig. 30: Cold abscess.

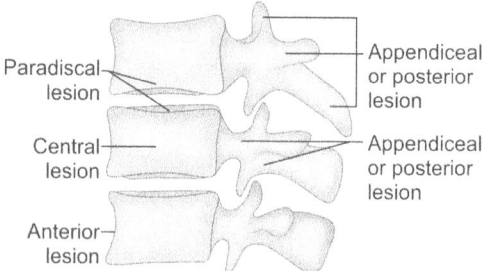

Fig. 31: Types of vertebral lesions.

- **Central lesion:** It is the lesion of the body of a single vertebra. This may lead to early collapse of weakened vertebra.
- **Anterior lesion:** It is the lesion localized to the anterior part of vertebral body. The infection may spread up or down under the anterior longitudinal ligament.
- **Appendiceal/Posterior lesion:** In this lesion the posterior complex of vertebra, i.e. the pedicle, lamina, spinous process or transverse process are affected.

Clinical Presentation in Active Stage
- **Typical attitude in skeletal TB**: Involvement of
  - Cervical spine causes wry neck.
  - Lower cervical causes military position.
  - Lower thoracic causes elder man's gait.
  - Upper lumbar causes prominent abdomen.
  - Lower lumbar causes increased lordosis.
- **Spine irregularity in TB:**
  - Kyphosis occurs in approximately 95% of cases.
  - Scoliosis may occur in approximately 5% cases.
  - Secondary/Compensatory lordosis may occur.
  - Paravertebral thickening.
- **Pain:**
  - Back pain is the commonest presenting problem.
  - Night cries: Severe pain at night.
  - Diffuse dull ache is present in early stage but later it becomes localized to the affected diseased segment.
  - Pain may be radiating along affected nerve root. So radicular pain may present depending on affected root, e.g.
    - Pain in arm is present when cervical nerve roots are affected.
    - Girdle pain is present when dorsal nerve roots are affected.
    - Pain in groin is present when lumbar nerve roots are affected.
- **Stiffness:**
  - Early symptom in TB.
  - It is due to the spasm of paravertebral muscles and is a protective mechanism.
- **Deformity:** Knuckle deformity (1–2 vertebras are collapsed)/Gibbus deformity (2–3 vertebras are collapsed)/Kyphus deformity (it is an angular kyphosis where more than 3 vertebrae are collapsed) (Figs. 32A and B).
- **Cold abscess:** Patient may initially present with a swelling or problem secondary to its compression.
- **Paraplegia in neglected cases.**
- **Constitutional symptoms** (only in 20% cases): Malaise, weight loss, loss of appetite, night sweats, evening rise of temperature.

Clinical Presentation in Healed Stage
- No systemic feature is present. However, the deformity that occurs during active stage persists.
- Stiffness of spine
- Restricted ROM of spine
- Neural deficits present in around 20% cases.

Complications
- Paraplegia
- Cold abscess
- Sinuses
- Secondary infection
- Amyloid disease
- Fatality.

Diagnosis
Laboratory Tests
- Blood test: Increased ESR and lymphocyte count
- Mantoux/Tuberculin skin test
- Ziehl-Neelsen staining.

X-ray findings: Findings are **"SADDER"** spine (Fig. 33).
- **Sclerosis.**
- **Abscess:** Evidence of cold abscess.

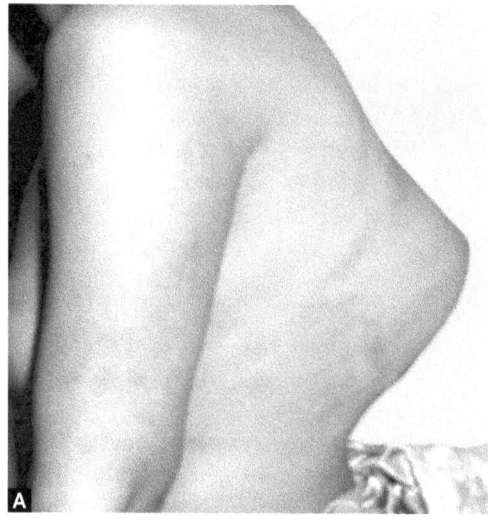

Figs. 32A and B: A. Gibbus deformity; B. Knuckle deformity.

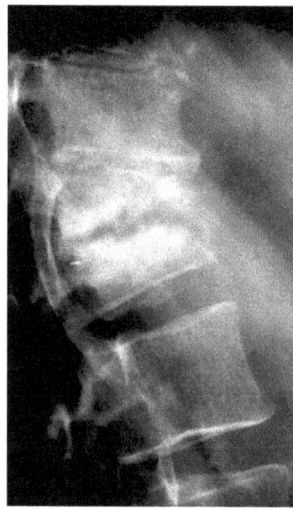

Fig. 33: X-ray finding of TB spine.

- **D**isc space reduction.
- **D**estruction of vertebral body.
- **E**rosion of end plates.
- **R**arefaction of the vertebra above and below the lesion.
- **K**yphosis/Gibbus (severe kyphosis).

Examination
- **Inspection:** To detect any active or healed primary lesion.
- **Palpation:**
  - Palpation to check the local rise in temperature
  - Palpation of all the spinous process for any abnormal prominence
  - Tenderness over the spinous process
  - Paraspinal muscle spasm or tenderness
  - Any swelling/cold abscess: Palpate for any fullness or swelling on the back along the chest wall and anteriorly.
- **Neurological examination:** of the limb to detect any neural deficit. It includes detailed:
  - Motor and sensory examination
  - Examination of reflexes
  - Bowel and bladder function.
- **Posture:** Spinal attitude and deformity should be examined.
- **Gait:** Patient walk with short step in order to avoid jerking the spine.

Management
- **General treatment:**
  - Rich protein diet, adequate sunlight, etc.
  - This treatment aims at building up the general resistance of the body.

- **Chemotherapy:**
  - 9 months regime: Rifampicin and isoniazide.
  - 6 months regime: First two months: Isoniazide, rifampicin and pyrazinamide.
  Next four months: Isoniazide and rifampicin.
- **Local treatment:** Aim is to prevent or correct the deformity by immobilizing the part with complete bed rest.

Surgical Treatment
Indication
- Neurological symptom.
- Kyphosis with several vertebral involvements.
- Resistance to chemotherapy.
- Recurrence of disease.
- Spinal instability.

Surgical Techniques
- Curettage of the lesion
- Joint debridement
- Synovectomy
- Salvage operation
- Spinal decompression
- Spinal fusion.

Physiotherapy Management
For the patient treated conservatively:
Patient is directed to prevent the complication arising due to prolonged immobilization.
- Patient should be educated on postural attitude which may further compress the cord.
- Gentle full active movements of spine.
- Slow and deep breathing in order to maintain vital capacity.
- Strength of the muscle group innervated by the spinal segment of affected vertebra.

After healing of the lesion:
- Deep breathing exercises should be made vigorously to improve mobility of thoracic spine.
- Begin spinal exercise with extension gradually increased.
- Mobility to be progressed further as small active free trunk movement.
- Ambulation to be initiated with spinal brace.

After surgical treatment:
- Chest physiotherapy.
- Education of positioning and movement.
- Methodology of safe bed activity.
- Technique of sitting from lying position.
- Mobility and strengthening exercise of spine.

Immediate postoperative phase:
- Care must be taken to avoid stress over the operated area.
- Breathing exercise.
- Prevention of DVT.
- Prevention of pressure sore.
- Simple resisted exercise to the unaffected area.

During mobilization:
- Gradual mobilization of spine.
- Log rolling, standing and ambulation are initiated.
- Strengthening of spinal extensors.
- Education about back care.
- Activities of daily living (ADL) are encouraged.
- Over straining activities should be prevented.

CHAPTER

6

Arthritis

■ OSTEOARTHRITIS

Osteoarthritis is a chronic degenerative joint disease (DJD) result from the breakdown of joint cartilage and underlying bone characterized by pain, swelling, stiffness and instability of the joint (Fig. 1).

Etiology

- **Primary/idiopathic osteoarthritis (OA):**
  - Mostly related to aging.
  - It could results from abnormal stresses on normal weight bearing joints or normal stresses on weakened joints.
- **Secondary OA:** This type of OA is caused by some other factors but the resulting pathology is same as in primary OA.
  - Post-traumatic.
  - Congenital or developmental diseases
    – **Localized:**
      - Mechanical or local factors: For example, unequal limb length, extreme valgus/varus deformity, scoliosis.
      - Hip disease: For example, Perthes disease, CDH, slipped femoral epiphysis.
    – **Generalized:**
      - Metabolic disease: For example, Gaucher's disease, osteoporosis.
      - Bone and joint diseases: For example, avascular necrosis, gouty arthritis, septic arthritis, Paget disease, osteochondritis.
      - Endocrine disease: For example, diabetes mellitus, acromegaly, hypo/hyperthyroidism.
      - Previous history of rheumatoid arthritis.
      - Obesity
      - Bone dysplasia: For example, epiphyseal dysplasia.

Predisposing Factors (Fig. 2)

- **Age:** The prevalence of OA increases significantly with increasing age.
- **Gender:** Between the age of 45 to 55 years, males are more prone as compare to females. Although after 55 years, females are more prone as compare to males.
- **Association with some systemic factors:** For example, elevated level of serum uric acid, C-reactive protein, hypertension.
- **Associated biomechanical factors:**
  - **Joint hyperlaxity:** Increased joint laxity frequently causes subluxation and injuries to joint due to malalignment.

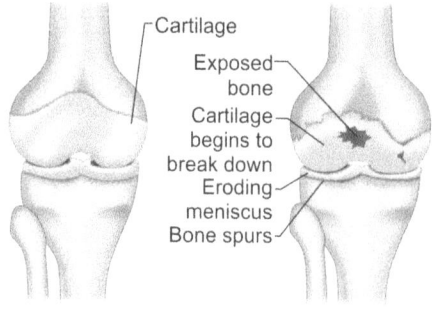

Fig. 1: Osteoarthritis of knee joint.

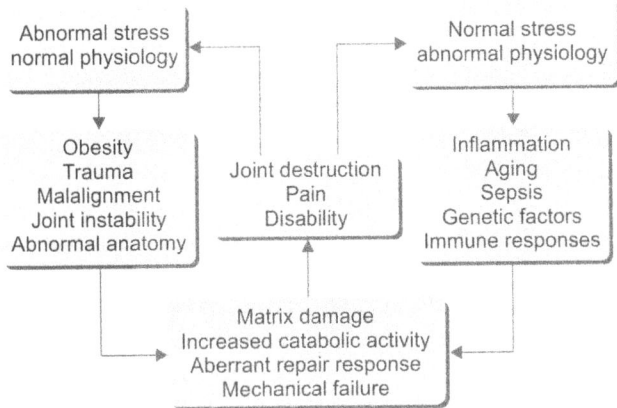

Fig. 2: Predisposing factors of osteoarthritis.

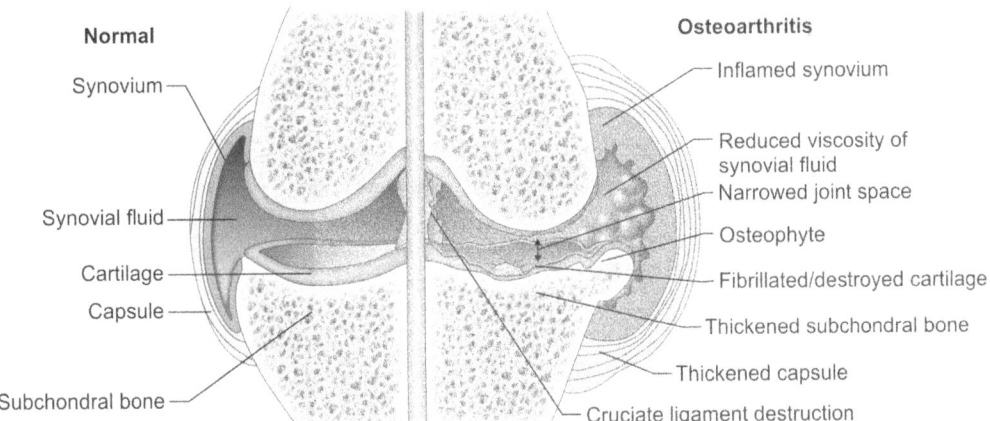

Fig. 3: Pathophysiology of osteoarthritis.

These recurrent injuries further leads to the destruction of periarticular structures and predates the arthritis.
- **Effect of mechanical overuse:** Repetitive mechanical stress can damage the periarticular structures and leads to degeneration of joint.
- **Obesity:** Excessive loading of joint due to obesity speeds up the breakdown of cartilage and increase the susceptibility to osteoarthritis.

Pathophysiology (Fig. 3)

Osteoarthritis is primarily a disease of cartilage. Cartilage is a unique tissue with viscoelastic and compressive properties which are imparted by its extracellular matrix, composed predominantly by type II collagen and proteoglycans.

Cartilage normally contains:
- Chondrocytes (cellular): 1–2%
- Liquid phase: 70–80%
- Solid phase: 20–30% collagen type II and other proteoglycans.

Normally, the matrix is constantly exposed to dynamic remodeling process. The volume of cartilage is maintained by the regular balance activities of degenerative and synthetic enzymes. However, in osteoarthritis the matrix degrading enzymes overpowers the synthetic enzyme and causes the loss of collagen and proteoglycans from the matrix.

In response to this loss, chondrocytes proliferates and synthesize enhanced amounts of proteoglycans and collagen molecules. As the disease progress reparative attempts are outmatched by progressive cartilage degradation. Fibrillation, erosion and cracking initially appears in the superficial layer of cartilage and progress over time to deeper layers resulting eventually in large clinically observable erosions.

Stages of Osteoarthritis (Fig. 4)

- **Changes in articular cartilage, i.e. loss of proteoglycans:** Decrease proteoglycans and water content in cartilage makes the cartilage less resilient.
- **Fibrillation:** Multiple, tiny cracks develops initially on the superficial layer and gradually to the deeper layer of articular cartilage.
- **Exposure of subchondral bone:** Synovial fluid flows through the cracks into the deeper tissue of cartilage. This leads to the break down and lodging of cartilage in synovium and gradually exposes the subchondral bone.
- **Secondary synovitis:** Presence of osteocartilagenous bodies in joint synovium or joint space triggers the inflammatory reaction and eventually the synovium becomes hyperemic and hypertrophied.
- **Changes in subchondral bone:** Exposed subchondral bone responds by neovascularization. This process causes the resorption of osteoclasts and formation of osteoblasts that progressively lead to the thickening of the subchondral bone in the exposed area.
- **Eburnation:** Exposed subchondral bone grinds the opposite joint surface as the joint moves. It becomes eburnated, shiny and smooth.
- **Subchondral bone cyst:** Subchondral bone cysts are formed due to the flow of synovial fluid into the bone marrow space following a crack in the eburnated subchondral bone.

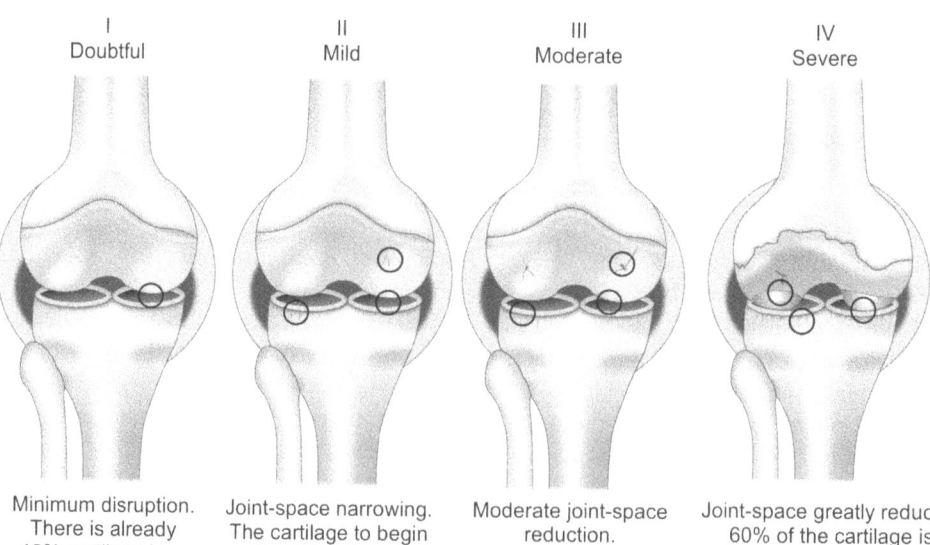

Fig. 4: Stages of osteoarthritis.

- **Development of osteophytes:** In later stages, bony spur develops at the edges of the bone. These bony spurs also known as osteophytes are the masses of bone and cartilage that forms due to the modulation of mesenchymal tissue of synovium into osteoblasts and chondroblasts.

Clinical Presentation
- **Pain:** Deep pain within or near the affected joint. Initially pain worsens with activity during the course of the day. But gradually with progression, pain occurs even at rest also.
- **Stiffness:** Stiffness usually occurs after period of rest and improved with activity. Morning stiffness usually lasts for about 30 minutes or less.
- **Swelling:** The swelling may be hard (caused by osteophytes or bony enlargement) or soft (caused by synovial thickening and extra fluid).
- **Crepitus:** Painful sensation, such as rubbing, cracking or grating within joint may be felt when performing specific activities, such as bending, kneeling and stair climbing.
- **Reduced ROM and disuse of joint:** As arthritis progress, movement of the affected joint is increasingly restricted due to pain and other biomechanical factors.
- **Nodules:** They are the bony enlargement in small joints. Usually they are not painful but sometimes they are painful, swollen and red. This condition is known as nodal OA. Heberden's nodes and Bouchard's nodes are developed in fingers at DIP and PIP joint respectively that significantly limits the movements of the fingers (Fig. 5).
- Osteoarthritis commonly affects the proximal weight bearing joints, such as hip, knees and spine. Although it may also affect hand and foot.

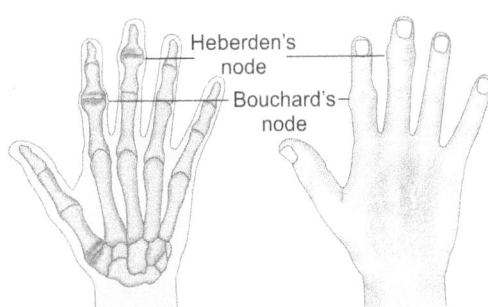

Fig. 5: Heberden's node and Bouchard's node developed at DIP and PIP joint.

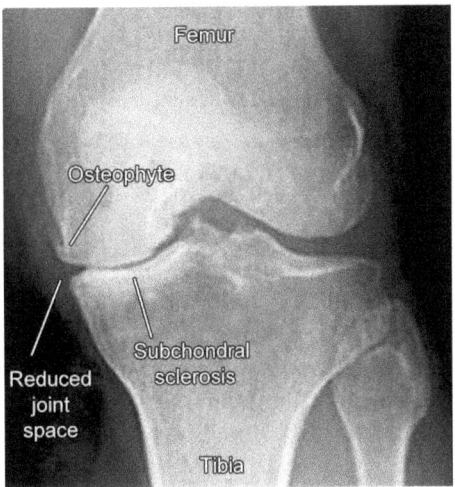

Fig. 6: X-ray finding of osteoarthritis.

Diagnosis
Imaging Studies
X- Ray Findings (Fig. 6)
- Narrowing of joint space
- Osteophytes at the margin of joint
- Subchondral cyst
- Subchondral sclerosis.

Physical Examination
- **Observation:** Swelling, redness and warmth, skin rashes over the involved joint.
- **Palpation:** Presence of swelling and tenderness along the joint line.
- **Muscle strength:** Decreased muscle strength of surrounding muscles of the involved joint.

- **ROM:** Painful and restricted ROM of affected joint.
- **Balance and coordination**
- **Functional impairment:** Inability to perform the ADLs.

Management

Medication

- **Analgesics:** For example, acetaminophen, aspirin are used to decrease the pain.
- **Nonsteroidal anti-inflammatory drugs (NSAIDs):** They are used to reduce associated pain and inflammation.
- **Muscle relaxants:** It is used to relieve muscle spasm that could contribute to patient's discomfort.
- **Intra-articular corticosteroid injections:** Used to reduce pain, swelling and inflammation.
- **Intra-articular injection of hyaluronic acid (hyalgan and synvisc)** known as visco supplements (lubricating substance found in normal joint fluid).
- **Nutritional supplements:** Glucosamine sulfate and chondroitin sulfate reported to "cure" arthritis. These are produced with in the body and are used in manufacture or repair of cartilage. It relieves pain and stiffness when combine with exercise, weight control and physiotherapy.

Physiotherapy Treatment

- **Pain relieving modalities:**
  - **Heat therapy:** To relieve pain, stiffness, swelling and relax muscles before exercises, e.g. moist hot pack, Paraffin wax bath, SWD.
  - **Cryotherapy:** It also relieves pain, stiffness and swelling, e.g. cryopack or ice massages.
  - **Low frequency modalities:** IFT, TENS.
  - **Ultrasound:** To decrease pain, inflammation and to promote healing.
  - **Therapeutic massage:** To decrease pain, swelling, muscle guarding and stiffness.
- **Joint taping/brace:**
  - It provides stability and support to the affected joint.
  - It reduces strain on inflamed soft tissue around the joint.
  - It helps to improve patient's awareness of joint position.
- **Strengthening exercises:** Strengthening may help to minimize adverse effect of weight on joints by reducing the amount of force that is transmitted across the affected joint. Therefore strengthening exercise of surrounding muscle of joint is necessary.
  It can be classified into further categories: Isometric, isokinetic and isometric exercises. Resistance exercise with single set of 15 repetitions twice a week. Gradually 2 sets of 10 repetitions.
  Lifting free weights, weighing machines and elastic theraband can be used for resistance.
- **To improve the flexibility:** In severe arthritis, prolonged disuse of muscle due to pain not only causes weakness but also results in alteration in its shape and length that further leads to tightness, shortening and gradually visible joint deformities. Therefore stretching exercises of surrounding muscle of the affected joint is necessary to prevent muscular and articular changes.
- **To improve joint ROM:** AAROM, PROM and AROM exercises of involved and proximal involved joints.
- **To improve cardiovascular conditioning:** Compromised functional abilities due to associated pain and restricted ROM leads to decrease cardiovascular fitness. Therefore general conditioning and endurance exercise should be implemented to improve the cardiovascular conditioning, e.g. aerobic exercises 30 minutes workout with proper warm up and cool down, walking, jogging, biking, cycling, swimming and rowing.

- **To control weight:** Weight control reduces the pain by decreasing stress on weight bearing joints and increases the self-esteem of the patient. Regular workouts with diet control should be practiced to decrease the body weight.

Surgical Treatment
Indications
- Severe pain not relieved by conservative treatment
- Marked joint instability
- Significant impaired functional abilities.

Surgical Techniques
- Osteotomy (realigning of joint)
- Scoping the joint (washing out the joint)
- Arthrodesis (fusion of joint)
- Arthroplasty (joint replacement).

■ RHEUMATOID ARTHRITIS

Rheumatoid arthritis is a chronic, autoimmune, progressive, systemic inflammatory disorder of unknown etiology characterized by symmetric synovitis, joint erosion and multisystem extra-articular manifestations.

Epidemiology
- **Age of onset:** Although it may occur at any age. It usually occurs between 30–50 years.
- **Gender:** Females are more affected than males.
- **Family history:** People having inherited genes are more susceptible to develop rheumatoid arthritis (RA).
- **Smoking:** Heavy long-term smoking is a strong risk factor for RA.

Etiology
Exact cause of RA is not known. RA is most likely triggered by combinations of factors:
- Abnormal autoimmune response.
- Genetic susceptibility, i.e. hereditary factor (HLA-DR4)
- Increased serum levels of immunoglobulins (Ig), e.g. IgM, IgA, IgG.
- Rheumatoid factor (RA factor) is present in over 70–80% of patients.
- **Environmental factors:** RA can be triggered by an infection (viral or bacterial) in people having inherited tendency for disease.

Pathophysiology
Stages of Rheumatoid Arthritis (Fig. 7)
- **Proliferative phase:** Proliferative inflammation of synovium occurs with increased exudates that gradually lead to the thickening of synovium.
- **Granulation tissue phase:** Granulation tissues (pannus) are formed that causes the erosion and destruction of the cartilage. Gradually it spreads to the contiguous areas that further lead to the destruction of joint capsule and muscles that control the joint.
- **Fibrous ankylosis phase:** Invasion of pannus by tough fibrous tissues leads to fibrous ankylosis.
- **Bony ankylosis phase:** Calcification of fibrous tissues causes bony ankylosis.

Clinical Presentation
- **Morning stiffness** that last for at least 1 hour.
- **Pain:** Pain in joints for at least 6 weeks before a diagnosis of RA is considered. Pain often occurs symmetrically and may be more severe on one side.
- **Swelling:** Inflamed joints are usually swollen and often warm and boggy when touched.
  - Swelling may occur in ankles.
  - In some cases fluid accumulates in the sac behind the knee and forms a cyst known as Bakers cyst.
- **Specific joint involvement:**
  - Small peripheral joints are more involved.
  - Almost always develops in wrist, MCP joint, knees and 1st MTP joint.
  - Cervical spine, shoulder, elbow, hip and TM joints and even joint between small bones inside inner ear.
  - DIP joint is usually not involved.

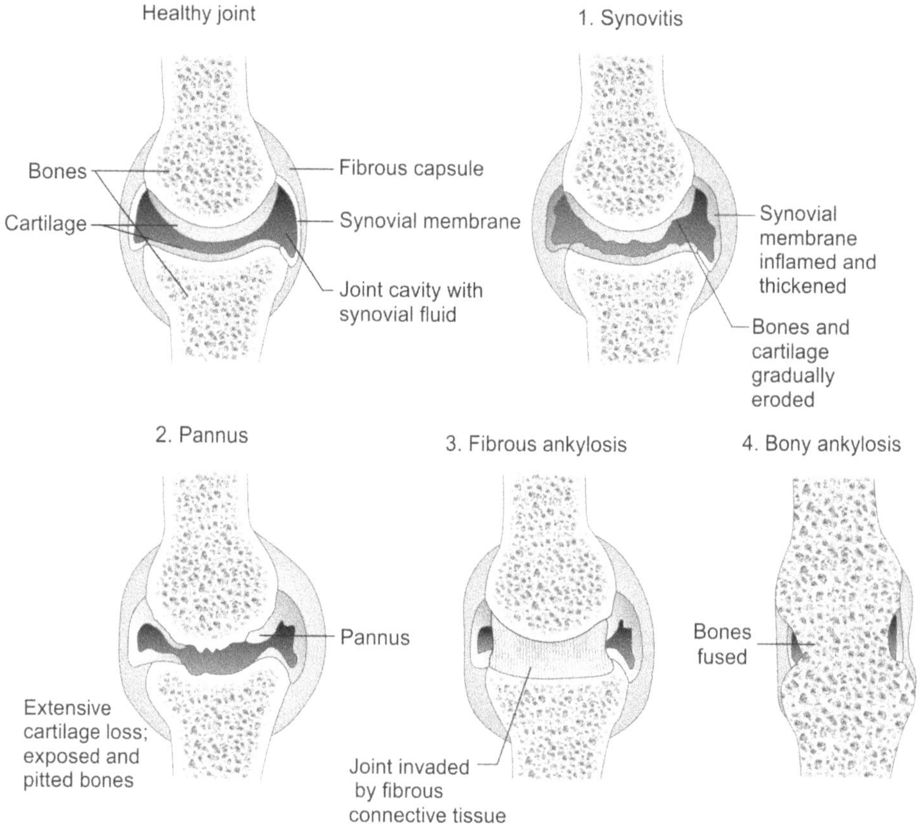

Fig. 7: Stages of rheumatoid arthritis.

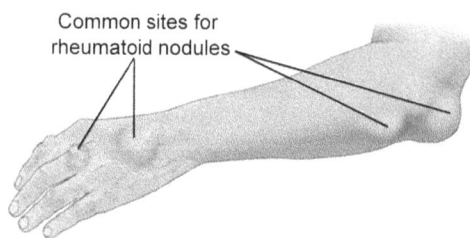

Fig. 8: Rheumatoid nodules.

- **Nodules:** In around 20% of RA patients, inflammation of small blood vessels causes the formation of nodules or lumps under the skin (Fig. 8).
  - Pea-sized or slightly larger.
  - Often located near elbow, although can occur anywhere.
- **Flu like symptoms** like fatigue, weight loss and fever.
- **Symptoms in children:**
  - Juvenile RA is also known as "Still's disease".
  - It is usually preceded by pink rashes, high fever, shaking, chills along with pain and swelling in multiple joints.
- **Extra-articular manifestation (Fig. 9):** Chronic lung diseases like interstitial fibrosis, pulmonary hypertension, etc.
- **Kidney failure:** Kidney is rarely involved but the drugs used for the treatment may damage the kidney.
- **Skin problems:** Rashes, ulcer, blisters and lumps occurs under the skin, particularly on the fingers and under the nails.
- **Heart disease:** RA patients are at increased risk of death from coronary artery disease.

Arthritis

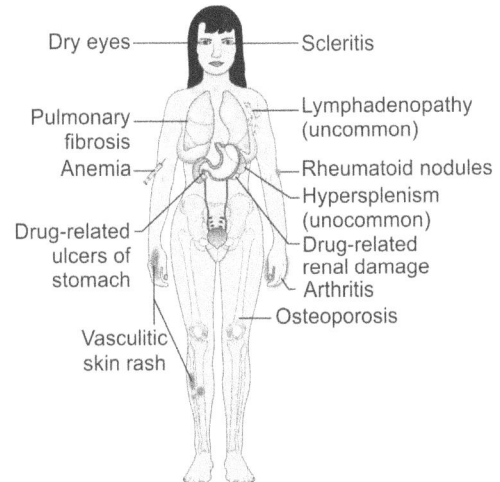

Fig. 9: Extra-articular manifestations.

- **Osteoporosis:** Decreased bone density more common in postmenopausal females particularly affecting the hip joint.
- **Vasculitis:** Autoimmune inflammatory abnormalities in small blood vessels. It may effect many organs of the body.
- **Eyes:** Inflammation of blood vessels of eye may lead to corneal damage, scleritis or episcleritis.
- **Peripheral neuropathy** causing tingling, numbness and burning sensation in hands and feet.
- **Lymphoma and other cancers:** More likely to develop non-Hodgkin's lymphoma.
- **Pregnancy:** Conceived mother with RA are at higher risk for premature delivery and more likely to develop hypertension in last trimester.
- **Hematological changes:** Decreased number of RBC, i.e. anemia.
- **Muscle weakness and ligament destruction.**

Diagnosis

Articular Manifestations

Rheumatoid arthritis (RA) is marked by bilateral, peripheral and symmetrical pattern of joint involvement. Common joint deformities in rheumatoid arthritis are:

- **Cervical spine:** Often involve atlantoaxial joint and midcervical region which leads to decrease ROM particularly in rotation. Also produce radiating pain due to nerve and cord compression.
- **Temporomandibular (TM) joint:** Involvement of TM joint causes the inability to open mouth, side glide or protrusion. Normal approximation of upper and lower teeth may be altered following persistent inflammation.
- **Shoulder joint:** Primary involvement of glenohumeral, sternoclavicular, AC joint and secondary involvement of scapulothoracic joint. Chronic inflammation of shoulder causes the distension and thinning of joint capsule and ligaments, erosion of joint surface and inflammation of tendon or bursa.
- **Elbow joint:** Capsular inflammation, ligamentous distension and joint surface erosion can lead to joint instability causes irregular and catching joint movements. Pain can cause persistent spasm that leads to flexion contracture of elbow.
- **Wrist joint:** Early synovitis between 8 carpal bones and radius leads to rapid development of flexion contracture which diminishes the power grasp.
  - Chronic inflammation of proximal row of capsule leads to volar subluxation of wrist and hand on radius. Accentuating the normal 10–15° of volar inclination of carpus on distal radius.
  - Chronic inflammation leads to loss of radius ligamentous support, destruction of ECU and fibrocartilage on distal side of ulna.
  - Attenuation of these restraining structures allow ulnar deviation of proximal carpals that further resulting in radial deviation of distal carpal row in the wrist. (5–10° of ulnar deviation occurs in normal healthy wrist).
- **Hand deformities (Fig. 10):**
  - **Metacarpophalangeal (MCP) joint:** Volar subluxation and ulnar drift of

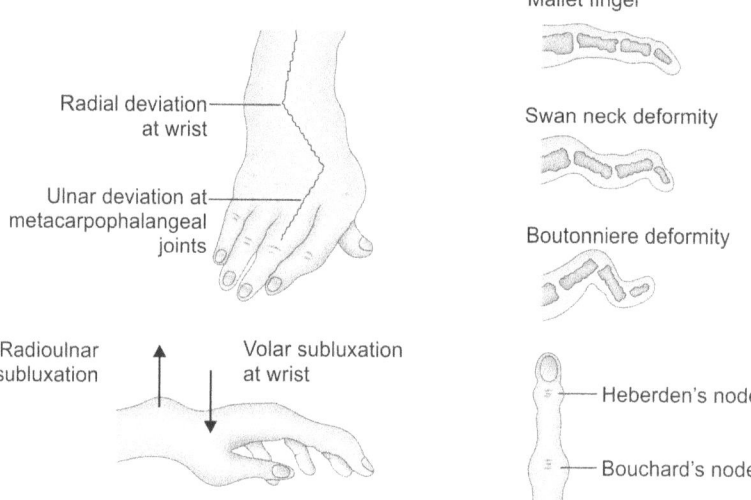

Fig. 10: Wrist and hand deformities in rheumatoid arthritis.

MCP joint occurs which tilt proximal phalanges in ulnar direction. This could be because of the summation of following reasons:
- Accentuation of normal anatomical placement of phalanges and pull of intrinsic muscles in ulnar direction also contribute to ulnar drift at MCP joint during hand motion.
- Weakened ligament cannot resist a pull toward volar subluxation during power pinch or grasp.
- When flexor tendons bowstring effect develops across the MCP joints due to synovitis of the joint and flaring of damaged tendon sheaths which causes the distal shift of fulcrum of the flexor tendons that further places an additional ulnar and volar pull on proximal phalanges.
- Radial deviation of carpals further enhances MCP ulnar drift at phalanges to compensate for loss of normal ulnar deviation at wrist. This is known as zigzag effect where forces in hand try to move index finger back into normal functional position in line with the radius.

- **Proximal interphalangeal (PIP) joint:** Two characteristic deformities are seen at PIP joint which are as follows:
  1. **Swan neck deformity:** Hyperextension at PIP joint and flexion at DIP joint.
     - **When synovitis occurs at MCP joint:** Pain due to chronic synovitis of MCP joint causes reflex muscle spasm of intrinsic muscle. Biomechanical force of intrinsic muscles combines with hypermobility of chronic inflamed joints results in volar subluxation and PIP hyperextension.
     - **When synovitis occurs at PIP joint:** Chronic synovitis of PIP joint leads to the stretching of volar capsule of PIP joint. Because of this, lateral bands moves dorsally. Now the tension placed on FDP by PIP flexes the DIP joint. FDS further predispose to PIP hyperextension.
     - **When synovitis occurs at DIP joint:** Chronic synovitis at DIP joint

causes the rupture of EDC at its insertion at DIP joint leads to DIP flexion and PIP hyperextension due to unrestrained pull by FDP.
2. **Boutonniere deformity:** Extension at DIP joint and flexion at PIP joint. As a result of chronic synovitis in PIP joint, insertion of EDC into middle phalanx also known as central slip lengthens and lateral bands slide volarly to force PIP into flexion.
- **Distal interphalangeal (DIP) joint:** Rarely involved in RA. DIP joints are involved only in the presence of co-existing MCP and PIP joints deformity. Occasionally tendon of EDC will rupture and unopposed pull of FDP will pull DIP into flexion known as Mallet finger deformity.
- **Thumb deformity:**
  - **Type I deformity:** MCP flexion and IP hyperextension without involvement of CMC joint.
  - **Type II deformity:** CMC joint subluxation and IP hyperextension
  - **Type III deformity:** CMC joint subluxation and MCP joint hyperextension. Most commonly occurring deformity.
- **Mutilans deformity (opera glass hand):** Grossly unstable thumb with severely deformed phalanges. X-ray finding shows severe bone resorption, erosion and shortening especially of MCP, PIP, radiocarpal and radioulnar joint.
- **Hip joint:** Less commonly involved in RA. In severe condition, inflammatory destruction of femoral head and acetabulum may push acetabulum into pelvic cavity known as **"protrusio acetabula"**.
- **Knee joint:** Most commonly involved because of having relatively large amount of synovium. Chronic synovitis leads to distension of joint capsule,

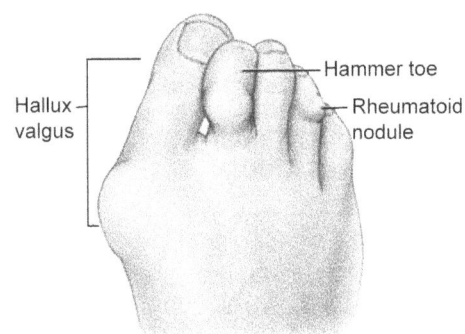

Fig. 11: Ankle and foot deformities in rheumatoid arthritis.

attenuation of collateral and cruciate ligament and destruction of joint surfaces. Slight flexed position due to pain cause flexion contracture.
- **Ankle and foot deformities (Fig. 11):**
  - **Hind foot pronation:** Chronic synovitis accentuates the natural tendency of talus to glide medially and in plantar direction resulting in pressure on calcaneus leading to hind foot pronation.
  - **Flat foot:** Plantar calcaneonavicular ligament is stretched leading to flattening of medial longitudinal arch.
  - **Bony spur:** Calcaneus may erode or develop bony exostosis known as spurs.
  - **Splay foot:** Synovitis weakens transverse arch leading to spreading of metatarsals and splay foot may develop.
  - **Hallux valgus:** It is characterized by medial deviation of first metatarsal and lateral deviation of great toe. Hallux valgus occurs due to the loss of integrity or subluxation of first MTP joint which in turn happens because of synovitis that causes distension of joint capsules and ligaments.
  - **Hammer toe:** It is the volar subluxation of MTP joint with PIP joint flexion and DIP joint hyperextension.

- **Cockup toes:** In this the volar subluxation of metatarsal head along with flexion of DIP and PIP joint.

Diagnostic Criterion of Rheumotoid Arthritis

1. Morning stiffness
2. Arthritis of 3 or more joints
3. Arthritis of hand joints
4. Symmetric arthritis.
5. Rheumatoid nodules
6. Serum rheumatoid factor
7. Radiographic changes.

Presence of at least 4 of these 7 criterions.
OR
Presence of one of the first four joint symptoms that last for at least 6 weeks is confirmatory diagnosis of RA.

Diagnosis

X-ray Findings

- **Swelling:** Presence of fusiform and periarticular swelling represents a combination of joint effusion, edema and tenosynovitis.
- **Osteoporosis:** Initially juxtra-articular and generalized osteoporosis occurs in advanced stage
- Joint space narrowing
- Marginal erosion
- Bony ankylosis.

Laboratory Findings

Blood Test

- Elevated ESR and C-reactive protein (CRP) in body indicates the presence of inflammatory process.
- RA factor (present in 70–80% of patient) and anti CCP antibodies (present in 60–80% patient).
- **Antinuclear antibody (ANA):** Identify the presence of autoimmune disorder.

Management

Medications

- **NSAIDs:** To decrease the pain and inflammation.
- **Analgesic:** To reduce pain, e.g. acetaminophen, tramadol.
- **Corticosteroids:** It quickly improves symptoms, such as pain, decrease joint swelling and tenderness and inflammation, e.g. Prednisolone, prednisone.
- **DMARDS (Disease-modifying antirheumatic drugs.**
  - It reduces inflammation.
  - It reduces or prevents joint damage.
  - It preserves joint structure and function, e.g. methotrexate, hydroxychloroquine, sulfasalazine.
- **Biologic DMARDS:**
  - It reduces the pain and stiffness.
  - It blocks the immune system messenger called cytokines.
  - A cytokine TNFα is known to be involved in causing AS.
  - Anti-TNFα agent block the effect of cytokines.
  - These agents can be injected in the skin or intravenously, e.g. etanercept, infliximab.

Physiotherapy Treatment

- **Rest:** Inflamed joint should be rested. However physical fitness should be maintained as much as possible.
- **Hot or cold therapy:**
  - **Hot therapy for chronic cases:** It relieves muscle spasm and obtains the elasticity of periarticular structures.
    Superficial heating modalities: Hot packs, IRR, fluidotherapy and hydrotherapy. 10–20 minutes once or twice a day.
  - **Cold therapy** preferred in acute conditions and in active involved joints where intraarticular heat is undesired.
- **Electrical stimulation:** To relieve pain and muscle spasm and decrease swelling.
  - TENS 15 minutes, 70 Hz for 3 times/week
  - Interferential therapy (IFT).
- **Orthosis or splinting:** It reduces the pain and inflammation.

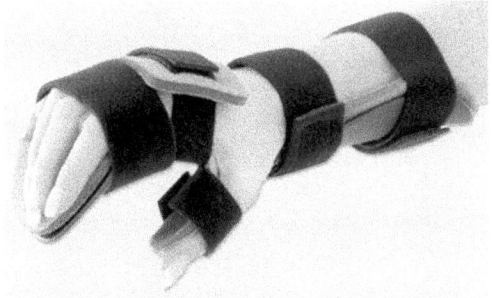

Fig. 12: Splinting of wrist and hand.

- It helps to support and minimize the stress over the affected joint
- It prevents the development of joint deformities
- The joint should be immobilized in functional position, e.g. Shoulder joint: 45° abduction
  Wrist joint: 20–30° DF (Fig. 12)
  Fingers: Slightly flexion
  Hip joint: 45° abduction without any flexion.
  Knee joint: Complete extension
  Ankle and feet: Neutral position.
- **Assistive devices and adaptive equipments:** For example, cane (can reduce 50% load on hip joint), elevated toilet seats, widened gripping handles.
  - It helps in joint protection and energy conservation.
  - It reduces the functional deficits.
  - It helps to maintain the self-efficiency and functional independence of patient.
- **Massage therapy:**
  - It helps in improving the flexibility and general well-being.
  - It helps to reduce the pain and swelling of inflamed joints.
  - It decreases the level of stress hormone and thus effective in depression and anxiety.
- **Therapeutic exercises:** Prolonged immobilization and functional disability gradually leads to muscle weakness. Therefore therapeutic exercises are required to maintain the normal muscle strength which is important for maintaining and improving the physical function, stabilization of joint and prevention of traumatic injuries.

Types and load of exercises depends on:
- Age of patient
- Stage of disease
- Compliance of patient with therapy
- Involvement of joints (local or systemic).

For acute and inflamed joints:
- Isometric exercises are used to maintain strength of muscle.
- Moderate contraction should be held for 6 seconds and repeat 5–10 times/day.
- Isometric contraction of more than 40% of maximal voluntary contraction may lead to impairment in blood circulation and fatigue after exercises.

For conditions where disease activity is low:
- Isotonic exercises with very low weight should be performed.
- Low intensity isokinetic exercise (50% of maximal volumetric contraction) is safe and effective.

For chronic and inactive arthritis conditions:
- Cardiovascular conditioning exercises with adequate rest period increases muscle endurance, aerobic capacity and improve functional ability of patients.
- ROM exercises to prevent contracture.

Caution: If the pain persists for more than 2 hours, too much fatigue, loss of strength or increase in joint swelling after exercises then exercises should be discontinued immediately and should be revised properly.

Avoid:
- Stair climbing
- Weight lifting
- Excessive stretch over tendon during stretching
- Ballistic stretching may damage tendons or joint capsule

Table 1: Difference between osteoarthritis and rheumatoid arthritis.

	Osteoarthritis	Rheumatoid arthritis
Age of onset	Most commonly occurs over the age of 50	Usually occurs between 20–40 years or can occur at any age
Speed of onset	Gradual onset over years	Rapid onset over weeks to months
Symptoms	Painful joints without swelling	Painful joints with swelling and stiffness
Joint involvement	• Asymmetrical joints involvement • Primarily affect proximal large weight bearing joints • **Hand:** PIP and DIP joints	• Symmetrical joints involvement • Primarily affects peripheral small joints. May involves large joints • **Hand:** MCP and PIP joints
Stiffness	• Morning stiffness for <30 minutes • Stiffness occurs after period of activity	• Morning stiffness for >1 hour • Stiffness occurs in period of rest
Systemic symptoms	Lack of systemic symptoms	Frequent fever, weight loss, fatigue, anorexia, muscle ache
Movement	Movement increases the pain	Movement decreases the pain.
Radiological findings	Loss of joint space and articular cartilage. Presence of osteophytes	Bony erosion, soft tissue swelling, periarticular osteopenia, angular deformities
Lab findings	RA factor negative, transient increase of ESR.	RA factor and anti CCP positive, marked increase of ESR, CRP and ANA.

(RA: rheumatoid arthritis; DIP: distal interphalangeal joint; PIP: proximal interphalangeal joint; MCP: metacarpophalangeal joint; ESR: erthrocyte sedimentation rate; CCP: cyclic citrullinated peptide; CRP: C-reactive protein; ANA: antinuclear antibodies)

- High impact activities
- Prolonged walking as it can increase intra-articular pressure in diseased joints.

Surgical Treatment

Indication: Significant joint damage with deformity and loss of function.

Surgical Procedures
- Arthroplasty (total joint replacement)
- Arthrodesis (fusion of joint).

The differential diagnosis between osteoarthritis and rheumatoid arthritis are shown in Table 1.

■ GOUTY ARTHRITIS

It is a chronic, progressive inflammatory disorder characterized by recurrent attacks of painful and inflamed joints due to the deposits of uric acid crystals in the synovial fluid and lining (Fig. 13).

Epidemiology
- Genetic predisposition.
- **Gender:** Males are more affected than Females.
- **Age:** Commonly occurs between 2nd to 4th decades of life.

Predisposing Factors
- Alcohol abuse
- **Diet:** High consumption of protein diet e.g. red meat and beans
- Obesity
- Endocrine disorders, e.g. diabetes, hyperlipidemia, hyperparathyroidism
- Hypertension
- **Medications:** Long-term use of diuretics or aspirin
- Chronic inflammatory systemic diseases, e.g. RA, SLE, multiple sclerosis, etc.
- Myeloproliferative disorders.

Arthritis

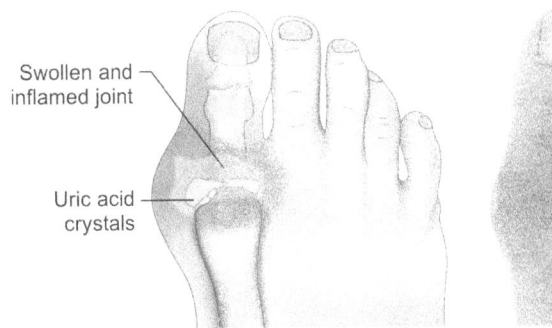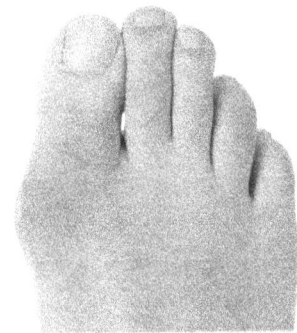

Fig. 13: Gouty arthritis.

Tissues affected by gout include:
- **Joints:** Gout frequently affects the 1st MTP joint. The condition is known as "Podagra". However it may also affect other small joints like joints hands and digits as well as large joints like knee or hip joint.
- **Bursae:** In gout, the most commonly inflamed bursa is olecranon bursa and prepatellar bursa.
- **Tendon sheaths:** The tunnels that protect and provide nutrition to tendons in hands and feet may be affected in gout.
- **Kidneys:** High uric acid levels may cause kidney stones and sometimes cause the kidney damage also. Around 15% of gout patient are suffering from kidney stones.

Pathogenesis

Sodium urate is deposited as crystal on the surface of articular cartilage causing the erosion of articular cartilage. Gradually the subchondral bone is replaced by crystalline deposit known as tophi. A pannus of granulation tissue grows over the articular surface that invades and replaces the cartilage. This granulation tissue bridges the joint to the opposite articular surface and produces fibrous ankylosis.

Clinical Presentation (Fig. 14)
- A typical gout attack is characterized by the sudden onset of severe pain, swelling, warmth and redness of a joint.
- Primary attack subsides within 3–10 days. However, recurrent attacks involve more joints and usually persist longer, i.e. up to 3 weeks.
- Nocturnal attack are common because accumulation of fluid during the day leaves the joint faster than the uric acid in lying position, making the uric acid more concentrated and thus more ready to form crystals.
- Exacerbation of pain on the movement and palpation of the affected joint.
- Systemic reaction like fever, malaise, tachycardia and chills.
- In chronic conditions, the hard lump of uric acid deposited around the joint and under the skin known as "tophi". They commonly develop in fingers, hands, feet, upper ear cartilage and around the elbow.
- If left untreated, tophi around the joint may burst and discharge chalky masses of uric acid crystals through the skin and eventually cause deformities and osteoarthritis.
- 1st MTP joint is the most commonly affected joint in gout.

Complications
- Joint deformity
- Osteoarthritis
- Tophi may produce draining sinuses that may become infected
- Renal stones, pyelonephritis, obstructive renal disease.

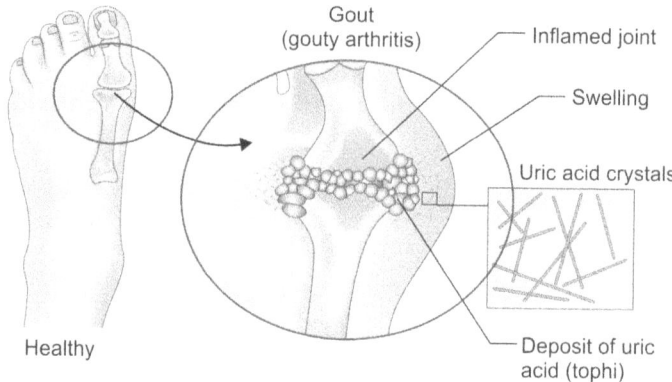

Fig. 14: Clinical presentation of gouty arthritis.

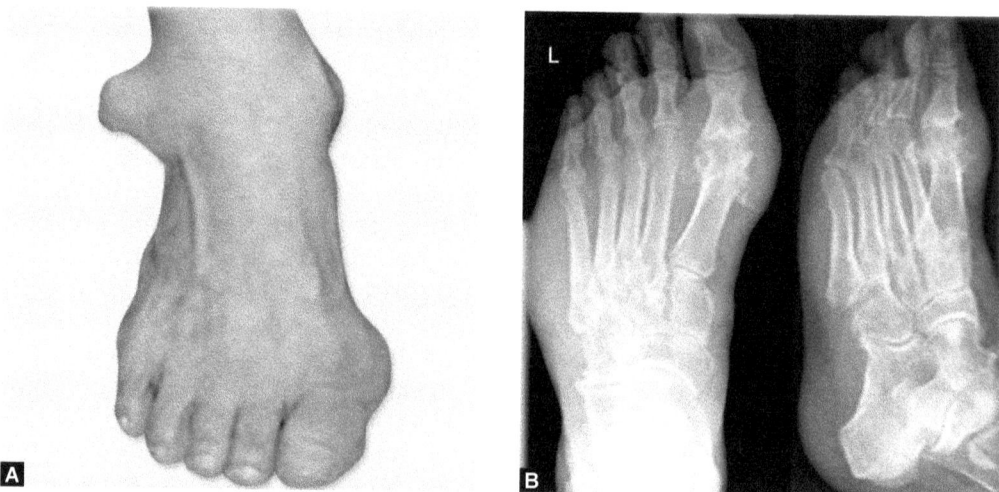

Figs. 15A and B: Gross appearance and X-ray findings of tophi.

Diagnosis

X-ray Findings (Figs. 15A and B)
- Tophi
- Normal mineralization
- Asymmetric polyarticular distribution
- Juxta-articular bony erosion associated with periarticular tophi.
- Subchondral erosions with overhanging bony edges.
  - **Arthrocentesis:** A clinical procedure in which synovial fluid is aspirated from joint cavity. Arthrocentesis reveals the presence of uric acid crystals in joint fluid.
- **Blood test:** Normal serum uric acid is 7.0 mg/dL in males and 6.0 mg/dL in females. More than this level is considered as elevated level of uric acid.

Management

Conservative Treatment

For acute attack
- Medication is used to reduce the pain and inflammation are: Colchicine, NSAIDs and intra-articular corticosteroid injection.
- Drugs used for lowering uric acid are: Allopurinol, febuxostat, lesinurad, probenecid, etc.

- Joint aspiration is used to aspirate the excess fluid from joint cavity and helps to decompress the joint.

Preventive Measures
- Weight reduction
- Healthy diet and optimal exercise
- Maintain the adequate intake of fluid, i.e. 2 L/day
- Cessation of smoking
- **Avoidance of alcohol:** Alcohol has diuretic effects that can contribute to dehydration and can precipitate acute attack of gout. Alcohol also affects the metabolism of uric acid that can cause hyperuremia.
- Avoidance of foods high in purines.
  High: Mussels, liver, kidney, meat soups, sweetbreads, beer and wine
  Moderate: Chicken, salmon, crab, mutton, pork, beef, ham.
- **Encourage:** Low fat dairy products, vitamin C, and coffee.

Physiotherapy Treatment
- **Cryotherapy:** To reduce pain and inflammation.
- **Pain relieving modalities:** Ultrasound/TENS/IFT, etc.
- **Therapeutic exercises:** Regular exercise helps to:
  - Prevent the recurrence of gout.
  - Strengthen and maintain the healthy bones, muscle and joints.
  - Improve mobility and flexibility.
  - Improve circulation.
- **Stretching exercises:** Stretching exercises are necessary to reduce joint stiffness and improve the circulation. Simple stretches, such as knee bends helps to relieve tension in the joint and reduce inflammation.
- **ROM exercises:** It helps to maintain the mobility of joints.
- **Endurance program:** It helps to improve the blood circulation and cardiovascular function. Low impact exercises like swimming and stationary cycling are recommended to avoid any additional strain on the lower extremities.
- **Strengthening exercises:** It helps to condition or tone the muscles and to promote circulation in the extremities.

Surgical Treatment
Indication: In chronic gout, that develops destructive gouty arthritic changes especially in 1st MTP joint.

Surgical Techniques
- **Removal of tophi:** Large nodules around the finger or toe joint, tendons or bursae are removed to reduce the pain. It is necessary to remove the inflamed and painful bursa because it may progressively become infected.
- **Joint fusion:** Joint fusion of smaller joints is indicated in case of permanent joint destruction in chronic gout to relieve the pain.
- **Joint replacement:** The goal of the surgery is to relieve the pain and maintain the mobility of the joint. The knee joint is the most common joint requiring replacement due to gout.

CHAPTER 7

Metabolic Bone Diseases

OSTEOPOROSIS

Osteoporosis means "porous bone" (Fig. 1). It is skeletal disorder characterized by decreased bone density with microarchitectural disruption and fragility resulting in increased risk of fracture.

Predisposing Factors

- **Non-modifiable factors:**
  - Women after menopause
  - Hereditary: Family history of osteoporosis
  - Advance age
  - Estrogen deficiency in females
  - Decrease testosterone level in males.
- **Modifiable factors:**
  - Excess alcohol consumption (more than 3 units/day)
  - Vitamin D deficiency
  - Tobacco smoking (it inhibits the activity of osteoblasts)
  - High protein diet (diet high in animal protein leads to increase urinary calcium loss from bones)
  - Caffeine (more than 2 cups/day)
  - Soft drink (may displace calcium containing drink from diet rather than directly causing osteoporosis)
  - Malnutrition (low dietary calcium, phosphorous, Mg, Zn, boron, fluoride, copper, vitamin A, C, E, K and D due to inadequate sunlight)
  - Underweight/inactivity: As bone remodeling occurs in response to physical stress, physical activity and weight bearing exercise.
  - Excess physical activity can lead to constant damage to bone.

Types of Osteoporosis

Primary Osteoporosis
- Type 1: Postmenopausal osteoporosis
- Type 2: Age-related osteoporosis.

Secondary Osteoporosis

Loss of bone is caused by an identifiable agent or disease process.
- **Diet and nutrition:** Calcium or vitamin D deficiency, malnutrition, high animal protein diet, high fat diet (it reduces calcium absorption in the gut), excess sugar (it depletes phosphorus)
- **Endocrine disorders:** Cushing syndrome, hypo or hyperthyroidism, diabetes mellitus, acromegaly, adrenal insufficiency, pregnancy and lactation causes reversible bone loss.

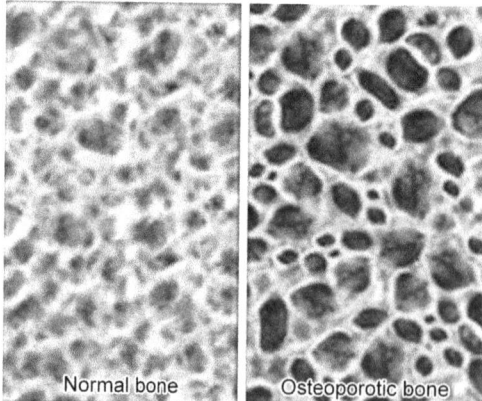

Fig. 1: Normal and osteoporotic bone.

- **Renal disease:** Renal insufficiency leads to osteodystrophy
- **Gastrointestinal or liver disease**, e.g. liver cirrhosis
- **Rheumatologic disorders:** Patient having rheumatoid arthritis (RA), systemic lupus erythematosus (SLE) or ankylosing spondylitis are at high risk of developing osteoporosis.
- **Medications:** Prolonged intake of steroid, barbiturates, antiepileptic, anticoagulants, immunosuppressant, etc.
- **Multiple myeloma and malignancy:** Bone marrow infiltration causes bone loss.
- **Prolonged immobilization** causes continuous release of calcium from bone into the blood that progressively leads to osteoporosis.

Pathogenesis

Underlying mechanism of osteoporosis is an imbalance between bone resorption and bone formation. There is constant matrix remodeling of bone. Bone is resorbed by osteoclast cells after which new bone is deposited by osteoblast cells.

Three mechanism of developing osteoporosis are:
1. Inadequate peak bone mass
2. Excessive bone resorption
3. Inadequate formation of new bone during remodeling.

Clinical Presentation

It is often known as "silent disease" as it is not recognized until fracture occurs. Usually, bone mass is lost over many years with no sign and symptoms.
- Generalized bone pain and tenderness
- Neck pain or discomfort in the neck
- Persistent back pain
- Rib pain
- Fatigue and abdominal pain
- Brittle nails
- Loss of height (patient may lose as much as 6" height)
- Tooth loss and periodontal disease.
- Spinal deformities like Dowager's hump or stooped posture.

Diagnosis

- **Conventional radiography:** It is relatively insensitive to detect early changes of disease process and requires substantial amount of bone loss (about 30%) to be apparent on X-ray image. X-ray findings of osteoporosis are:
  - Cortical thinning
  - Increased radiolucency.
- **DEXA scan (Dual energy X-ray absorptiometry):** It is most accurate test as it can detect changes even after a percentage changes and there is comparatively less exposure to radiations than standard chest X-ray. It is also known as BMD (bone mineral density) test. There are two types of DEXA scanning.
  1. **Central scanning:** It is most preferred method because it measure bone density at hip and spine where bone loss occurs most rapidly.
  2. **Peripheral test also known as screening test:** It is used when central test cannot be done. It measures bone density in lower arm, radius, wrist, finger or heel.

Results are reported in 2 ways:
1. **T-score:** It compares the patient's bone density with optimal peak bone density of young healthy adult of same gender. It is reported as number of standard deviation below average (Fig. 2).

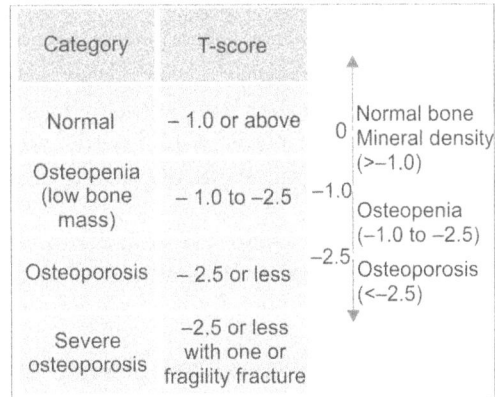

Fig. 2: DEXA T-score.

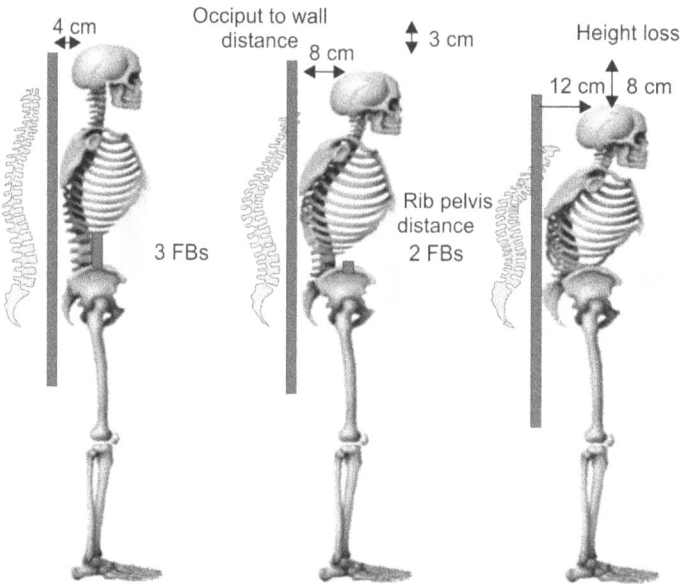

Fig. 3: Rib pelvis and occiput to wall distances.
(FB: finger breadth)

2. **Z-score:** It compares patient's bone density with the bone density of the average person of same age, weight and gender. The finding of Z-score less than –1.5 represents osteoporosis.

Physical Examination
- Decreasing height greater than 1.5 inches.
- Low body weight. Weight loss ≥10% since age 25 is significant
- Dorsal kyphosis/humped back
- Exaggerated cervical lordosis
- Tooth loss
- Skin fold thickness
- Assess for localized pain, muscle spasm, neurologic deficit (risk of spinal cord compression), loss of strength, ROM in affected area.
- **Flesche test or occiput to wall distance:** Patient stand against the wall and asked to touch the back of head to the wall without the upward movement of chin, i.e. to maintain the neutral position of spine. Test is considered to be positive if the patient is not able to touch the occiput to the wall. Normal occiput to wall distance should be zero. Degree of kyphosis can be measured by this test. A measurement more than 7 cm correlates strongly with thoracic fracture (Fig. 3).
- **Rib pelvic distance:** Occult anterior lumbar fracture can be revealed by measuring rib pelvic distance. Patient standing with arm outstretched at 90° angle. Examiner places the fingers in the gap between inferior costal margin and the pelvis. Test is considered to be positive if the distance is less than 2 finger breadths at the midaxillary line (Fig. 3).

Preventive Measures (Fig. 4)
- **Lifestyle modification:**
  - Smoking cessation
  - Moderation of alcohol intake
- **Exercise and nutrition:** Studies have found that regular exercise with proper diet delays the degeneration of bone. According to these studies jogging, walking

Metabolic Bone Diseases

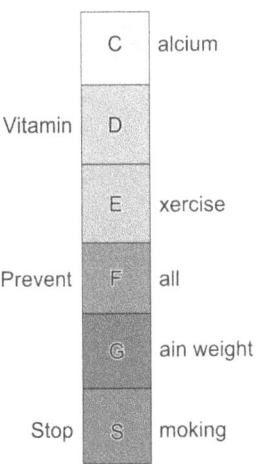

Fig. 4: Basic prevention of osteoporosis.

or stair climbing at 70–90% of maximum effort thrice a week along with 1500 mg of calcium per day increases the bone density of lumbar spine by 5% over 9 months.
- **Nutrition:** Diet sufficient in calcium such as milk, cheese, yogurt, almond, broccoli, cauliflower and vitamin D.
- **Calcium and vitamin D supplements**: Adolescents need around 1200 mg calcium daily and postmenopausal women may need 1500 mg calcium daily. Elderly should be advised to take 400–800 units of vitamin D daily.

Management

Medications

Antiresorptive Agents
- Biphosphates, e.g. sodium alendronate, risedronate, ibandronate.
- Estrogen replacement therapy.
- Raloxifene (selective estrogen receptor modulator) slows bone resorption.
- **Calcitonin:** Inhibits osteoclast activity.

Bone Anabolic Agents
- Teriparatide stimulates the activity of osteoblasts
- Calcium salt
- Sodium fluoride.

Physiotherapy Management

Aims
- Fracture prevention by improving the bone health and reducing the risks of fall.
- To improve posture and reduce deformity.
- To reduce and control pain.
- To provide education in order to facilitate self-management.

Treatment
- **Pain Management**
  - TENS
  - Hot therapy
  - Hydrotherapy
  - Relaxation therapy
- **ROM exercises**: Free active mobility exercises such as spinal extension exercises (quadruped position to strengthen the back), chin tucks, scapular retractions, hip extension, knee extension and ankle movement. All these exercises improve posture, balance and strength.
- **Weight bearing exercises:** Studies have found that weight bearing exercises helps to maintain bone mass and can increase it by 1 to 2%. Low impact activities such as walking outdoors or on treadmill, gentle non-pounding forms of dance and stair climbing, etc. All these activities help in loading the bones, encourage an upright posture, improve cardiovascular fitness and bone density.
- **Flexibility exercises**: Improved flexibility helps to
  - Decrease the stress induced by the tight muscles over the bones.
  - Improve the ability to maintain good posture.
  - Improve the body mechanics. Good flexibility also reduces the risk of fall by:
    – Improving overall physical function and postural control.
    – Improving the mobility, this in turn improves the balance.
    – Gentle stretching of tight muscles that occurs due to the occurrence

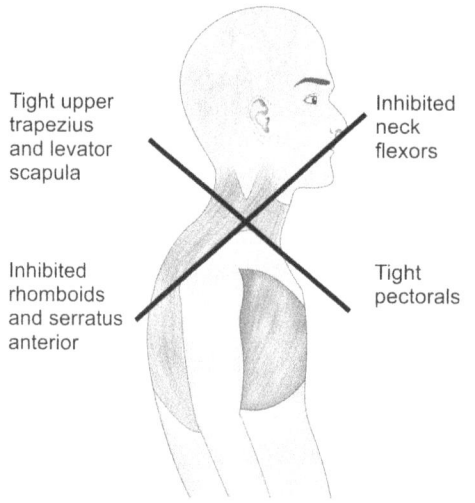

Fig. 5: Upper cross syndrome.

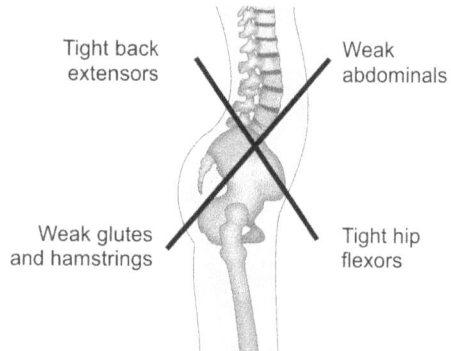

Fig. 6: Lower cross syndrome.

of upper cross syndrome in thoracic kyphotic posture such as upper trapezius, levator scapula and pectoralis major and minor (Fig. 5).
  – Gentle stretching of tight muscles that occurs due to the presence of lower cross syndrome in increased lordotic posture such as trunk extensors, quadratus lumborum and hip flexors, particularly the iliopsoas muscle (Fig. 6).
- **Strengthening exercises:** Gentle strengthening exercises using weight or resistance band. Strengthening of postural muscles that weakens due to bad posture in osteoporotic patients causing upper and lower crossed syndromes mentioned above. Strengthening of serratus anterior, rhomboids, neck flexor, abdominals (isometrics), hip extensors, i.e. hamstring gluteal maximus. Patient should begin with isometric exercise and gradually progress to resistance exercises.
- **Closed chain exercises** of lower limb such as cycling, leg press and upper limb exercises such as arm press.
- **Postural exercises:** These exercises are used to prevent the structural deformity and maintain good posture. Postural exercise program should include spinal extension, chin tucks, scapular retractions and hip extension, etc.
- **Balance exercises:** Poor balance may lead to fall that can easily fracture an osteoporotic bone.
  Exercises to improve balance—standing with feet close together, standing with one foot in front of the other, performs these exercises with closed eyes, tandem walking and frenkel exercises.
  All exercises should be progressed gradually in terms of impact and intensity.

Avoid:
- Spinal flexion exercises. As anterior compression forces to the vertebra caused by flexion movement can cause compression fractures
- Manipulation
- Ballistic stretching
- Undue compressive strain on spine
- High risk movement pattern
- High impact activities like running, jumping and pounding forms of dance
- High intensity training at onset
- Combined flexion and rotation of trunk to reduce stress on the vertebra
- Exercise or activities that may involve quick changes of direction like some sports could result in falls or bone shearing.

RICKETS AND OSTEOMALACIA

Rickets is the softening of bones in childhood due to defective bone mineralization as a result of inadequate intake of vitamin D and insufficient exposure to sunlight, also associated with impaired calcium and phosphorus metabolism (Fig. 7).

Osteomalacia is softening of bones due to defective bone mineralization in adults.

Etiology

Occurs due to the deficiency of vitamin D, calcium or phosphorous.

Vitamin D is a fat soluble vitamin that is essential for the normal formation of bones and teeth and necessary for the appropriate absorption of calcium and phosphorous from the bowel which is essential for bone mineralization. Therefore inadequate vitamin D leads to the deficiency of calcium and phosphorous that progressively results in the demineralization of bones.

- Poor exposure to sunlight
  - Dark skin (black children)—darker skin pigmentation produces vitamin D more slowly and hence requires greater sun exposure.

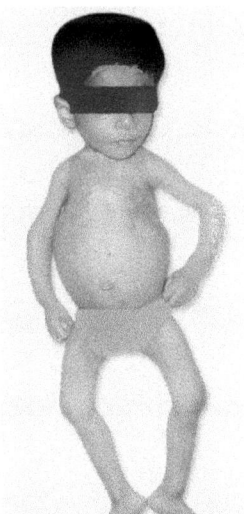

Fig. 7: Rickets.

- Improper feeding:
  - Inadequate intake of vitamin D
  - Improper calcium and phosphorous ratio
- Fast growth, increased requirement that cause relative deficiency.
- Disease that lead to malabsorbtion
  - Liver diseases
  - Renal diseases
  - Gastrointestinal disease, e.g. celiac disease, pancreatitis
  - Cystic fibrosis
- Medications
  - Antacids reduces the absorption of calcium and phosphorous
  - Anticonvulsants lead to increase vitamin D catabolism and also inhibit its absorption.
  - Corticosteroids.
  - Loop diuretics.

Types of Rickets

- **Hypophosphatemia rickets** (vitamin D resistant ricket): It is caused by chronically low levels of phosphates in the blood. In this the absorption of calcium and phosphorous is normal but the phosphate is lost through the kidney into the urine.
- **Renal rickets:** It is caused by kidney disorder. Excessive loss of calcium and phosphate occurs due to the decreased ability of kidney to regulate the amount of electrolytes lost in the urine.
- **Nutritional rickets:** It is caused by dietary deficiency of vitamin D, calcium or phosphate. Infants and children are at greater risk of developing nutritional rickets. It most commonly includes
  - Dark skinned infants
  - Exclusively breastfed infants
  - Infants born to vitamin D deficient mothers
  - Older children who kept out of direct sunlight
  - Children having strict vegetarian diet.

Vitamin D Metabolism

Vitamin D is naturally synthesized by the body in the presence of sunlight and stored in liver. Vitamin D is produced in the skin by the action of ultraviolet rays of sunlight on its precursor, 7-dehydrocholestrol. Vitamin D is also absorbed from the diet such as fortified milk, fish oil etc. Following the conversion of 7-dehydrocholestrol in cholecalciferol (vitamin D3), it is absorbed in gastrointestinal tract. This vitamin D3 is transported through the blood to liver and converted to calcidiol (25-hydroxyvitamin D). Calcidiol is then transported through the blood to kidneys, where it is metabolized to calcitriol (1, 25-dihydroxy vitamin D). Calcitriol maintains the level of calcium and phosphorus in the body by stimulating the small intestine, bone and kidney to absorb calcium, phosphate and magnesium (Fig. 8).

Pathophysiology

Deficiency of vitamin D decreases the absorption of calcium and phosphorous in blood and serum. Low serum calcium concentration in serum prompts the secretion of parathormone from parathyroid. This parathormone liberates the calcium from the bone to restore the normal serum concentration and also increase the release of phosphorous from the urine. This collectively causes decrease in the level of calcium and phosphorous in body that leads to softening of the bone (Fig. 9).

Clinical Presentation of Rickets (Fig. 10)

- Pain or tenderness in bones
- Stunted growth and short stature
- Delayed milestone
- Irritable child
- Lethargy and hypotonia
- Baby is floppy
- Decreased muscle tone (loss of muscle strength)
- Muscle cramps
- Dental deformities:
  - Delayed formation of teeth
  - Defects in the structure of teeth or holes in the enamel

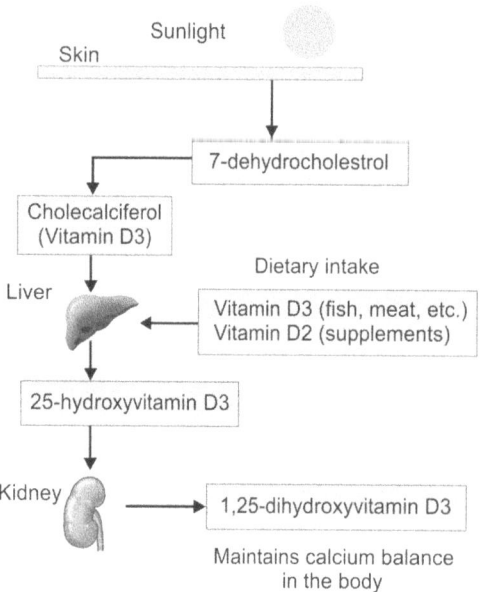

Fig. 8: Synthesis, absorption and metabolism of vitamin D.

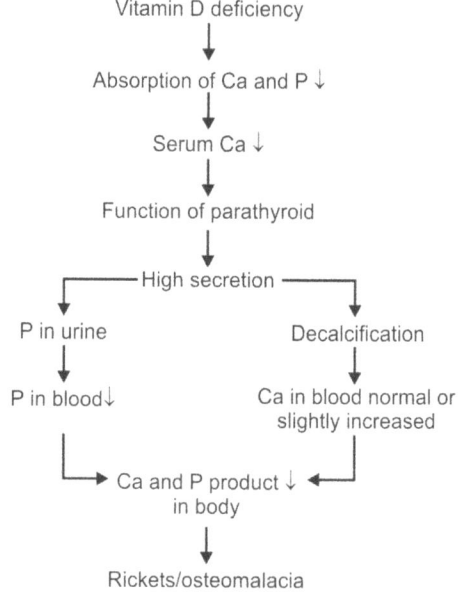

Fig. 9: Pathophysiology of rickets and osteomalacia.

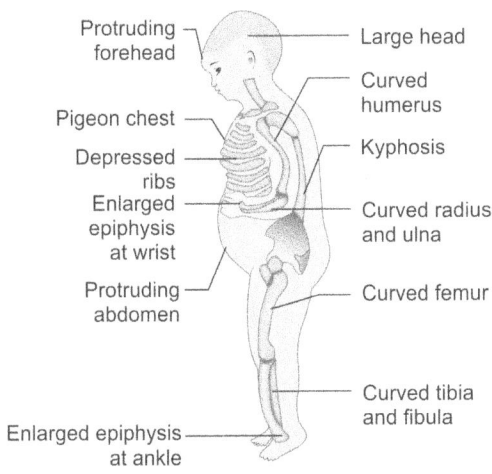

Fig. 10: Clinical manifestations in rickets.

- Increased cavities in teeth
- Progressive weakness of teeth
- Skeletal deformities, including
  - An oddly shaped skull
  - Soft skull usually around the suture line (craniotabes)
  - Bowlegs in toddlers
  - Older children may have knock knees.
  - Bumps in the rib cage known as rachitic rosary
  - Protruding breastbone, i.e. pigeon chest
  - Spine deformities like scoliosis or kyphosis
  - Pelvic deformities
  - Widened wrist

Clinical Presentation of Osteomalacia
- Backache.
- Diffuse skeletal pain
- Proximal muscle weakness and wasting
- Vertebral collapse may lead to loss of height.
- Difficult walking often with waddling gait.
- Pelvic flattening
- Insufficiency fracture of tibia/femur.

Stages of Rickets
There are 3 stages of vitamin D deficiency:
1. Hypocalcaemia due to poor intestinal absorption and reduced bone resorption.
2. Normal calcium and low phosphate state due to secondary hyperparathyroidism.
3. Severe bone disease with recurrence of hypocalcemia.

Diagnosis
X-ray Findings
- Widening or abnormally shaped metaphysis (most actively growing part of bone below the growth plate)
- Obvious bowing of femurs
- Osteopenia (bones are not dense)
- Rib flaring (rachitic rosary)
- Multiple fractures at different healing stages.
- Looser zones.

Laboratory Investigations
- Decrease in serum calcium level, serum phosphorous, calcidol, calcitriol and urinary calcium level.
- Increase in parathyroid hormone, alkaline phosphate and urinary phosphate.

Physical Examination in Rickets
Head (Figs. 11A and B)
- Craniotabes
- Frontal and parietal bossing
- Flat occiput
- Anterior fontanelle is large with delay in closure.

Chest (Fig. 12)
- **Rachitic rosary:** Costochondral swelling—prominent knobs on bone between ribs and sternum.
- **Harrison's sulcus or groove:** A horizontal line visible on the chest where the diaphragm attaches to the ribs.
- **Pigeon chest:** Protrusion of sternum.

Extremities (Fig. 13)
- Widening of wrist and ankle.
- Bowing of legs or knock knee.

Spinal Deformities
Scoliosis, kyphosis or lordosis.

270 Simplified Approach to Orthopedic Physiotherapy

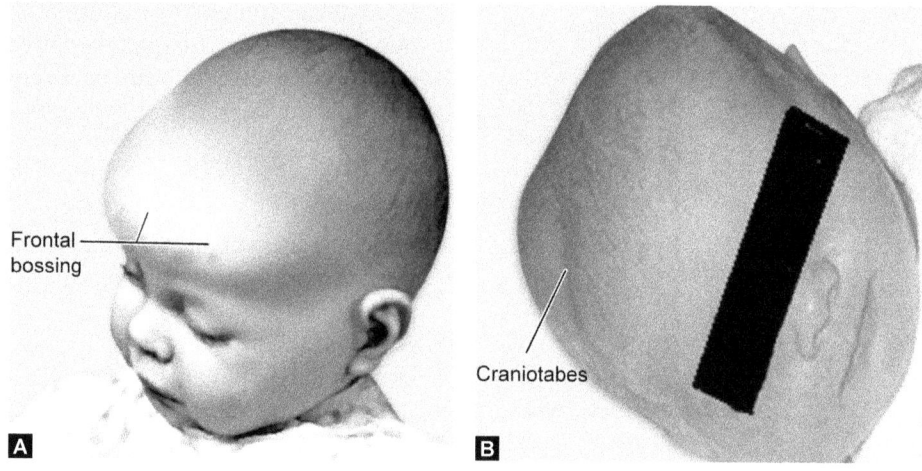

Figs. 11A and B: A. Frontal bossing; B. Craniotabes.

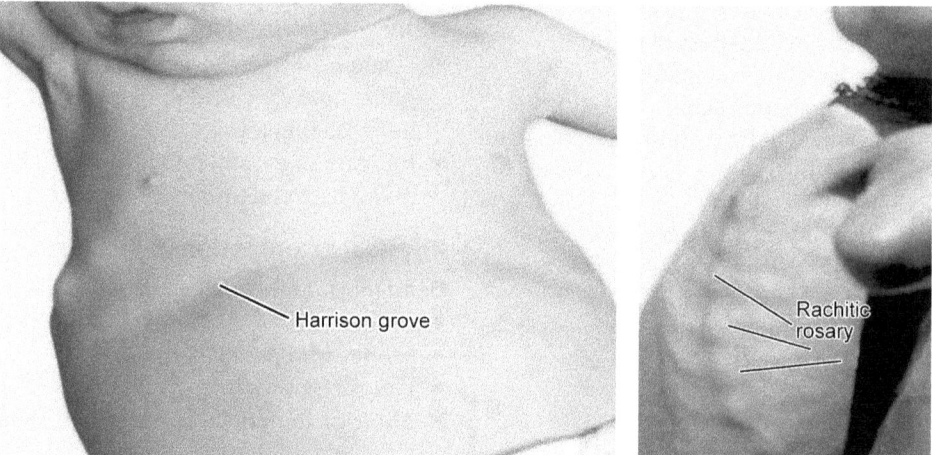

Fig. 12: Harrison grove and Rachiltic rosary.

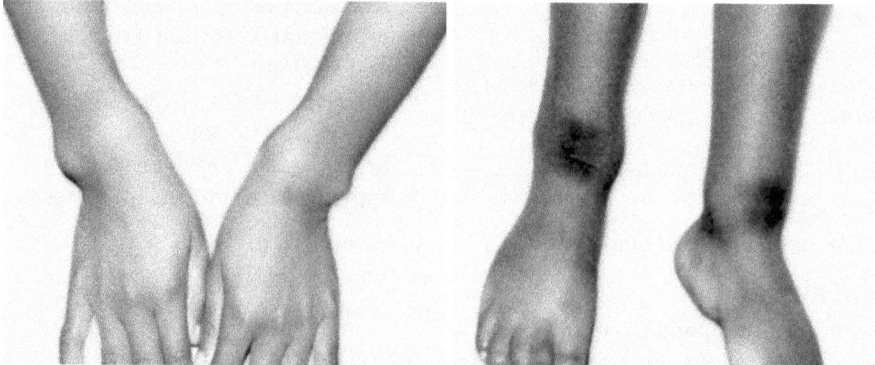

Fig. 13: Widening of wrist and ankle due to rickets.

Pot Belly due to
- Hypotonia of abdominal muscles and intestine.
- Downward displacement of the liver and spleen.

Physical Examination in Osteomalacia
- Bone tenderness
- Proximal muscle weakness
- Proximal muscle wasting
- Hypotonia
- Gait disturbances-waddling gait.

Management

Special Treatment: Vitamin D Therapy
- **Oral therapy:** Vitamin D 2000–4000 IU/day for 2–4 weeks, then continue with preventive dosage-400 IU/day.
- **Intramuscular therapy:** A single large dose: For severe case, rickets with complication or patient who cannot bear oral therapy. Vitamin D3 200000–300000 IU. Continue with preventive dosage after 2–3 months.

General Treatment
- **Diet:** Increase dietary intake of calcium, phosphate and vitamin D including cod liver oil, halibut liver oil and viosterol.
- **Sunlight:** exposure to ultraviolet B light (most easily obtained when the sun is highest in the sky)
- **Supplementation:** Dosage 1–3 g/day. Vitamin D3 (cholecalciferol) is the preferred form because it is more readily absorbed than vitamin D2. According to the American Academy of Pediatrics, all infants, including those who are exclusively breastfed, may need vitamin D supplementation until they start drinking at least 500 ml of vitamin D fortified milk.

Physiotherapy Treatment
- If left untreated, the child can develop spinal curvatures, seizures, and osteoporosis. Once the child becomes older and still cannot absorb vitamin D, it is very important for them to try and increase bone growth as much as possible. Exercises while standing or weight bearing can help to increase bone growth but due to osteoporosis, they may also are at high risk for fractures. Physiotherapy may also help to reduce any skeletal or muscular pain through stretching and strengthening exercises as well as hands on manual techniques.
- Braces may be used to reduce or prevent bony deformities.
- Patient should avoid contact sports until the complete recovery from rickets. There are no direct physiotherapy interventions for vitamin D deficiency. Patients are referred to physiotherapy treatment for the treatment of the impairments caused by vitamin D deficiency like muscle weakness, decline in physical functioning or to prevent the falls.
- Physiotherapy of rickets and osteomalacia is same as discussed for osteoporosis.

CHAPTER 8

Arthroplasty

Surgical reconstruction or replacement of a malformed or degenerated joint is used to relieve pain and restore range of motion (ROM).

Indications
- Severe joint pain with weight bearing or motion.
- Gross instability and limitation of motion.
- Traumatized and malaligned joint.
- Failure of previous joint surgery.
- Extensive destruction of articular cartilage of joint secondary to arthritis (rheumatoid arthritis or osteoarthritis)
- Severe pain and disabling joint stiffness.
- For correction of deformity of joint.

Contraindications
Absolute Contraindications
- Neuropathic arthropathies.
- Malignant tumor.
- Systemic infection or sepsis (joint sepsis).
- Active infection in joint.
- Severe vascular disease.

Relative Contraindications
- Severe osteoporosis.
- Debilitated poor health.
- Obesity for lower limb.
- Marked muscle weakness
- Localized infection especially bladder, chest or skin.
- Any skin condition within the field of surgery, e.g. psoriasis.
- Past history of osteomyelitis around the joint.

Implant Fixation
Types of fixation used to connect implants to the bones are:
- **Cemented fixation:** Implant is fixed to the bone by fast curing bone cement. Usually polymethylmethacrylate cement is used.
- **Cement less fixation:** Implant can be press onto the bone, this type of fixation relies on new growing bone into the surface of implant. In this, the implant surface are coated or textured with a porous material (hydroxyapatite coating) so that the new bone grows into the surface of implant. Screws may be used to stabilize the implant until the bone growth occurs. Hydroxyapatite coating also allows a strong chemical bonding between the bone and the implant in order to enhance a proper fixation. Cementless fixation is not indicated in osteoporotic patients.
- **Hybrid fixation**: It is the combinations of both cemented and cement less design, e.g. in total knee replacement, femoral component is inserted without cement whereas tibial and patellar components are fixed with cement.

Implant Material
- Metal parts are made up of titanium or cobalt chromium based alloy.
- Plastic parts are made up of ultra-high molecular weight polyethylene.

Properties of Material Used
- **Biocompatible:** They are non-toxic, non-irritant, non-allergic and non-carcinogenic.

- High compression, bending and torsional strength.
- Low friction and wear rate.
- Good shock absorbing capacity.
- Good corrosion resistant in synovial fluid.
- Ability to move smoothly against each other.
- Ability to retain their strength and shape for long time.

■ TOTAL KNEE REPLACEMENT (TKR)

The surgical replacement of knee joint with prosthetic implants is known as TKR (Fig. 1).

Implant Component (Fig. 2)
- **Tibial component:** The flat part that attaches to the top of the resurfaced proximal end of tibia. This part is usually made up of a flat metal platform with a cushion of strong and durable plastic known as polyethylene.
- **Femoral component:** The largest and metallic curved part that attached to the distal end of resurfaced femur. It is grooved to facilitate the smooth movement of patella during the flexion and extension of the knee.
- **Patellar component:** It is a domed shape piece of polyethylene that replaces the damaged knee cap.

Surfaces Replaced in TKR
- Distal end of femur.
- Proximal end of tibia.
- Posterior surface of patella.

Types of Knee Replacement
- **Posterior cruciate retaining design:** In this, anterior cruciate ligament is removed but the posterior cruciate ligament is preserved to prevent the femur from sliding off the anterior edge of the tibia. The femoral and tibial components have notches to accommodate the ligament. It is indicated in patients having healthy posterior cruciate ligament (PCL).
- **Posterior cruciate substituting design:** In this both anterior and posterior cruciate ligament are removed and parts of implants substitute for PCL. Tibial component has a raised surface that is cushioned with a raised sloping cam or post which compensates for the missing PCL to provide knee stability in the absence of ligament.
- **Bicruciate retaining design:** In this design, both ACL and PCL are preserved that helps the operated knee to function like a non-replaced knee.
- **Unicompartmental implants design:** In this design, only one compartment (lateral or medial) of knee joint is replaced (Fig. 3).

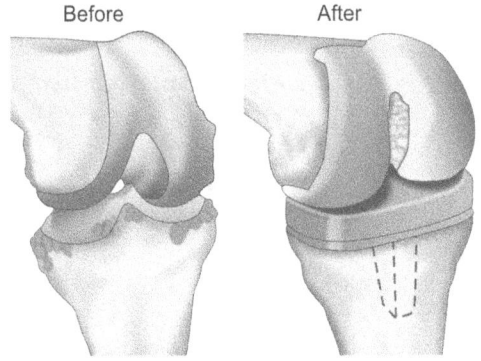

Fig. 1: Total knee replacement.

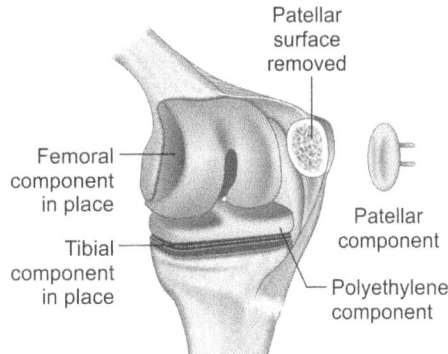

Fig. 2: Implant components in TKR.

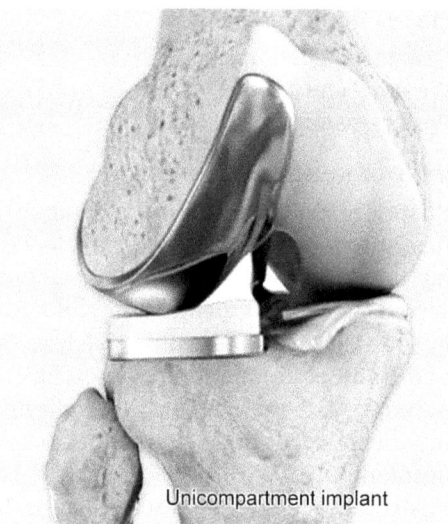

Fig. 3: Unicompartment implant design.

Physiotherapy treatment: Postoperative physiotherapy treatment protocol for TKR.

Phase I	Immediate postoperative phase: Day 1–10
Goals	Active quadriceps muscle contraction
	Independent ambulation
	Passive knee extension to 0°
	To reduce pain and inflammation
Day 1–2	WBAT
	Knee immobilizer with pillows under ankle to encourage passive knee extension
	Cryotherapy
	DVT prophylaxis (TED hose anti-embolism stocking)
Exercises	Ankle pumps with elevation
	Passive knee extension
	SLR if not contraindicated
	Quadriceps isometrics
	Knee extension exercises 90–30°
	Gentle knee flexion exercises
Day 4–10	Weight bearing as tolerated
	CPM: 0–90° as tolerated

Contd...

Phase I	Immediate postoperative phase: Day 1–10
Exercises	Same as above
	AAROM knee flexion
	Hip adduction-abduction
	Knee extension exercises 90–0°
	VMO exercises
Phase II	**Motion phase: Week 2–6**
Goals	Improve ROM (0–110°)
	Independent ambulation
	Increase strength and endurance
	Reduce swelling and inflammation
	Return to functional activity
Week 2–4	WB with assistive device
Exercises	Same as above
	Terminal knee extension 45–0°
	SLR (flexion-extension)
	Prone lying exercises
	Hamstring curls
	Stretching: hamstring, calf and quadriceps
	Squats
Week 4–6	WB: Independent ambulation
Exercises	Front and lateral step ups
	Front lunges
	Same as above
Phase III	**Immediate activit phase: Week 7–12**
Goals	Progression of ROM (0–115°)
	Increase strength and endurance
	Cardiovascular fitness
	Strengthening 85% of contralateral limb
	Eccentric-concentric exercises of limb
	Functional activity
Exercises	Same as above
	Progressive walking program

Contd...

Contd...

Phase III	Immediate activit phase: Week 7–12
	Endurance program
	Eccentric-concentric knee control
Phase IV	Advanced activity phase: Week 14–26
Goals	Maintain and improve strength and endurance of lower limb
	Return to ADLs
Exercises	Same as above
	Passive stretching into flexion
	Stationary bicycle
	Backward walking
	Eccentric extension

(WBAT: weight-bearing as tolerated; DVT: deep vein thrombosis; TED: thrombo-embolic deterrent; SLR: straight leg raising; CPM: continuous passive motion; AAROM: active assistive range of motion; VMO: vastus medialis oblique; ADLs: activities of daily living)

- **When the patient has difficulty in obtaining full knee extension: Therapist should include**
  - Backward walking
  - Passive extension
  - Eccentric extension
  - Standing kicks
  - Electric muscle stimulation and VMO biofeedback
  - Place towel beneath ankle.

- **In case of delayed knee flexion: Therapist should include**
  - Passive stretching into flexion
  - Wall slides for gravity assistance
  - Stationary bicycling.

■ TOTAL HIP REPLACEMENT (THR)

It is the surgical replacement of hip joint by prosthetic implant (Fig. 4).

Implant Components (Fig. 5)

- **Acetabular component (socket):** Bowl or cup shaped piece that fits into resurfaced socket. It is usually made of metal but is occasionally made of ceramic or combination of plastic and metal.
- **Acetabular liner:** The plastic liner fits into the acetabular component and allows the femoral head to glide easily and more naturally in socket.
- **Femoral head:** The ball that fit directly into plastic lined socket and attached to femoral stem. These are made of durable metal, plastic, ceramic or combination of materials.
- **Femoral stem:** It is a metal stem attaches to the ball and supports the new hip joint.

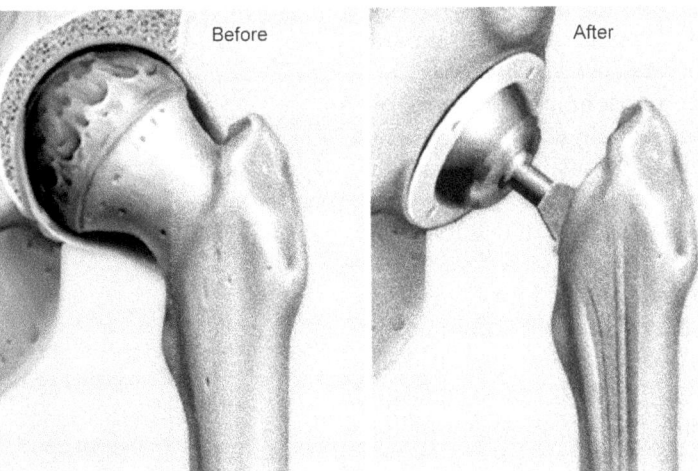

Fig. 4: Total hip replacement.

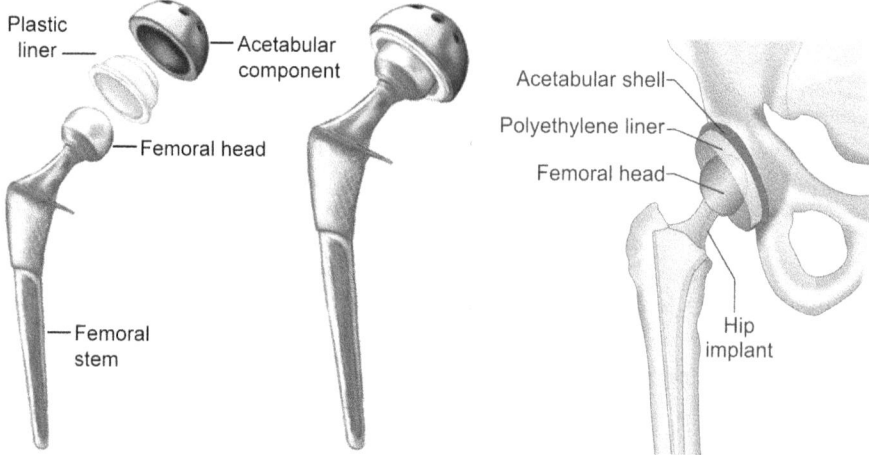

Fig. 5: Implant components of THR.

Types of Hip Replacement

- **Stem type with acrylic cement fixation:** In this technique, both the femoral and acetabular components are secured to the bones with an cement (acrylic polymer) called polymethyl methacrylate (PMMA).
- **Stem type without cement fixation:** In this technique, implants are attached to the bone without cement. These cement less implants are textured or have porous surface coating that allows new bone to grow into the surface of the implant.
- **Stem type with hybrid fixation:** In hybrid fixation, the acetabular component is fixed without cement and the femoral component is attached with cement.
- **Hemi surface replacement/hemiarthroplasty:** In this technique, only one component of the hip joint (usually femoral head) is replaced. It is indicated in case of AVN of femoral head and fracture of femoral neck.
- **Surface replacement of hip:** It involves the shaving and capping a few millimeters of joint surface and reshaped it with prosthetic shell rather than replacing the entire hip joint. It reduces the risk of postoperative dislocation and leg length discrepancy.

Physiotherapy treatment: Postoperative physiotherapy treatment protocol for THR.

Precautions	For 6 weeks
	Posterior approach: Avoid hip flexion more than 90°, internal rotation or adduction beyond neutral. Patient must use hip chair and abduction pillow
	Direct anterior approach: Avoid passive hip extension and external rotation
	Lateral approach: Avoid passive and active hip extension and external rotation
	Wear TED hose
	Pillow under ankle and NOT under knee
Phase I	**Protective phase: Week 0–1**
Goals	Reduce pain, swelling and inflammation
	Independent bed mobility and transfer
	Independent ambulation 100 feet
Treatment	Cold pack to reduce pain, inflammation and swelling
	Bed mobility and transfer training including sit stand

Contd...

Arthroplasty

Contd...

Phase I	Protective phase: Week 0–1
	Exercises: Ankle pump, quadriceps and gluteal isometrics
	Gait training using appropriate assistive device
Phase II	**Transitional phase: Week 1–3**
Goals	Reduce pain, swelling and inflammation.
	Increase ROM and strength.
	Improve functional independence
	Normal gait pattern using appropriate assistive device
Treatment	*Exercises:* • Ankle pumps • Heel slides • Passive/active assisted and active ROM exercises in supine position. • Hip adduction/abduction, flexion/extension, IR/ER only to be performed within ROM precaution guidelines. • Passive, active assisted and active ROM exercises in sitting: long arc quads, ankle pumps
	Strengthening exercises: • Quads sets in full extension • Gluteal sets • Short arc quads
	Gait training: • Continuing training with assistive device • Wean from walker to crutch to cane without any gait deviation
	Modalities: Cold packs to reduce pain and swelling
Criteria for progression to next phase	
	Minimal pain, inflammation and swelling
	Patient ambulates with assistive device without gait deviation
Phase III	**Outpatient early phase: Week 3–6**
Goals	Increase ROM
	Increase lower limb and trunk strength

Contd...

Contd...

Phase III	Outpatient early phase: Week 3–6
	Balance and proprioceptive training to assist with functional activities
	Gait training: Wean off assistive device when patient can ambulate without deviation
	Functional activity training
Treatment	*Exercises:* • Stationary bike • Initiate transverse abdominus and level 1 trunk stabilization • 3 ways SLR (flexion, abduction, extension – No extension for lateral approach until 6 weeks) • Closed chain weight shifting activities including side stepping • Balance exercises: single leg stance, alter surfaces, eye open or closed • Lateral step up and step down with eccentric control • Front step up and down
	Functional activities: • Sit to stand activities • Lifting and carrying • Ascending/descending stairs
	Gait training
Criteria for progression to next phase	
	Minimal pain and swelling
	Patient ambulate without assistive device without gait deviation
	Good voluntary quadriceps control
Phase IV	**Outpatient intermediate phase: Week 6–12**
Goals	Increase overall strength of lower limb
	Return to all functional activities
	Begin light recreational activities
Treatment	Progress Phase III exercises by increasing resistance and repetitions
	Progressive trunk stabilization exercises
	Front lunges and squat activities
	Progressive balance and proprioceptive activities
	Initiate overall exercise and endurance training (walking, swimming, biking, etc.)

CHAPTER 9

Arthrodesis

Arthrodesis is referred to the fusion of a joint which has been damaged/destructed due to disease/trauma beyond repair or reconstruction with marked instability and severe functional handicap.

Indications

- To relieve severe pain, e.g. in secondary osteoarthritis (OA) and rheumatoid arthritis (RA).
- In paralytic conditions, e.g. poliomyelitis where muscles are paralyzed partially or completely
- Infection and tumor
- Arthritic disease unsuitable for arthroplasty
- Recurrent dislocation of joint
- Stabilization after resection of neoplastic lesions
- After failure of joint replacement.

Contraindications

- Osteonecrosis
- Neuropathic arthropathies
- Ipsilateral (other) joint fusion
- Contralateral (same) joint fusion.

Types

- **Intra-articular arthrodesis:** Articular cartilage is removed from both the opposing body ends and shaped to fit in an optimum functional position. Fusion is secured by internal fixation, external fixator, plaster cast or by combination of these methods.
- **Extra-articular arthrodesis:** Joint surfaces are not denuded of its cartilage but fusion is achieved in position of optimum function by bone graft placed outside but adjacent to the joint. Bone to bone fusion is obtained above and below the joint.
  Indications:
  - Useful in treating children because much of their joint surfaces are cartilage
  - Patient who have large amount of necrotic bone
  - Active infection as in tuberculosis (hip, shoulder and spine)
  - When there is no risk of reactivating or spreading infection as the joint itself is not opened.
- **Combined arthrodesis:** This includes the combination of above two procedures.

■ SHOULDER ARTHRODESIS

Indications

- Massive unreconstructable rotator cuff tear
- Post-traumatic brachial plexus palsy
- Recurrent dislocation
- Shoulder paralysis/paralytic disorder
- Failed shoulder athroplasty
- Stabilization after resection of neoplastic lesions.

For shoulder fusion, serratus anterior, trapezius and muscles of forearm and hand should be functional to control scapulothoracic movement after fusion.

Contraindications

- Progressive neurologic condition
- Ipsilateral elbow fusion

- Contralateral shoulder fusion
- Charcot arthropathies (nonunion rate is very high).

Position of joint fusion: Shoulder abduction 20-30°, forward flexion 20-30°, internal rotation 20-30°.

Complications
- Malpositioning of shoulder, i.e. excessive shoulder abduction or flexion may results in periscapular pain
- Traction neuritis
- Pseudoarthrosis/nonunion.

ELBOW ARTHRODESIS

Indications
- Infectious arthritis
- Failed elbow arthroplasty
- Post-traumatic arthritis
- Arthritic disease incompatible for arthroplasty
- Severely comminuted intra-articular fracture.

Position of Joint Fusion
- Unilateral: Elbow flexion 90°
- Bilateral:
  - One elbow: Elbow flexion 110° (permit patient to reach mouth)
  - Other elbow: Elbow flexion 65° (to aid in personal hygiene).

Complications
- Neurovascular injury
- Wound infection
- Delayed union
- Nonunion/malunion

Postoperative
- External fixator (for 12 weeks) or a long arm cast (for 6 weeks) is applied until bones ends fuse together
- Stiches are removed after 10-14 days
- Keep the arm elevated above heart level to avoid swelling and throbbing.

WRIST ARTHRODESIS

Indications
- Post-traumatic arthritis
- Neoplastic lesion
- Severely comminuted intra-articular fracture
- Rheumatoid arthritis
- Wrist and hand paralysis
- Spastic hemiplegia
- Failed total joint arthroplasty
- Failed limited arthrodesis.

Contraindications
- Open physis of distal radius (it closes approximately at age of 17)
- Elderly patients with sedentary life-style, especially if non-dominant wrist is involved
- RA patient where tendon transfer and joint replacement may be more appropriate.

Position of Joint Fusion
- **Wrist joint:** 10°–20° dorsiflexion, 5° ulnar deviation to neutral
  - In bilateral wrist joint fusion one joint 20° dorsiflexion and other in slight flexion.
- **Hand:** MCP joint: 20-30° flexion
  - **PIP joint:** Fixed from 25° flexion in index finger to almost 40° of little finger (i.e. less flexion at radial fingers than at ulnar fingers)
  - **DIP joint:** 15-20° flexion.

Complications
- Tendon adhesions/ruptures
- Distal radioulnar joint pain/instability
- MCP joint stiffness
- Carpal tunnel syndrome
- Reflex sympathetic dystrophy
- Nonunion.

Postoperative
- Elbow length cast applied for 6 weeks
- Stiches are removed after 10-14 days
- Keep the arm elevated above heart level to avoid swelling and throbbing.

HIP ARTHRODESIS

Indications
- **In young adults**
  - Post-traumatic degenerative disease
  - Avascular necrosis
  - Septic arthritis
- **For failed arthroplasty:** Due to infection or mechanical failure
- **In skeletally immature person**
  - Tuberculosis (TB) and septic arthritis
  - Painful ankylosis following slipped capital femoral epiphysis
  - Congenital coxa vara
  - Aseptic necrosis of head of femur.

Contraindications
- Systemic inflammatory disease (RA/SLE)
- Bilateral hip disease
- Patient with stiff spine
- Patient on long-term corticosteroid
- Ipsilateral knee involvement
- Occupation required long period of sitting/bending/squatting/climbing
- Severe degenerative changes in lumbosacral spine.
- Active sepsis of hip (infection should be manifested inactive for 12 months before arthrodesis is considered).

Position of joint fusion: Hip flexion 30°, adduction 0–5°, external rotation 0–15°.

Complications
- Malposition which hampers function and put unwanted strain on other joints
- Nonunion
- Leg length discrepancy
- Degenerative joint disease or ipsilateral knee/back/contralateral hip (after 15–25 years)
- Low back pain (due to excessive motion at lumbar spine and ipsilateral knee)
- Malposition of hip, i.e. excessive flexion may cause compensatory lumbar lordosis that may lead to back pain
- More than 10° of hip adduction or abduction may lead to varus or valgus knee instability.

Postoperative
Hip spica cast applied for 8 weeks.

KNEE ARTHRODESIS

Indications
- Painful ankylosis after infection, TB or trauma.
- Severe joint instability
- Salvage after an unsuccessful reconstructive procedure
- Severe deformity in paralytic condition (polio or any other neuromuscular disease)
- Neuropathic arthropathies (diabetes, syphilis)
- Severe post-traumatic or degenerative arthritis
- Congenital dysgenesis of femur
- Marked angular deformity.

Contraindications
- Bilateral knee disease
- Ipsilateral hip and ankle pathology
- Severe segmental bone loss
- Generalized involvement with condition such as RA or epiphyseal dysplasia
- Contralateral lower limb amputation.

Position of joint fusion: Full extension or 15° flexion, 5° valgus, 10° external rotation.

Complications
- Leg length discrepancy
- > 20° flexion cause marked increase in energy expenditure
- Back pain related to abnormal pelvic tilt and pelvic motion during gait.
- Activities like boarding bus, train and other forms of activity of daily living (ADL) is difficult.

ANKLE ARTHRODESIS

Triple arthrodesis: Arthrodesis of subtalar, calcaneocuboid and talonavicular joint.

Indications
- Severe foot deformity (plano valgus, equino valgus, equino varus, cavo varus)
- Post-traumatic arthritis
- Rheumatoid arthritis with severe deformity
- Infectious arthritis, e.g. tubercular arthritis
- Neuromuscular deformity
- Salvage of failed total ankle arthroplasty
- Bone tumor around ankle
- Neuropathic arthropathies with severe deformity.

Position of Joint Fusion
- Ankle joint: 0° flexion, 0–5° valgus, 5–10° external rotation
- Subtalar joint: neutral position
- Great toe: MTP joint in few degree of extension and slight valgus.
  - IP joint in neutral position and rest of toes in neutral position.

Complications
Limited hind foot motion that makes walking on uneven surfaces difficult.

Postoperative
- Short leg cast for 6–8 weeks.
- Nonweight bearing (NWB) for 0–4 weeks, partial weight bearing (4–8 weeks) and full weight bearing (after 8 weeks) as per condition of the patient allows.
- Recovery occurs in around 12–14 weeks.

Physiotherapy Management
Basic aim of treatment is to train the patient to functionally use the arthrosed joint and the limb.

During immobilization phase:
- Prevent and manage postoperative complications like deep vein thrombosis (DVT).
- Maintain the proper position of operated joint.
- Strengthening as well as range of motion (ROM) exercises of joints free from immobilization.
- Initiate early weight bearing in lower extremity arthrodesis.
- Initiate early functional use in upper extremity arthrodesis.

During mobilization phase:
- Whole extremity is exercised in functional pattern of movement.
- Several repetitions are required for the improvement of function of upper extremity.
- Gradual weight bearing, weight transfer and balancing exercises with assistive device should be initiated in lower extremity.
- Strengthening of surrounding muscles.

Optimal functions should be regained by 4 weeks following mobilization.

CHAPTER 10

Amputation

Amputation: Amputation is the surgical, congenital or spontaneous removal of a limb or projecting body part.

Disarticulation: Surgical removal of the whole limb or a part of limb through joint.

Causes

- **Circulatory disorders:** Circulatory disorders that cause irreversible loss of blood supply to extremity resulting in ischemia, ulceration or gangrene such as peripheral vascular diseases, e.g. Buerger's disease, atherosclerosis, thromboembolism, diabetes, arteriovenous aneurysm etc.
- **Neoplasm:** Primary malignant tumors that cannot be resected or irradiated, e.g. osteosarcoma, chondrosarcoma, fibrosarcoma.
- **Trauma:** Any traumatic condition that causes extensive loss of bone, soft tissue and blood supply where gangrene is in evitable or reconstruction is impossible, e.g. blast injuries crush injuries, road traffic accidents, industrial accidents, etc.
- **Congenital deformities:** Absence or abnormality of a limb present since birth with unknown etiology, e.g. polydactyl, congenital pseudoarthrosis, syndactyl, congenital absence of long bones.
- **Thermal, chemical or electrical injuries:** Injuries following excess exposure of heat, cold, current that creates extensive tissue destruction and deformity, e.g. acid burn, electric burn or frostbite due to extreme cold exposure.
- **Infection:** In acute or chronic infections that cannot be controlled by any medical or other possible treatment, e.g. chronic osteomyelitis, gas gangrene, etc.

Indications of Amputation

Three **"Ds"** are the indications of amputation:
- **Dead:** When there is complete tissue death, e.g. peripheral vascular disease, frostbite, severe trauma or burn, etc.
- **Dangerous:** When preserving the damaged or diseased body part may risk the life of patient, e.g. malignant tumor, potential lethal sepsis, etc.
- **Damned nuisance:** When it is better to remove the body part to improve the functional ability and independence of patient, e.g. gross malformation, recurrent sepsis, congenital deformities, severe intolerable pain.

■ LEVEL OF AMPUTATION

Selection of the Level of Amputation

The appropriate level is determined on the basis of following factors:
- **Viability of tissues:** Amputation should be aimed to eradicate the pathology completely for which the amputation is performed.
- **Adequate blood supply to skin flaps and stump:** It is important that the stump should be well healed and nontender.
- **Optimal length for the prosthetic fitting:** Length of stump should be optimal for the proper fitting of prosthesis because too short stump increases the chances of slipping out of prosthesis and too long stump

increase the chances of pain, ulceration, etc.
- **Joint** must always be preserved whenever possible.

Levels of Lower Limb Amputation (Fig. 1)

- **Hemipelvectomy:** Amputation of whole lower limb and ipsilateral hemi pelvis.
- **Hip disarticulation:** Amputation of whole lower limb through the hip joint.
- **Above knee amputation/transfemoral:** Amputation through the femur.
- **Knee disarticulation amputation:** Amputation through the knee joint.
- **Below knee amputation/transtibial:** Amputation through the tibia and fibula.
- **Ankle disarticulation (Syme's amputation):** Amputation through the ankle joint.
- **Midtarsal (Chopart amputation):** Amputation between talus and calcaneus proximally and cuboid and navicular distally.
- **Tarsometatarsal (Lisfranc amputation):** Amputation of forefoot at tarsometatarsal line.
- **Transmetatarsal amputation (partial foot amputation):** Amputation through the metatarsals.
- **Amputation of digits (toes):** Amputation through metacarpophalangeal (MCP); proximal interphalangeal (PIP) or distal interphalangeal (DIP) joints.

Levels of Upper Limb Amputation (Fig. 2)

- **Forequarter amputation:** Amputation of whole upper limb with ipsilateral scapula and a portion of clavicle.
- **Shoulder disarticulation:** Amputation through the surgical neck of humerus.
- **Above elbow amputation/transhumeral:** Amputation through the humerus.
- **Elbow disarticulation:** Amputation through elbow joint.
- **Below elbow amputation/transradial:** Amputation through radius and ulna.
- **Krukenburg's amputation:** It is a type of below elbow amputation involves the separating of radius and ulna to provide a pincer like grasp.
- **Wrist disarticulation:** Amputation through the wrist joint.
- **Transmetacarpal amputation:** Amputation through metacarpals.
- **Amputation of digits/transphalangeal:** Amputation through MCP, PIP or DIP joints.

■ CHARACTERISTICS OF IDEAL STUMP

- **Ideal stump length:** Ideally the most distal level that will heal without any complications and provide functional stump should be selected.
  - **Hip disarticulation:** In case of hip disarticulation, it is advisable to keep the head and neck of femur to provide a horizontal weight bearing surface.
  - **Transfemoral amputation:** Stump should be as long as possible.
    - Optimal length of stump should be approximately 7.5 to 10 cm from superior border of patella and 23 to 27 cm from greater trochanter. It helps in the better fitting of the knee mechanism in prosthesis.
    - Minimum length of 8 cm from crotch line is required for prosthetic fitting otherwise stump slips out of socket during flexion.
  - **Knee preservation:** It is important to preserve the knee joint as knee retains the proprioceptive sensation and thus amputee is able to sense the positioning of foot even in darkness.
  - **Transtibial amputation:** Ideal level should be at the musculotendinous junction of gastrocnemius. Ideal length of stump should be 12–17 cm from knee medial joint line for better prosthetic fitting.
  - **Syme's amputation:** In ankle disarticulation, 6 cm ground clearance is

284 Simplified Approach to Orthopedic Physiotherapy

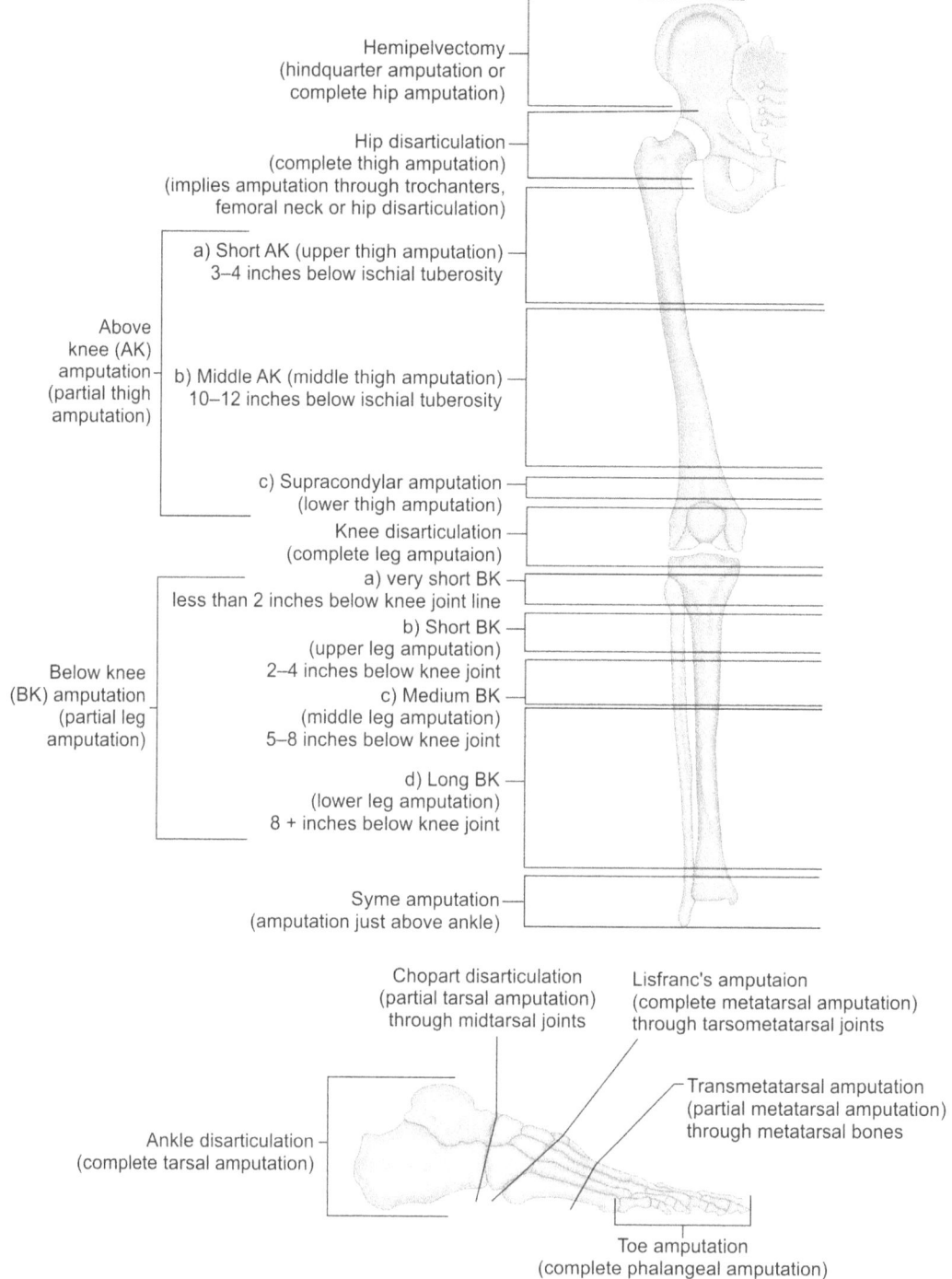

Fig. 1: Lower limb amputation.

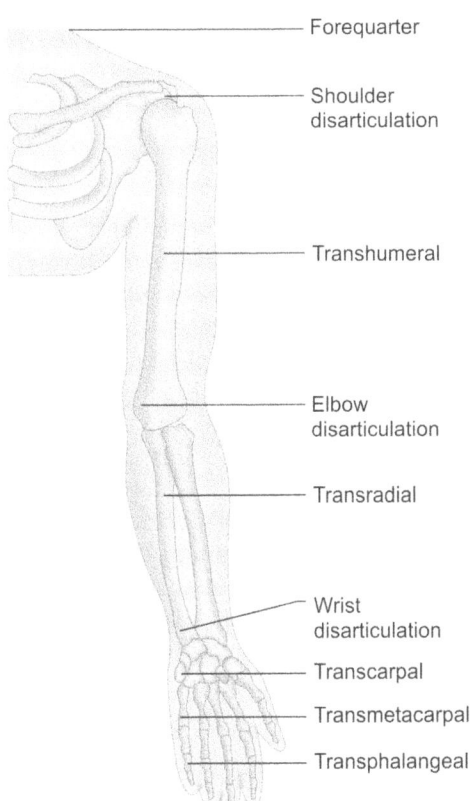

Fig. 2: Upper limb amputation.

required for prosthetic fitting, otherwise contralateral limb become shorter and will require height compensation.
- **Partial foot amputation:** In midtarsal amputation and other distal amputations, sole of skin should be retained otherwise stump will fail to bear weight and will have frequent breakdown.
- **Shoulder disarticulation:** In case of shoulder disarticulation it is advisable to retain the head and neck of humerus to provide a horizontal support for prosthetic fitting.
- **Transhumeral amputation:** The stump size should be as long as possible. Ideally 20 cm from acromion or 8 cm clearance from elbow joint is advisable for fitting of elbow prosthesis.
- **Transradial amputation:** In Transradial amputation, at least 3 cm length from the crease line at cubital fossa is required for better prosthetic fitting. An ideal length is 18 cm from olecranon processor or 5 cm clearance from wrist is required for fitting of wrist unit.
- **Suture line or scar:**
  - Scar should be supple and non-tender.
  - Scar should not be on high pressure zone.
  - Scar should be non-adherent: Scar adherent to subcutaneous tissue, neuroma or bone usually causes ulceration and pain.
- **Musculature around the stump:** Stump should be well padded, i.e. bone should be well covered by muscles.
  There should be good muscle power.
  Antagonistic muscles should be sutured together to maintain muscle tone.
- **Range of motion (ROM)** of proximal joints to stump should be complete and pain free for optimal use of prosthesis.
  Proximal joints should be supple with no fixed deformity.
- **Skin over the stump:** Healthy sensate skin is essential to withstand the extra load associated with prosthetic fitting. It can also give a positional feedback of prosthesis.
- **Tip of bone:** It should be smooth particularly the tibial tip should be beveled and smoothened with a file.
- **Ideal shape:** The stump should be conical in shape.

STUMP MANAGEMENT

- **Measures to control edema:** Immediate postsurgical—plaster cast mold is applied as primary dressing which forms a protective cover over the stump, preventing infection from outside.
  Secondary dressing is applied over the primary dressing to prevent edema, speed up the heeling process and maintain the

size and shape of stump optimal for prosthetic fitting.

Other measures to control stump edema:
- Stimulation with limb in elevation with elastic bandage.
- Resisted exercises to stump and rest of the joints.
- Bed end should be elevated 30°.
- Use of stump board in wheelchair.
- **Flowtron therapy:** It uses intermittent compression therapy to treat edema. In this stump is placed in invigilated plastic bag in which air pressure varies rhythmically to reduce edema.
- **Pressure environment treatment:** In this device, limited pressure control is maintained to aid the healing process of stump but there has no temperature control.
- **Controlled environment therapy:** Dressing free stump is placed in a clear, sealed plastic sleeve attached to a pressure cycle machine. Temperature, pressure, sterility and humidity in device are controlled to give an ideal environment for stump healing.

- **Stump bandaging:** Bandaging usually applied when stitches are removed (after 2–3 weeks) for conditioning of stump, shaping the stump by reducing stump edema and accustomed the stump to pressure.

  Principles of stump bandaging:
  - All turns of bandage should be diagonal (circular turns may produce tourniquet effect) (Fig. 3)
  - Pressure should grade from very firm at the end of stump to moderate proximally
  - Extra pressure is necessary over the corner to obtain the conical shape of stump
  - Skin should not be remaining uncovered after bandaging except for the joint. Joints should not be bandaged to allow their free movements
  - Bandage should not be too tight to be painful and restrict blood flow.
  - If bandage becomes too tight or loose, take it off, re roll and reapply it.
  - Stump should be bandaged 24 hours/day before getting prosthesis.
  - In above knee amputation, bandage must not extend up to the groin to prevent the formation of a roll of flesh over the adductor tendon that may lead to the infection of follicles due to continuous friction with the socket of prosthesis. Some of the turns should also be applied around the waist to act as an anchor.
  - In above knee amputation, short-sized stump should be bandaged with hip in extension and adduction.
  - In below knee stump amputation should be bandaged with knee in slight flexion.

- **Shrinker socks:** can be applied after a week of suture removal.
  - It should not be too tight to be painful and restrict blood flow.
  - Top of shrinker does not roll. As the rolled shrinker may give a tourniquet

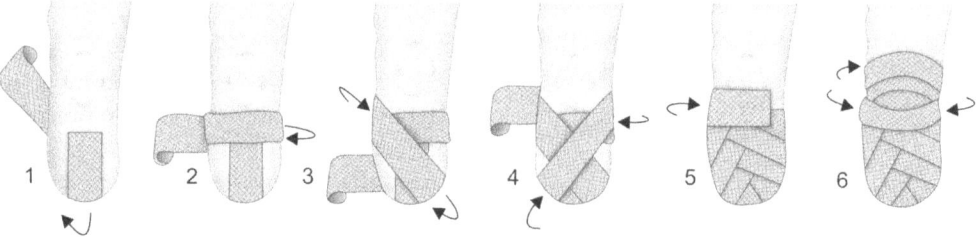

Fig. 3: Bandage wrapping technique.

effect that can reduce the blood supply to the stump.

- **Stump hygiene**
  - Stump should be washed at night as this will minimize swelling and allows the natural skin oil to be replaced overnight.
  - Do not soak the stump in bath water as this will soften the skin on the stump and make it prone to injury.
  - Use mild antiseptic, fragrance free, unmedicated talcum, this will absorb perspiration.
  - Do not use astringent, surgical spirit or other drying preparation on the stump that can reduce natural protective oil of skin.
  - Use mildly abrasive like loofah.
  - Wearing socks may help to draw perspiration from skin, provide padding and have a cooling effect for stump.
  - Stump sock should be changed every day and should be washed with warm water with mild soap and should be rinsed and dried properly.
  - Antiperspirant may be used to control perspiration build up in the socket.
  - Antibacterial cleansers may be used on stump to limit skin problems causing bacteria.
  - Silicon based lotion or gel should be preferred.
  - Once abrasion occurs use medicated lotion, zinc oxide as healing agent.
  - Socket should be cleaned every day to remove the stock of dried perspiration on the inner surface of socket.
  - Socket should be washed with warm water and mild soap and wiped with damp cloth to clean and dry it thoroughly before donning it.

POSTOPERATIVE PHYSIOTHERAPY MANAGEMENT

Physical Examination

- **Past medical history:** A detailed medical history should be taken.
- **Mental status:** cognitive function of patient should be examined.
- **Sensation:** Sensation of stump should be checked. As decrease in awareness of pain, temperature and light touch can increase the potential for injury and tissue breakdown.
- **ROM:** ROM of upper limbs, sound lower limb and residual limb should be evaluated.
  Common contractures:
  - In transfemoral amputation: When stump size is long, hip flexion, ER and adduction.
  - In transtibial amputation: Knee flexion. Soft tissue contracture or tightness should be assessed.
- **Strength:** Strength of all the limbs including trunk and residual limb should be assessed.
- **Balance and coordination:** Ability to maintain the COG over BOS should be assessed.
- **Bed mobility:** Ability of bed mobility should be assessed as early bed mobility helps to prevent contracture and pressure, i.e. excessive friction of sheets against the suture line.
- **Transfer:** Ability to transfer from wheelchair to bed, toilet seat or car and vice versa.
- **Wheelchair propulsion:** Ability to stop, turn and control wheelchair should be assessed.
- Assessment of the ambulation with assistive device with or without prosthesis.

Preprosthetic Training

- **Prevention of postoperative complication:** Respiratory and circulatory complications: Breathing exercises and ankle toe movement to prevent DVT.
- **To prevent deformities:**
  - **Positioning of residual limb:** The proper positioning of residual limb is necessary to prevent tightness and contracture that may affects the proper fitting of

prosthetic socket and functional ability of the patient. Bilateral amputee is more prone to have hip and knee contracture due to decreased mobility.

Commonly occurring contractures in amputations are:
- In above elbow amputation: Shoulder adduction and rotation contracture.
- In below elbow amputation: Elbow flexion contracture.
- In above knee amputation:
  - Hip flexion and abduction contracture: When stump size is short.
  - Hip flexion and adduction contracture: When stump size is long.
- In below knee amputation: Knee flexion contracture.
- In partial foot amputation: Plantar flexion contracture.

Proper positioning of residual limb (Fig. 4):
- **In above knee amputation:**
  - Stump should be parallel to unaffected leg using pillow laterally along the stump without resting on pillow to maintain the neutral rotation with no abduction in supine position.
  - Short period of prone lying by placing the pillow anteriorly under the stump maintain the hip extension and prevent the flexion contracture of hip.
  - Avoid prolonged sitting and use of soft mattresses that can predispose the development of hip flexion contracture.
- **In below knee amputation:**
  - Do not use pillow below the knee.
  - Use stump board while sitting in wheelchair.
- **Gentle stretching:** Slow, gentle, repetitive sustained manual stretching should be initiated. In acute injuries gentle PROM twice daily is sufficient to maintain the mobility.
- **Traction:** Sustained sessions of gentle traction should be given to stretch the contracture developing areas.
- **Corrective splint:** Static splinting should be used as an adjunct to passive ROM to prevent contracture and deformity.

■ **To control stump edema:**
- Stimulation with limb in elevation with elastic bandage.
- Resisted exercises to stump and rest of joints.
- Bed end should be elevated 30°.
- Stump board in wheelchair.
- **Pressure environment treatment:** In this device, limited pressure control is maintained to aid in the healing process of stump but there has no temperature control.

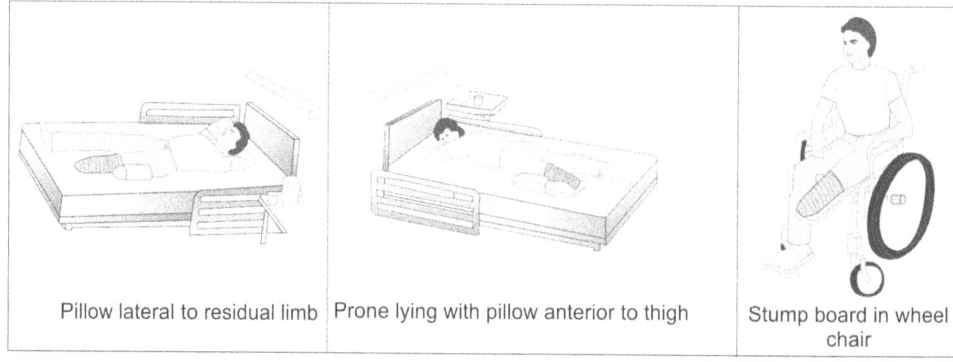

| Pillow lateral to residual limb | Prone lying with pillow anterior to thigh | Stump board in wheel chair |

Fig. 4: Proper positioning of residual limb.

- **Controlled environment therapy:** Dressing free stump is placed in a clear, sealed plastic sleeve attached to a pressure cycle machine. Temperature, pressure, sterility and humidity in device are controlled to give an ideal environment for stump healing.
- **Flowtron therapy:** It uses intermittent compression therapy to treat edema. In this stump is placed in invigilated plastic bag in which air pressure varies rhythmically to reduce edema.
- **To strengthen the muscles:** Following muscles should be strengthened along with trunk muscles and muscles of the unaffected extremities to improve the functional ability and early ambulation of the amputee.
  - **Shoulder disarticulation:** Shoulder elevators, depressors, protractors and retractors. Mobility exercises of neck and trunk are also important.
  - **Above elbow amputation:** Flexors, abductors and extensors of shoulder along with scapular elevators and retractors of the unaffected side.
  - **Below elbow amputation:** Elbow flexors, extensors, pronators and supinators of forearm.
  - **Hip disarticulation:** Pelvic rotators and elevators.
  - **Above knee amputation:** Hip flexors, extensors, abductors, and shoulder girdle muscles.
  - **Below knee amputation:** Knee flexors, extensors, hip abductors and extensors.
  - **Syme's amputation:** Knee flexors and extensors, hip abductors and extensors.
  - **Stump exercises:** Gradually progress from isometric to active and then resistive exercises.
  - **Trunk muscle:** Abdominals and back extensor strengthening is required for transfers, ambulation, to decrease the risk of back pain and to assist in the reduction of gait deviations associated with the trunk.
- **To maintain range of motion:** Active range of motion (AROM) exercise of whole body including the residual limb.
  - For prevention of decreased ROM and contractures.
  - Restricted ROM may result in difficulties with prosthetic fitting, gait deviation or inability to ambulate with prosthesis.

  When restriction of ROM is established: Passive ROM, contract relax stretching, soft tissue mobilization, myofascial techniques, joint mobilization and other methods are used to restore the complete ROM.
- **Bed mobility**
  - Use of trapeze, side rail or human assistance should be taught to severely involved patient.
  - Mat activities including log rolling, side lying to sitting, supine lying on elbows to long sitting, etc.
- **Transfers:** Patient should be taught about the transfer techniques, e.g. transfer from bed to chair or wheelchair, wheelchair to toilet or car seat and vice versa.
  - **In unilateral amputation:**
    - **Slide board transfer:** Wheelchair is placed closed to the bed on the unaffected side and slide board is placed between the two surfaces. The patient is taught to use his upper body to scoot himself along the board toward the wheelchair (Fig. 5).

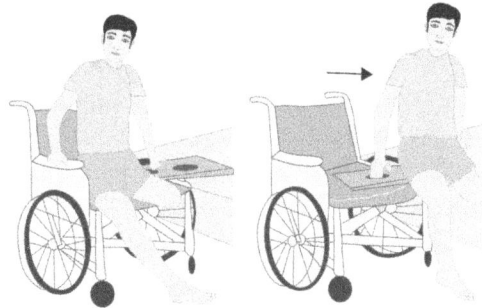

Fig. 5: Sliding board transfer amputee.

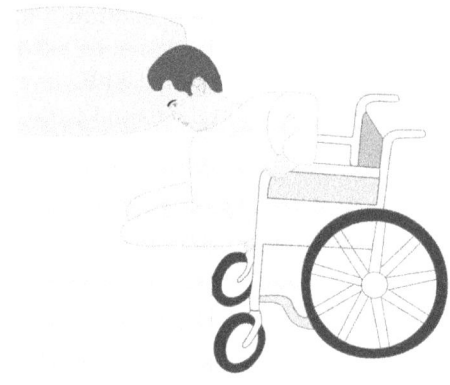

Fig. 6: Head on transfer technique.

- **Pivot transfer technique:** Wheelchair is placed closed to the bed on the unaffected limb side. The patient is taught to pivot over the unaffected limb while placing one hand on the armrest of chair and other hand on the bed.
- In bilateral amputation:
  - **Lateral sliding board transfer:** It is used initially before attaining the good strength of lattismus dorsi and triceps required for the lifting of body and pushing forward with both hands.
  - **Head on transfer technique (Fig. 6):** It is practiced after attaining the good strength of lattismus dorsi and triceps. Wheelchair is positioned with the front of the chair towards the transferring surface of bed. The patient slides forward onto the desired surface by lifting the body and pushing forward with both hands.
- **Wheelchair propulsion:** Wheel propulsion should be taught to amputee to increase the level of independence and for early ambulation.
  - Initially the patient should be taught about the basic skills like forward propulsion, turns, preparation for transfer such as braking or parking.
  - Later on advanced wheelchair skills should also be taught to the patient like ascending and descending ramps, floor to wheelchair transfer and curb jumping, etc.
- **Unsupported standing balance:**
  - Initially single limb balance should be taught to gain confidence during stand pivot transfer, ambulation with assistive devices, hopping and other activities depending on the level of skill of amputee.
  - Ambulation training should be initiated in parallel bars using support of both hands. After gaining the confidence with double arm support, the patient should shift towards single arm support by withdrawing the hand of the amputated side from bars and subsequently standing without support should be practiced.
  - Balance and righting skill should be improved by challenging activities like tapping the shoulders in different directions or tossing a ball back and forth, etc.
  - After attaining the full confidence in parallel bars, patient should be trained to perform these skills outside the parallel bars.
- **Ambulation with assistive device:**
  - Amputee needs an assistive device in many conditions like when they cannot wear the prosthesis due to skin irritation, poor prosthetic fitting, and edema.
  - Amputee should select the appropriate assistive device on the basis of following points:
    - Unsupported standing balance
    - Upper limb strength
    - Coordination with assistive device
    - Level of cognition
  - For example walker is preferred for the amputee having poor balance, strength

and coordination and forearm crutches may be used in case of good balance and strength.

Postprosthetic Training in Lower Limb Amputation

Proper gait training, donning and doffing of prosthesis, maintenance of prosthesis and its components are necessary parts of the prosthesis training.

Pre-Gait Training

The aim of gait training is to attain the maximal level of functional independence. Gait training should be initiated immediately after 5 days of surgery. It should include the following:

- **Preprosthetic exercises:** It helps to maintain ROM and improve muscle strength of whole body along with the residual limb.
- **Balance and coordination exercises:** After amputation center of gravity (COG) of amputee shift towards the unaffected lower limb, that shifts again after getting the prosthetic limb. Therefore the amputee has to learn to maintain COG and entire body weight over prosthesis. Once comfortable with weight bearing equally on both limbs, the amputee may initiate independent standing and eventually ambulation.
- **Orientation to COG and base of support (BOS):** The following are the techniques to rehabilitate the orientation. Initially the ambulation program starts in parallel bars.

Pre-Gait Training Techniques

Lateral weight shifting
- Stand between the parallel bars using double arm support. Shift the body weight from sound leg to the prosthesis.
- Progress to single arm support with contralateral hand.
- Progress to weight bearing with finger tips support.
- Progress to weight bearing without support.

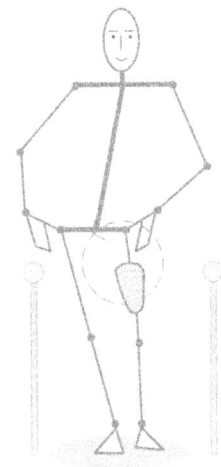

Fig. 7: Pelvic rotation.

Forward and backward weight shifting
- Stand between parallel bars using double arm support. Shift the pelvis forward and backward without moving shoulders.
- Progress to single arm support with contralateral hand.
- Progress to weight bearing with finger tips support.
- Progress to weight bearing without support.
- **Pelvic rotation:** Stand between parallel bars with or without support and rotate the pelvis (Fig. 7).
- **Sideward walking:** Stand between the parallel bars with double hand support and walk sideways toward the prosthetic side and back.
- **Full weight shift:** Stand between the parallel bars with or without hand support with one leg in front of the other. Shift the body weight from one leg to other by moving the pelvis and trunk from front to back.
- **Heel strike (Fig. 8):** Stand between the parallel bar with or without hand support and step forward with prosthesis by keeping the knee straight and pushing the heel downwards.

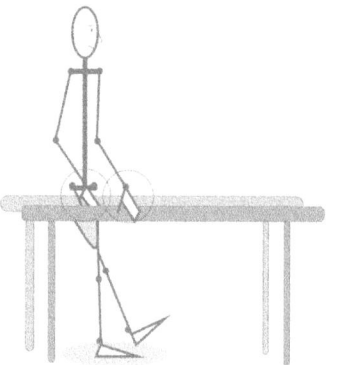
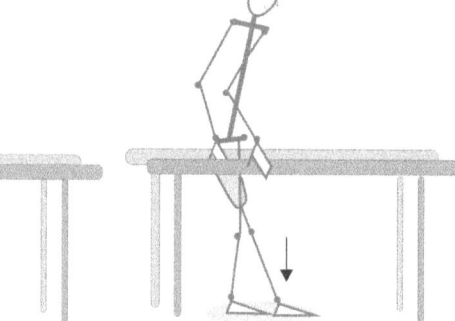

Fig. 8: Heel strike.

- **High stepping (single limb standing) (Fig. 9):** Stand between the parallel bars with hand support by placing sound leg on a raised object, e.g. stool of 4–8 inches. Progression can be made by increasing the height of stool and reducing the hand support.
- **Balance board (Fig. 10):** Stand between the parallel bars on a balance board using double hand support and shift the body weight from one limb to other. Progression can be made by shifting the body weight anteriorly and posteriorly.
- **Football:** Stand between the parallel bars with or without hand support and kick a ball with sound leg.
- **Upper limb activity:** Stand between the parallel bars and catch and throw the ball.

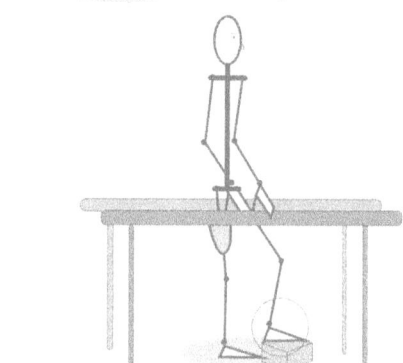

Fig. 9: Single limb standing.

Gait Training

When the amputee is able to bear full weight on the prosthesis and expertise in performing balance activities in parallel bar then Gait training should be initiated for proper ambulation and increasing the functional ability of the subject.

Gait Training Techniques

Sound Leg Step Forward

Stand between the parallel bars with double hand support and step forward with sound leg by keeping the hand parallel to prosthesis.

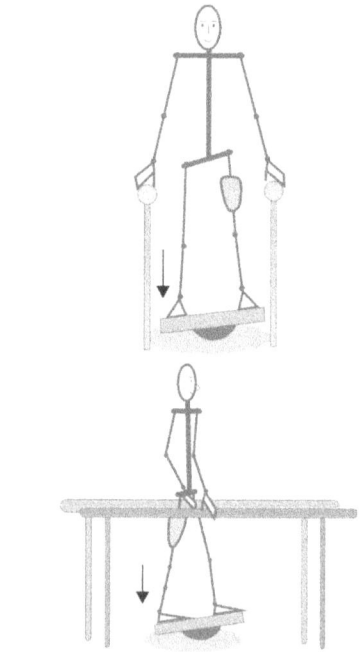

Fig. 10: Balance board.

Sound Leg Step Backward
Stand between the parallel bars with double hand support and step backward with sound leg by keeping the hand parallel to prosthesis.

Sound Leg Step Through
- Stand between the parallel bars with double hand support and step forward and backward with sound leg by keeping the hand parallel to prosthesis by maintaining an upright position, allowing the trunk and shoulders to move backward and forward without lateral flexion.
- Progress the exercises to one hand support and then to without support.

Prosthetic Leg Step Forward then Backward and then Step Through
These exercise are performed in the same manner as with sound leg.

Walking between the Parallel Bars
- Stand between the parallel bars and walk between them without any lateral flexion of trunk or uneven step length.
- Progression can be made with single arm support and then to without support.

Advance Exercises
- When the patient gain full confidence in walking without support in the parallel bar, the therapist proceed to other advanced exercises outside the parallel bar to improve balance, coordination and proprioception.
- Bouncing a ball while standing then walking, balancing a stick upright on the hand, balancing on prosthetic limb, walk on uneven surface going up and down a slope, and finally running.

Functional Exercises
To re-educate the functional training to increase the functional independence of amputee in daily activities. For above knee amputee:
- **Rising from a chair:** Stand up by placing the sound leg under the chair and flexing the trunk (Fig. 11).

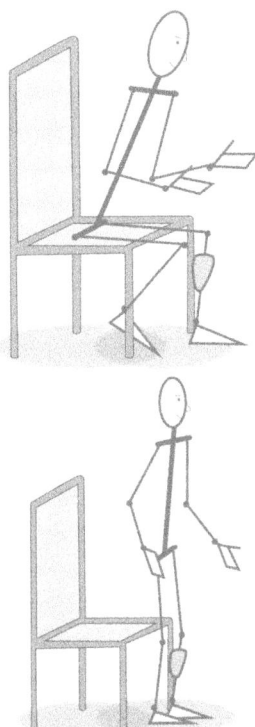

Fig. 11: Rising from a chair.

- **Climbing a staircase:** Climb a staircase by ascending the sound leg first followed by the prosthetic leg.
- **Descending a staircase:** Descend a staircase by descending the prosthetic leg first followed by the sound leg.
- **Sitting down and getting up from floor:**
  - **Method 1:** Place the prosthesis in retroflexion, abduction and external rotation. Bend the trunk by supporting on both hands and one knee then turn and sit on the floor. Do the reverse for getting up (Fig. 12).
  - **Method 2:** Move the prosthetic limb forward and bend the sound knee by supporting on both hands. Do the reverse for getting up (Fig. 13).

Analysis of Amputee Prosthetic Gait
Following components are necessary for the analysis of amputee gait:

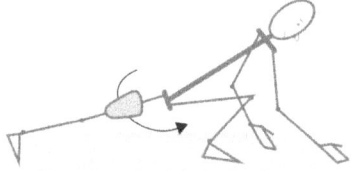

Fig. 12: Sitting down on floor: Method 1.

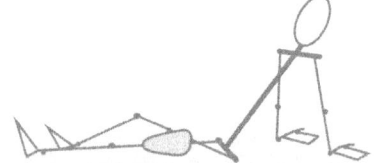

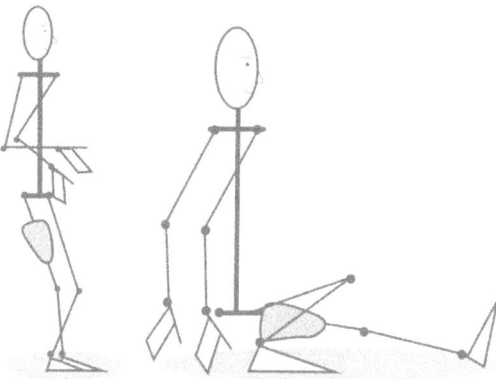

Fig. 13: Sitting down on floor: Method 2.

- **Observation:** It is essential to observe the motion from both the planes, i.e. sagittal plane motion and frontal plane motion.

- **Identification of gait deviation:** Any gait characteristics that differs from the normal pattern is known as gait deviation (Table 1).
- **Determination of causes:** It is very essential to determine the possible causes of gait deviations which could be prosthetic or patient cause.
  - **Prosthetic cause:**
    – Prosthetic malalignment
    – Poorly fitted prosthetic socket
    – Prosthetic manufacturer defect.
  - **Patient causes:**
    – Restricted ROM of one or more joints
    – Muscular weakness
    – Contracture
    – Pain
    – Excessive fear
    – Any collateral medical condition
    – Old habitual pattern.

Table 1: Types and causes of possible gait deviation.

Gait phase	Name	Description	Prosthetic causes	Amputee causes
Transfemoral amputation				
Heel strike to midstance	Knee instability	Knee flexion 'jerky' in presentation during heel strike to foot flat	• Inadequate flexion in socket limiting active hip extension • Too hard heel cushion less shock absorption also producing flexion moment at knee	• Hip flexion contracture not accommodated in socket • Hip extensor weakness
	Terminal impact	Rapid forward movement of shank that lead to maximum knee extension before heel strike	Insufficient knee friction	As habit by assuming to keep knee in full extension before heel strike

Contd...

Amputation

Contd...

Gait phase	Name	Description	Prosthetic causes	Amputee causes
Transfemoral amputation				
	Foot slap	Forefoot descends too rapidly like slapping the ground	• Plantarflexion resistance is too soft • Heel lever arm is too short	Forcibly driving foot into quick flat to assure extension of knee
At midstance	Lateral trunk bending	Trunk flexes towards prosthesis during prosthetic stance phase	• Prosthesis too short • Lack of prosthesis lateral wall • High medial wall causing discomforts so lateral bending to avoid discomfort	• Very short stump that fails to provide sufficient lever arm for pelvis • Weak abductors in the prosthetic side • As a habit pattern
	Abducted gait	Increased BOS during mobility, prosthetic foot placement is lateral to normal foot placement during gait cycle	• Too long prosthesis • High medial wall pressure on pubic region so keep the prosthesis abducted	• Abduction contracture • Habit pattern
	Excessive trunk extension	Hyperextend the trunk from heel strike to midstance	Insufficient socket flexion leads to lumbar hyperextension	• Hip flexion contracture • Weak hip extensors • Habit pattern
Midstance to toe off	Drop off	Sudden downward movement of trunk as anterior support is lost prematurely	• Socket placed too far anterior • Toe break placed posteriorly	
	Inadequate heel off/anterior trunk bending	Heel may not come off floor till the whole body is brought forward	Uneven steps between two legs	Hip flexion contracture
	Circumduction gait	The prosthesis swings laterally like an arc during swing phase	• Too long prosthesis • Difficult knee flexion due to too much friction in knee • Locked knee	• Abduction contracture • Not confident of flexing knee • Fear of stubbing the toe
	Vaulting	Patient rises on toe of the sound foot to swing the prosthesis through in little knee flexion	• Too long prosthesis • Inadequate suspension • Excessive knee friction • Locked knee	• Socket discomfort • Fear of stubbing of toe • Habit pattern

Contd...

Contd...

Gait phase	Name	Description	Prosthetic causes	Amputee causes
Transfemoral amputation				
	Medial or lateral whip	Medial whip is present when heel travels medially on initial flexion at the beginning of swing phase. Lateral whip exists when heel moves laterally	• Lateral whip result from excessive internal rotation of prosthetic knee • Medial whip due to excessive external rotation of prosthetic knee • Too light socket • Excess valgus, varus in prosthetic knee	Applying prosthesis in internal or external rotation
	Uneven arm swing	Arm on prosthetic side held close to body rather than freely swinging	Improperly fitted socket or unstable knee	• Improper training • Habit pattern
	Uneven timing	Steps of unequal duration and length with short stance phase in prosthetic side	• Improperly fitted socket causing discomfort • Insufficient knee flexion	
Transtibial gait deviations				
Heel strike to midstance	Absent knee flexion	Knee fully extended at heel strike	• Faulty suspension of the prosthesis • Too soft heel cushion	• Foot placement too far forward on stepping • Lack of preflexion of the socket • Discomfort/pain • Quads weakness
	Excessive knee flexion	Increased knee flexion at heel strike or mid stance, patient feels as though walking downhill	• Faulty suspension of prosthesis • Prosthetic foot set in too much DF • Stiff heel cushion	Flexion contracture of knee
At midstance	ER of foot at heel strike	ER of prosthesis/foot at heel strike	• Heel to hard • Loose socket	
	Knee instability	Knee flexion 'jerky' in presentation during heel strike to foot flat		Weak quadriceps
	Valgus/varus movement/ excessive lateral thrust of prosthesis	Knee shifts medially or laterally during prosthetic stance phase	• Loose socket • Abducted prosthesis • Excessive medial displacement of prosthetic foot	

Contd...

Contd...

Gait phase	Name	Description	Prosthetic causes	Amputee causes
Transfemoral amputation				
Midstance to toe off	Drop off/early knee flexion	Heel off occurs too early causing early knee flexion	• Excessive anterior displacement of socket over foot • Excessive DF of foot on prosthesis • Soft DF bumper	
	Knee hyperextension/delayed knee flexion	Delayed heel off causing hyperextension of knee, walking up hill sensation	• Excessive posterior displacement of socket over the foot • Hard DF bumper • Too much PF on foot	
	Whip	During swing phase foot 'whips' laterally or medially	• Poor suspension • Knee internally or externally rotated.	
	Pistoning	Amputee drops into socket as the foot moves into flat foot, tibia moves vertically during alternately WB and NWB period of gait cycle	• Lack of prosthetic socks • Suspension loose • Too large or faulty socket	

(BOS: base of support; ER: external rotation; DF: dorsiflexion; PF: plantarflexion; WB: weight-bearing; NWB: nonweight-bearing)

CHAPTER 11

Legg-Calvé-Perthes Disease

Legg-Calvé-Perthes disease (LCPD) is juvenile idiopathic osteonecrosis of proximal femoral head secondary to the disruption of its blood supply (Fig. 1).

It is also known as ischemic necrosis of hip, coxa plana, and osteochondritis and avascular necrosis of femoral head.

Epidemiology

- Most oftenly it occurs in children between 4–10 years.
- Male are more affected than female with ratio of 5:1.
- Both unilateral or (10–20% cases) bilateral involvement may present.

Etiology

Although it is an idiopathic disease, but a variety of theories about the underlying cause have been proposed. According to these various theories, LCPD may be linked to the following causes:

- Slipped capital femoral epiphysis.
- Direct trauma to femoral head.
- Prolonged use of steroids.
- Sickle cell anemia.
- Congenital dislocation of hip.

Predisposing Factors

- Impaired and disproportionate growth (delayed bone age).
- Second hand smoker (increased risk of ischemia leading to avascular necrosis).
- Children who are more active than average.
- Attention deficit hyperactivity disorder.

Anatomy

Branches of profunda femoris artery, i.e. medial and lateral circumflex femoral arteries supply the femoral head. The top of femoral head is supplied by a small artery in ligamentum teres which is the branch of posterior division of obturator artery (Fig. 2).

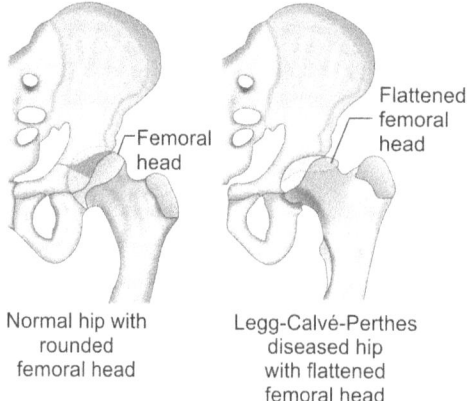

Fig. 1: Legg-Calvé-Perthes diseased hip.

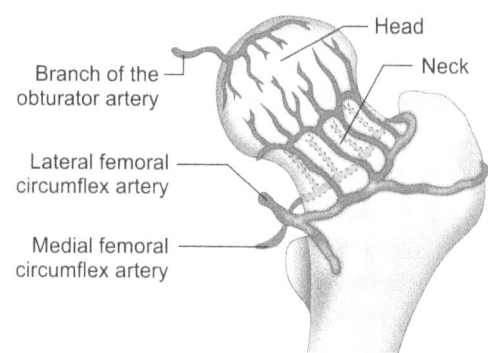

Fig. 2: Blood supply to head and neck of femur.

Legg-Calvé-Perthes Disease

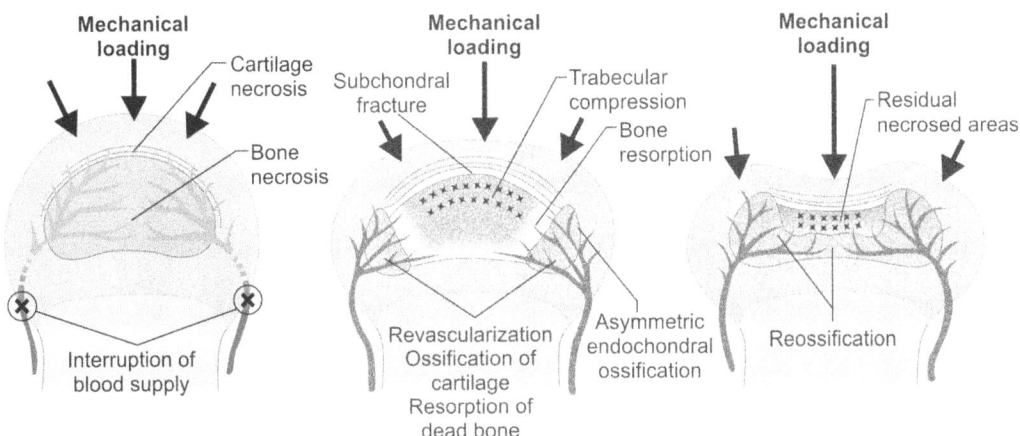

Fig. 3: Pathogenesis of LCPD.

Pathogenesis (Fig. 3)

Four phases of disease are:

Phase 1: Necrosis: Last for Several Months to 1 Year
- Ischemia or loss of blood supply to femoral head.
- Avascular necrosis, i.e. portion of bone turns into dead tissues.

Phase 2: Fregmentation: Last for 1–3 Years
- Resorption of dead bone cells lead to femoral head collapse.

Phase 3: Reossification: Last for 1–3 Years
New bone (healthier bone cell) regrows to reshape the femoral head.

Phase 4: Remodelling: Last for Few Years
Normal bone cells replace the new bone cells and femoral head reshapes itself into normal spherical shape.

Clinical Presentation

- **Limp:** Abductor lurch or psoatic limp present secondary to the weakness of abductor and psoas major muscle respectively.
  - Limp worsens after physical activity and improves following the period of rest.
- **Pain:** Pain occurs due to necrosis of bone.
  - Mild and intermittent pain in hip, knee, groin and anterior thigh.
  - Pain worsens with activity.
  - Nocturnal pain is frequent.
  - Referred pain on the medial aspect of ipsilateral knee or lateral thigh.
- **ROM:** Decrease in AROM of internal rotation and abduction
- **Gait:** Antalgic gait with limited hip movement.
  - Trendelenburg gait may present due to pain in gluteus medius or combination gait pattern.
- **Leg length discrepancy:** Premature closure of the epiphyseal and physeal plates due to avascular necrosis can lead to the shortening of the affected leg.
- **Unusual high activity level:** Usually affected children are physically very active and significant percentages of them have attention deficit hyperactivity disorder.
- **Abnormal growth patterns:** Forearms and hands are relatively short as compare to the upper arm. Similarly feet are relatively short as compare to tibia.
- Quadriceps muscle and adjacent thigh muscle atrophy.
- Hip may develop adduction-flexion contracture.

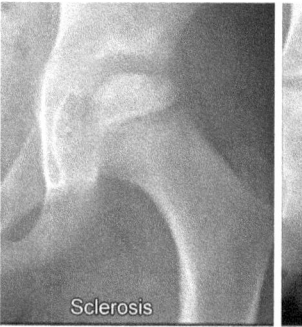 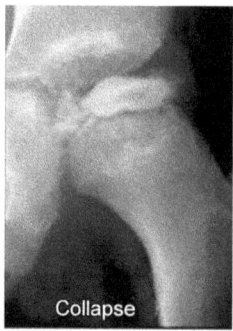 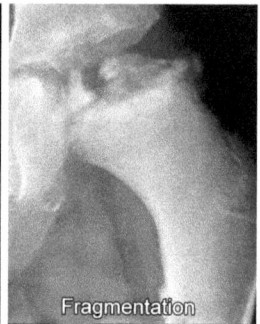 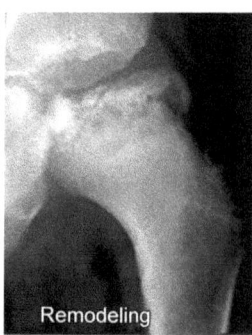

Fig. 4: X-ray findings of Legg-Calvé-Perthes disease.

Diagnosis

Imaging Studies: X-ray Findings (Fig. 4)

Early Findings
- Widening of joint space
- Flattening, loss of height of femoral epiphysis
- Radiolucency of bone
- Sclerosis and fragmentation.

Late Findings
- Broad, overgrown femoral head, i.e. known as coxa magna
- Short femoral neck
- Regular articular margins.

Physical Examination
- **Gait:** Usually antalgic gait
  - Trendelenburg gait
  - Duchenne gait.
- **Pain** occurs during acute stage on groin, anterior hip area or around greater trochanter or referred to knee.
- **ROM:** Restriction of hip abduction and Internal rotation.
- **Atrophy** of gluteus, quadriceps, and hamstring muscles.
- **Muscle strength:** Muscle strength of hip and knee muscles should be evaluated using manual muscle test.
- **Balance:** Examination of balance and co-ordination of patient should be done.

Management

Goals
- To reduce hip irritability.
- To restore and maintain hip mobility.
- To prevent the extrusion and collapse of femoral head
- To regain the spherical shape of femoral head.

Conservative Treatment

As Perthes disease is a self-limiting disease, head of femur should be minimally deformed to prevent long-term problem.

- **Children < 6 years age**
  - Need no intervention.
  - Refrain the child from contact sports which impact the hip.
  - **"Scottish rite brace"** may be used to provide containment of femoral head in acetabulum by maintaining hip flexion and abduction. It also allows the child to walk and be more independent (Fig. 5).
- **When onset of disease occurs after age of 6–8 years.**
  - Prolonged period without weight bearing is advisable.
  - Indicated for surgical treatment like osteotomy (femoral, pelvic).
  - Hip distraction by external fixator is used to relieve the hip from carrying weight of body and allows room for the top of femur to regrow.
  - Exercises: Activities that decrease mechanical stress on hip, e.g. swimming, cycling should be initiated.
  - Avoid high impact activities or running.
  - Treatment is aimed at minimizing damage during the course of disease.

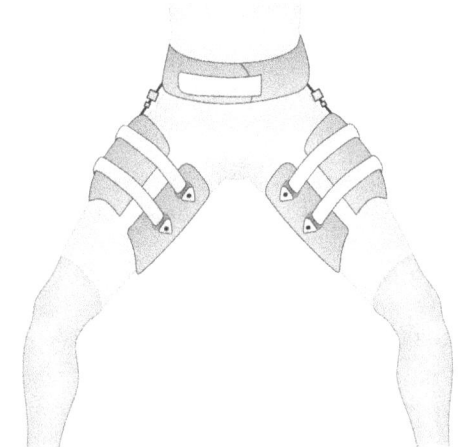

Fig. 5: Scottish rite brace.

Physiotherapy Treatment

Indications
- Children with necrosis of less than 50% of femoral head.
- Children with necrosis of more than 50% of femoral head, below 6 years having more than 80% of femoral head cover.
- Patient with mild course.

Treatment

- **To reduce pain:**
  - Cryo pack or hot pack.
  - Pain relieving modalities: Transcutaneous electrical nerve stimulation (TENS), interferential therapy (IFT), high voltage pulsed galvanic stimulation (HVPGS).
- **To increase and maintain ROM:**
  - Static stretching exercises of lower limb muscles
  - AROM and AAROM exercises of hip including internal rotation, external rotation, abduction, flexion and extension following passive stretch to retain newly gained ROM.
- **To increase strength:** Begin with isometric exercises then gentle isotonic exercises initially in gravity eliminated position and gradually progress to against gravity position.
  - Concentric and eccentric exercises
  - Strengthening of hip internal and external rotator, abductors, flexors and extensors
  - Strengthening of gluteus medius is necessary to decrease intra-articular pain and for pelvic control during single limb activities and ambulation.
- **To improve balance:** Exercises to improve balance—standing with feet close together, standing with one foot in front of the other, perform these exercises with closed eyes, tandem walking and other frenkle's exercises.

All exercises should be progressed gradually in terms of impact and intensity.

- **Gait training:** It should be initiated with appropriate assistive device as per the condition of patient.

Avoid
- Single limb weight bearing or activities as they may increase the intra-articular pressure in the hip joint.
- High impact activities.

Surgical Treatment

Indication
- When the child is of more than 6 years at the time of diagnosis.
- Children with necrosis of more than 50% of femoral head.

Surgical Techniques

Pelvic Osteotomy or Femoral Osteotomy

Goals of surgical treatment are:
- Realignment of hip bones
- To keep head of femur in acetabulum until healing is complete
- To eliminate hip irritability.
- To restore and maintain good hip mobility.

After the procedure the child is placed in cast for 6 to 8 weeks to protect the alignment.

CHAPTER 12

Edema

An abnormal accumulation of fluid in interstitial spaces of tissues is known as edema.

Causes
- **Deep vein thrombosis:** Thrombosis in deep veins of leg impairs the venous return and results in the pooling of blood in the affected leg.
- **Medication:** Calcium channel blocker, oral contraceptives, corticosteroids, antidepressants, etc. Calcium channel blocker causes dependent edema in feet and ankles whereas steroids cause non-pitting edema over face.
- **Heart disease:** Heart disease causes fairly symmetrical, dependent, pitting edema of ankle and feet that is more pronounced in evening.
- **Kidney failure:** In this condition, kidney loses the ability to eliminate enough salt and water that leads to the accumulation of fluid in feet, hands, abdomen, over face and around the eyes.
- **Liver disease:** Inability of liver to produce enough protein to maintain osmotic concentration of blood results in the movement of fluid towards the tissues and causes edema particularly in legs and abdomen.
- **Myxedema:** An underactive thyroid causes non-pitting edema over face, hand, feet and lower legs.
- **Minor frequent causes:** Local injury, varicose veins, insect bite or burn.

Types of Edema
- **Pitting edema (Fig. 1):** It is a type of edema in which an indentation is left behind, after the release of pressure applied to the swollen area, e.g. in cardiac failure, liver cirrhosis, DVT, nephrotic syndrome, pregnancy, etc.
- **Non-pitting edema:** In non-pitting edema the pressure induced indentation does not persist, e.g. in lymphedema and myxedema.

Classification on the basis of area involved:
- **Localized edema:** It occurs due to venous or lymphatic obstruction that may result from trauma or infection. It tends to be limited to localized area of body.
- **Generalized edema:** It occurs due to systemic process that occurs with chronic illness like cardiac, kidney or liver failure.

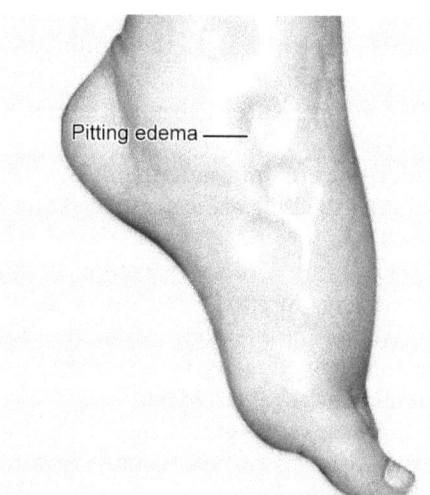

Fig. 1: Pitting edema.

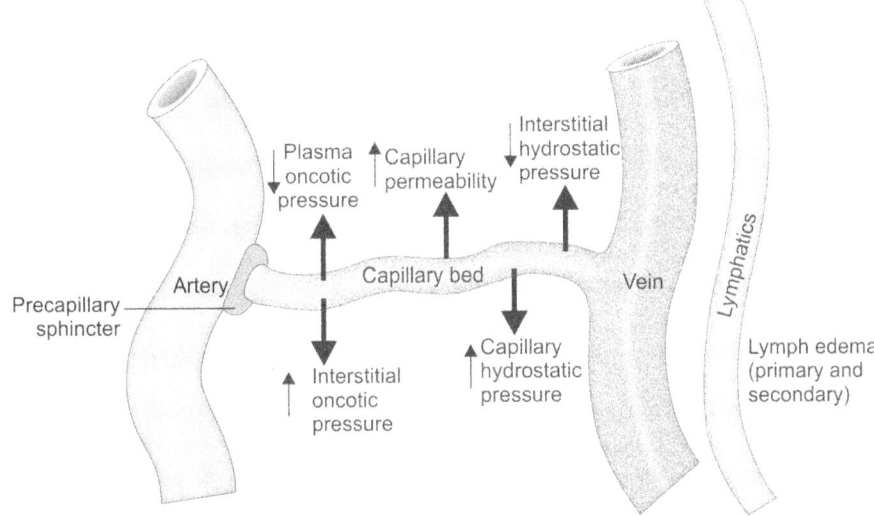

Fig. 2: Mechanisms that may cause edema.

Usually apparent in lower extremity, groin, abdomen or may exhibit whole body.

Etiopathogenesis

Edema is caused by mechanisms that interfere with the normal fluid balance of plasma, interstitial fluid and lymphatic flow. The following six mechanisms may cause edema (Fig. 2):
1. Decreased plasma oncotic pressure
2. Increased capillary hydrostatic pressure
3. Lymphatic obstruction
4. Tissue factor (increased oncotic pressure of interstitial fluid and decreased tissue tension)
5. Increased capillary permeability
6. Sodium and water retention.

Complications of Edema

- Restriction of ROM, limitation of function or pain.
- Disfiguring and disabling contractures and deformities—chronic edema particularly lymphedema having high protein level cause collagen laid down in the area leading to subcutaneous tissue fibrosis and hard induration of skin that may progressively leads to contracture and deformities.
- Infection—chronic lymphedema provides protein rich environment for bacterial growth and reduced tissue oxygenation that leads to infection.
- Chronic venous or lymphatic obstruction may result in cellulitis, ulceration and if unmanaged can lead to partial limb amputation.
- Chronic venous insufficiency causes itching due to stasis dermatitis and brown pigmentation of skin due to hemosiderin deposition.

Diagnosis

Physical Examination

- **Infection:** Assessment should be done with skin thermometer and both the sides should be compared.
- **Circumferential measurements:** To measure the circumference of limb, measurement should be taken at designated landmarks that should be compared with the contralateral side.
- **ROM and MMT:** ROM and muscle strength of the affected limb should be assessed.

- **Neurological assessment:**
  - Assessment of sensation including temperature, touch and pain
  - Assessment of reflexes
  - Observation of tissue quality like color, changes in hair growth, skin texture, presence of any wound or rashes.
- **Grades of pitting edema:**
  - **Grade 1:** A pit of 2 mm or less with no distortion and indentation disappears immediately.
  - **Grade 2:** A pit between 2 mm to 4 mm with negligible distortion and indentation disappears in 10–15 seconds.
  - **Grade 3:** A deep pit between 4 mm to 6 mm with swollen affected area and indentation takes 1 minute to disappear.
  - **Grade 4:** A deeper pit between 6 mm to 8 mm with gross distortion and indentation between 2 to 5 minutes to disappear.

Management

It depends on the causative factor of edema.

Preventive Measures

- **Reduce sodium intake:** High sodium intake aggravates the fluid retention.
- **Maintain proper weight:** Being overweight slows the body fluid circulation and put extra pressure on veins.
- **Travel breaks:** Regular break should be taken during long traveling to avoid the pooling of fluid in feet and ankle.
- **Standing or walking:** Stand and walk 'worth of stretching' for atleast 3–5 minutes after every hour to stimulate the blood circulation.
- **Elevation of limb:** Placing the limb at least 12 inches above the heart level for 10–15 minutes, 3 or 4 times a day stimulates the movement of excess fluid back into circulatory system.

Medication includes 3 "Ds": The 3D's are usually prescribed for medical conditions that causes excess fluid accumulation in body.

1. **Diuretics:** It promotes urination of sodium and water.
2. **Digoxin:** It controls the heart rate and increase the strength of heart's contraction to improve the blood circulation and reduce swelling in patients with heart problem.
3. **Dietary:** Less sodium and adequate protein intake.
   - **Foods that worsen edema:** Alcohol, caffeine, sugar, dairy products, soya sauce, animal protein, chocolates, olives and pickles, etc.

Physiotherapy Management

- **RICE therapy:** When edema occurs due to any injury, RICE therapy should be given in initial 24–72 hours after injury.
- **Massage therapy:** Massage helps in reducing the edema by facilitating the blood circulation, increasing the level of oxygen and nutrients to the involved tissue, removal of waste products and also by accelerating the forward movement of venous blood and lymph to the heart and lymph nodes respectively.

A wide range of massage can be used to reduce swelling:
  - **Effleurage:** It involves pushing the excess fluid toward different glands within the body using gentle long direction strokes. It is used when the area is tender.
  - **Deep strokes:** In this firm pressure is applied to get deeper within the muscles to push and remove excess fluid from the swollen area. It is used in chronic case of edema when the area is not tender.
  - **Lymphatic drainage:** It is a special type of massage that involves applying pressure towards the direction of glands. It stimulates the lymphatic system to increase lymph flow that picks up the metabolic waste and remove them through the glands.

- **Therapeutic exercises:** Exercises helps to enhance venous and lymphatic flow.
  - Exercise in combination with compression like isometric exercises during intermittent compression pumping or walking with compression bandage on lower limb.
  - Elevating the limb during exercises further facilitates the edema reduction.
  - Aquatic exercises are beneficial for patient with lower extremity edema and a stable cardiovascular system.
- **Non-mechanical compression:** Static or intermittent compression therapy increases the pressure surrounding the extremity to counterbalance any increased osmotic and hydrostatic pressure causing the fluid to flow out of the vessels into the extravascular space.
  If sufficient pressure is applied the hydrostatic pressure in interstitial space is more than in veins and lymphatic vessels reducing outflow from the vessels and causing fluid in interstitial space to return back into the vessels. Non-mechanical compression is given using:
  - Compression bandaging
  - Compression garments.
- **Mechanical compression device:**
  - **Intermittent pneumatic compression pump:** It helps to facilitate the edema reduction. It provides compression therapy by using a gradient pump that pushes air into a multi-chambered pneumatic sleeve fitted on the affected limb. It may apply in sequential or non-sequential manner. If sequential then pushes the air from distal to proximal.
  - **Inflation parameters:** Set the pressure below the diastolic pressure of patient to avoid the occlusion of arteries. So inflation pressure of 30–60 mm Hg for upper limb and 40–80 mm Hg for lower limb is optimal.
- **Electrical stimulation:** It facilitates the blood circulation by producing rhythmic contraction of muscles.
- **Contrast bath:** Alternate hot and cold application, rhythmically dilates and contracts the blood and lymphatic vessel which is used to pump and move the stagnant fluid out of the area.
- **Therapeutic modalities:** Modalities helps to improve the circulation that aids in reduction of accumulated fluid.
  - Ultrasound
  - LASER
  - Interferential therapy.

CHAPTER 13

Complex Regional Pain Syndrome

Complex regional pain syndrome (CRPS) is a chronic and progressive neuroinflammatory condition that is characterized by a group of symptoms including severe burning pain, tenderness, swelling, warmth or coolness, stiffness and discoloration of the skin of an extremity. Initially it may affect a single extremity but gradually it spreads throughout the body (Fig. 1).

It is also named as reflex sympathetic dystrophy, causalgia, shoulder-hand syndrome, Sudeck's reflex neurovascular dystrophy, post-traumatic pain syndrome, algodystrophy, neurodystrophy, post-traumatic dystrophy and transient migratory osteoporosis.

Epidemiology

- Females are more affected than males with the ratio of 3:1.
- Usually appears between 40 and 60 years.
- It may affect any region but extremities are more oftenly affected. In adults, upper limb is more affected than lower limb.
- It may appear unilateral or bilateral.

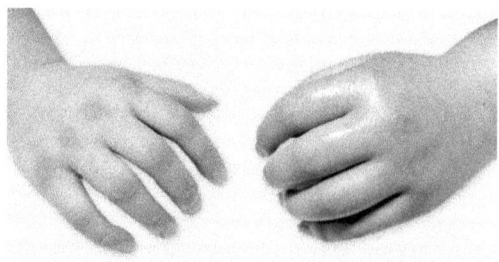

Fig. 1: Complex regional pain syndrome on hand.

- In Type I CRPS, 91% cases occur post-surgically and only 5% cases are post-traumatic.

Etiology

Exact cause is not known but the symptoms usually appear after:
- **Trauma:** Any accidental injuries, e.g. sprain, fracture, crush injuries and cut.
- **Surgical injury,** e.g. excision of tumor, scar, manipulation of organ.
- **Disease:**
  - Visceral disease, e.g. myocardial infarction.
  - Neurological disease, e.g. tumor, brachialgia, cerebrovascular accidents, nerve entrapment.
  - Infection.
  - Vascular disease, e.g. atherosclerotic conditions.
  - Musculoskeletal disease, e.g. injury to muscles, degenerative conditions of muscles and bones.
  - Drugs for tuberculosis and barbiturates.

Pathophysiology

There is no single pathophysiological mechanism that can explain the diversity and heterogeneity of symptoms. Therefore, it is now accepted that multiple mechanism are involved and the presentation depends on the relative contribution of each mechanism. The different pathophysiological mechanisms that are thought to contribute to CRPS include

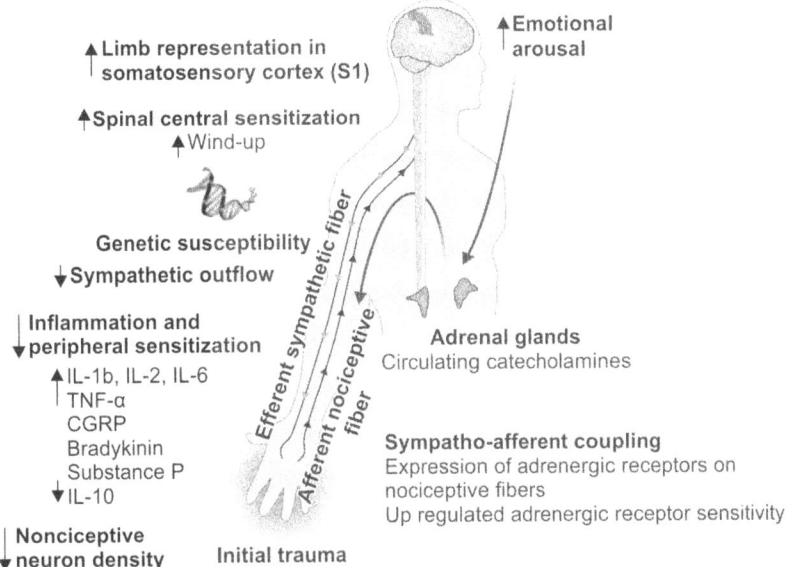

Fig. 2: Multifactorial process involving both central and peripheral mechanisms.

altered cutaneous innervation, central and peripheral sensitization, neurogenic inflammation, increased level of local and systemic inflammatory cytokines, lower systemic level of anti-inflammatory cytokines, overactivity of sympathetic nervous system, genetic and psychological factors (Fig. 2).

Types of CRPS

CRPS type I: It comprises 90% cases. It is traumatic in nature without any nerve damage and occurs after an initiative noxious event such as fracture, sprain, etc. It has two subtypes:
1. **Major:** It occurs after any skeletal injuries like fracture.
2. **Minor:** It occurs after soft tissue injuries like sprain, strain, etc.

CRPS type II: It is also known as "Causalgia". It develops after nerve injury. It is of two subtypes:
1. **Major:** It occurs due the involvement of mixed nerves.
2. **Minor:** It occurs due to the involvement of sensory nerves.

Clinical Presentation (Fig. 3)

- **Due to sensory disturbances:**
  - **Hypersensitivity:** Allodynia (pain from stimulus that normally does not provoke pain), hyperalgesia (increased pain from stimulus that normally provoke pain), hyperpathia, paresthesia (abnormal sensation either spontaneous or evoked), hyperesthesia (increased sensitivity to stimulus)
  - **Pain:** Severe constant, burning pain
    - Pain is disproportionate in intensity to the inciting event.
    - Pain increases with dependent position, activities, physical conditions or emotional disturbances.
- **Due to autonomic dysfunction:**
  - **Swelling:** Localized or generalized, fusiform or hard.
  - **Asymmetry of skin temperature:** Skin becomes warm and sweaty at times and cold and clammy at others.
  - **Asymmetry of skin color:** Ranging from pale to pink or even bluish color.

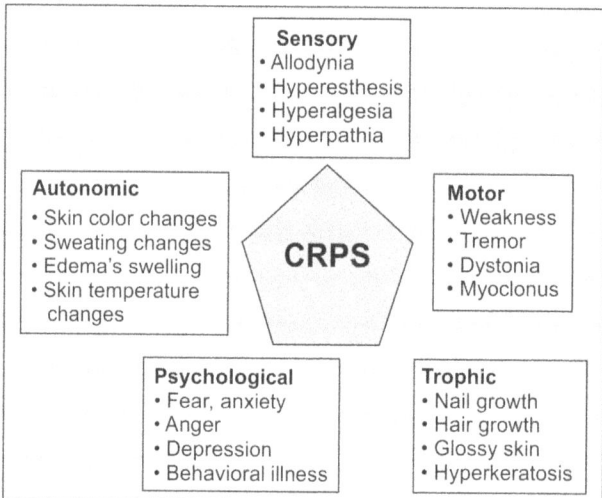

Fig. 3: Symptoms of CRPS.

- **Asymmetry of sweating:** Hyperhidrosis or dryness.
- **Due to motor dysfunction:**
  - Muscle weakness or atrophy
  - Tremor, dystonia and coordination deficits
  - Decreased ROM.
- **Trophic changes:**
  - Thick, brittle or rigid nails
  - Skin becomes thin and glossy
  - Increased or decreased hair growth.

Stages of Progression

Stage I: Acute Inflammatory Phase (Last for 0–3 Months)

- Constant burning and severe pain along with hypersensitivity
- Soft and localized edema
- Asymmetry of skin temperature switching between warm or cold
- Skin progressively becomes blotchy, purple, pale or red, thin and shiny and becomes sweaty
- Faster hair and nail growth.
- Presence of muscle spasm and joint pain.
- **X-ray:** Patchy bone thinning.

Stage II: Dystrophic Phase (Last for 3–9 Months)

- More marked pain and sensory disturbances
- Edema becomes hard that cause joint stiffness
- Continued skin changes
- Thin and rigid nails that cracks or breaks easily
- Slower hair growth
- Muscles weakness and joint stiffness
- **X-ray:** Cortical thinning and subchondral bone erosion represents osteoporosis.

Stage III: Atrophic Phase (Last for 9–18 Months)

- Pain spreads proximally and occasionally to the entire body
- Hardening of edema occurs gradually
- Skin becomes dry, cooler, thin, shiny and cyanotic
- Finger tips and toes become atrophic and possible contracture may present
- Restricted joint ROM because of tightened muscles and tendons (contracture)
- Muscle wasting
- **X-ray:** Demineralization and ankylosis of bones.

Diagnosis
Clinical diagnosis is based on patient's sign and symptoms.

Budapest Diagnostic Criteria
- Continuing pain, which is disproportionate to any inciting event.
- Must report 1 symptom in 3 of the 4 following categories:
  1. **Sensory:** Report of hyperesthesia and/or allodynia.
  2. **Vasomotor:** Report of temperature asymmetry and/or skin color changes and/or skin color asymmetry.
  3. **Sudomotor/edema:** Report of edema and/or sweating changes and/or sweating asymmetry.
  4. **Motor/trophic:** Report of decrease ROM and/or motor dysfunction (weakness, tremor, dystonia) and/or trophic changes (hair, nail, skin).
- Must display at least 1 sign at the time of evaluation in 2 or 3 or more following categories:
  1. **Sensory:** Evidence of hyperalgesia (to prick) and/or allodynia (to light touch and/or deep somatic pressure and/or joint movement).
  2. **Vasomotor:** Evidence of temperature asymmetry and/or skin color changes and/or skin color asymmetry.
  3. **Sudomotor/edema:** Evidence of edema and/or sweating changes and/or sweating asymmetry.
  4. **Motor/trophic:** Evidence of decrease ROM and/or motor dysfunction (weakness, tremor, dystonia) and/or trophic changes (hair, nail, skin).
- When there is no other diagnosis that better explains the signs and symptoms.

Management
Conservative Treatment
- **Medications:**
  - **NSAIDs (ibuprofen) and COX-2 (celecoxib) inhibitors:** They are used to reduce pain and inflammation in acute stage.
  - **Analgesics like opioids (acetaminophen):** It is used in severe pain.
  - **Antidepressants (amitriptyline) or anticonvulsants (dilantin):** They help to manage nerve pain and sleep disturbances.
  - **Corticosteroids:** Helps to reduce pain and inflammation.
  - **Bone loss prevention medications**, such as calcium modulating drugs (calcitonin), biphosphonates (alendronate), etc.
- **Regional anesthesia technique:** It is used in patient with moderate to severe pain that do not respond to pharmacological treatment. It includes sympathetic nerve block. Stellate ganglion block is done in upper extremity and lumbar sympathetic block is done in lower extremity.
- **Spinal cord implantation:** Tiny electrodes implanted along the spine and mild electric impulses are delivered to the affected nerves.
- **Surgical repair or release:** It is indicated in case of neural diagnosis like neuroma, neuroma in continuity and secondary compression neuropathies. In compression neuropathies, release of affected nerve from avascular scar tissues is performed. In nerve transection or neuroma in continuity, repair of affected nerve or nerve graft is preferred.
- **Sympathectomy:** Surgical or chemical sympathectomy: It is indicated in case of reappearance of symptoms after sympathetic block.

Physiotherapy Treatment
Acute Phase
Immobilization and contralateral therapy should be initiated in the acute phase because of the presence of marked pain and hypersensitivity. Intensive active therapy in the acute phase may lead to deterioration of the condition.

Chronic Phase
- **For pain relief:** Pain must be controlled before progressing to other treatment technique.
  - TENS
  - Heat or cold application
  - Contrast bath
  - Whirlpool therapy gives soothing and relaxing effect and controls the vasomotor function
  - Relaxation technique.
- **To decrease edema:**
  - Ultrasound: To decrease inflammation and adhesion
  - Elevation of limb: To decrease arterial hydrostatic pressure and assist lymphatic and venous draining
  - Light self-adhesive compression wraps or compression garments
  - Active ROM exercises
  - Caution: Passive retrograde massage and passive ROM should be avoided initially as they may stimulate an inflammatory response that can worsen the condition.
- **To maintain joint ROM and to prevent stiffness:**
  - Active ROM activities should be geared towards improving function with the affected hand (such as drinking from a cup, turning the knob of door, using a knife) and with affected leg (such as walking or stair climbing).
  - After the restoration of ROM and decreased muscle guarding, therapist should initiate strengthening exercises.
- **Sensory integration training:**
  - **Left right discrimination:** In CRPS, ability to recognize left and right is progressively compromised. To rehabilitate, images of different body parts at rest and during movements are shown and asked to recognize left and right side.
  - **Motor imagery program:** It is a mental process by which an individual rehearses or simulates a given action in his mind without actually performing the movement. It helps to reduce pain, improve ROM and strength.
  - **Mirror visual feedback therapy:** In this therapy, mirror is used to get visual feedback. For example for hand therapy, the affected hand is placed behind the mirror. The non-affected hand is then moved and the patient receives the visual feedback that the both the hands are moving without pain. This therapy helps in cortical reorganization. In CRPS, reduced movement of affected limb due to pain, altered the sensory feedback from the limb resulting in cortical reorganization of body's representation in brain that causes pain. In mirror therapy, this reorganization is changed by alternative sensory input using visual illusion thereby decreasing pain (Fig. 4).
  - **Body perception awareness:** In CRPS, patient has lack of awareness about the affected part of body. Due to severe and continuous pain in affected limb, patient represents neurological neglect like symptoms in which patient describes their affected limb with

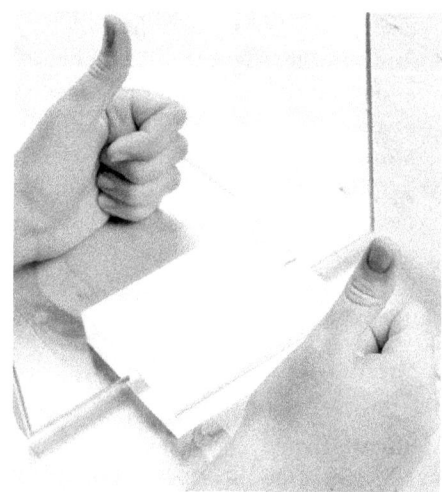

Fig. 4: Mirror visual feedback therapy.

negative emotional feeling, pay little attention to the limb as if it is not a part of his body. Body perception awareness therapy encourages the patient to look at, touch and think about the affected limb to increase the awareness of the affected limb and to perceive affected limb as a normal body part.

- **For desensitization of hypersensitive area:**
  - Touch stimulation—giving stimuli of different pressure (light or deep), temperature (hot or cold), and with different fabrics (cotton, silk, etc.).
  - Dipping the affected area in the bowl of dry rice, sand, kidney beans, etc.
  - Electrical stimulation—initiate with mild intensity and gradually progress to more intense to decrease the sensitivity of the area.
  - Massage like tapping or percussion.
  - Contrast bath: Place the painful part in cold water for 30 seconds then warm water for 2 minutes and repeat the process for 5 minutes.
  - **Stress loading program:** It is comprised of two components: Scrubbing and carrying. These activities load the affected limb that provides inhibitory proprioceptive input to the nervous system. In this technique, the affected limb is loaded to tolerance and progressive increase the frequency and duration that enable the nervous system to acclimate to the stimuli. This acclimation progressively desensitizes the hypersensitivity and allows nervous system to remodel itself and perceive the stimulus as normal sensation.
    1. **Scrubbing:** It applies constant force to the affected area for progressively increasing period of time. Scrubbing for upper limb is given using towel or scrub brush and scrubbing of lower limb is given by wearing socks or by deck brush fixed by a strap.
    2. **Carrying:** It involves loading the affected limb by carrying weighted object for extended period of time. For upper limb carrying heavy bag is effective here as for lower limb loading can be done by weight bearing and walking.

CHAPTER 14

Fibromyalgia

Fibromyalgia composed of Latin word *fibro* (fibrous tissue), Greek word *myo* (muscles) and *algos* (pain). It is a chronic disorder characterized by widespread musculoskeletal pain accompanied with cognitive impairment that severely affecting the quality of life and normal functioning of the patient (Fig. 1).

Epidemiology

- Females are seven times more affected than males.
- Typically develops between ages of 25-55 years.
- About 1 in every 25 people develop fibromyalgia at some satge in their lives.

Etiology

There are many hypotheses for the development of fibromyalgia but the exact etiology is not known.

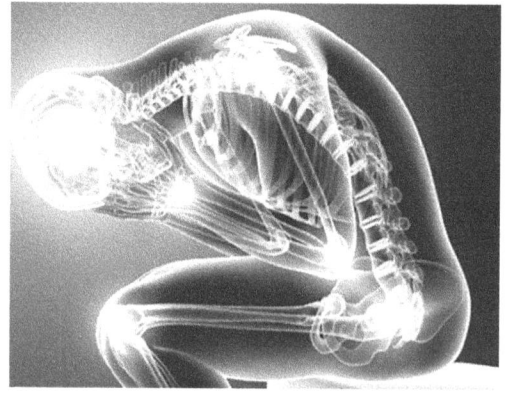

Fig. 1: Fibromyalgia.

There are several potential causes or risk factors:

- **Hereditary:** Some people are more likely to develop fibromyalgia because of their genes.
- **Accidents and injuries (surgical or traumatic):** Fibromyalgia may be triggered by an injury or trauma.
- **Autoimmune disorders:** Such as rheumatoid arthritis, systemic lupus erythematosus (SLE), ankylosing spondylitis, etc. in which the body's immune system perceives its own tissues as foreign body and release antibodies against them.
- **Infectious diseases** like hepatitis, parvovirus, Epstein-Barr virus or Lyme disease may be linked to fibromyalgia.
- **Hormonal changes:** Like decrease in the level of serotonin, noradrenaline and dopamine and increase the level of cortisol (released when the body is under stress) may trigger the fibromyalgia.
- **Psychological and emotional stress:** Anxiety, mood and sleep disturbance may alter the hormonal level that may further linked with fibromyalgia.

Clinical Presentation (Fig. 2)

- **Pain:** Widespread pain may be present throughout the body. It may be deep, sharp, dull, throbbing or aching pain in muscles, tendons and ligaments around the joints.
- **Fatique:** Whole body fatigue or malaise that makes the ADLs difficult.

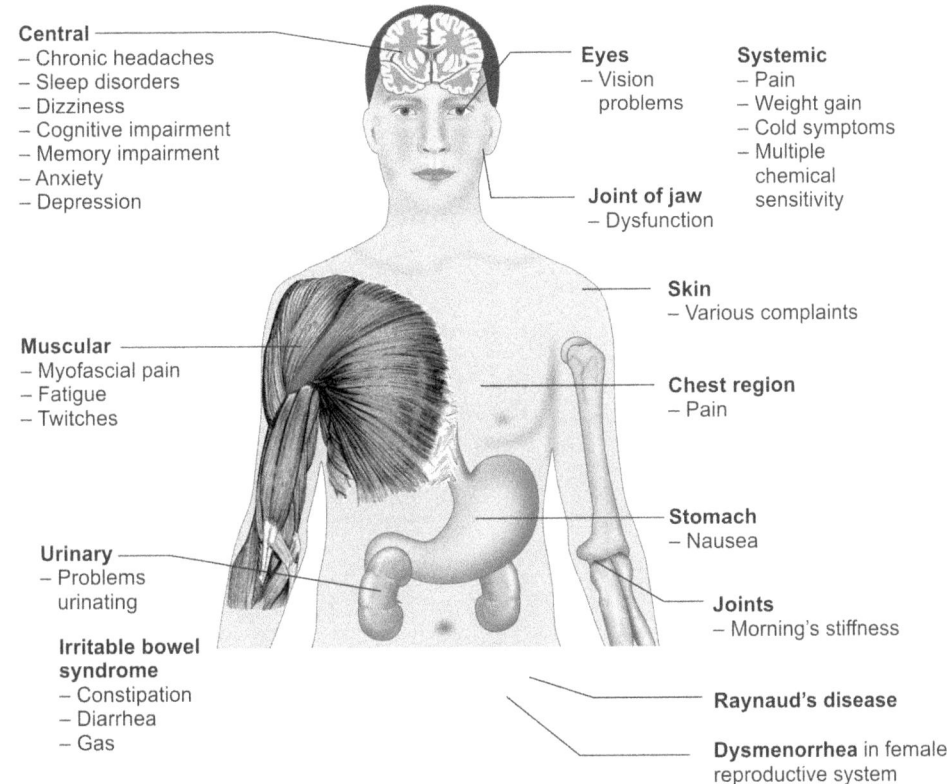

Fig. 2: Symptoms of fibromyalgia.

- **Stiffness:** Especially in the morning or after long period of inactivity.
- **Sleep:** Patient may have insomnia, sleep disturbances, or sleepiness.
- **Muscular pain:** Patient may complain of muscle tenderness, restless leg, muscle spasms or joint stiffness.
- **Sensory disturbances:** Cold sensitivity, hyperalgesia, sensation of coldness, pins and needles or tingling sensation in peripherals may be present.
- **Cognitive problems:** Forgetfulness or lack of concentration may present.
- **Psychological problems:** Depression, flare, headache, irritability, dizziness, anxiety or mood swings may present.
- **Dysmenorrhea in females:** Menstrual cramps may occur.
- **Chest pain:** Palpitation.
- **Urinary bladder irritability:** Painful urination.
- **Irritable bowel syndrome:** It is a digestive disorder that is characterized by pain and bloating in stomach and can lead to constipation, diarrhea, abdominal gas or acid reflux.
- **Raynaud's syndrome:** It consists of spasm of small arteries in the peripherals due to exposure to cold or stress that causes the pain, paleness or bluishness of the hands or feet.
- **Sensitivity to environmental factors:** Patient becomes sensitive to changes in weather, bright light, noise, smell, medication or some food.

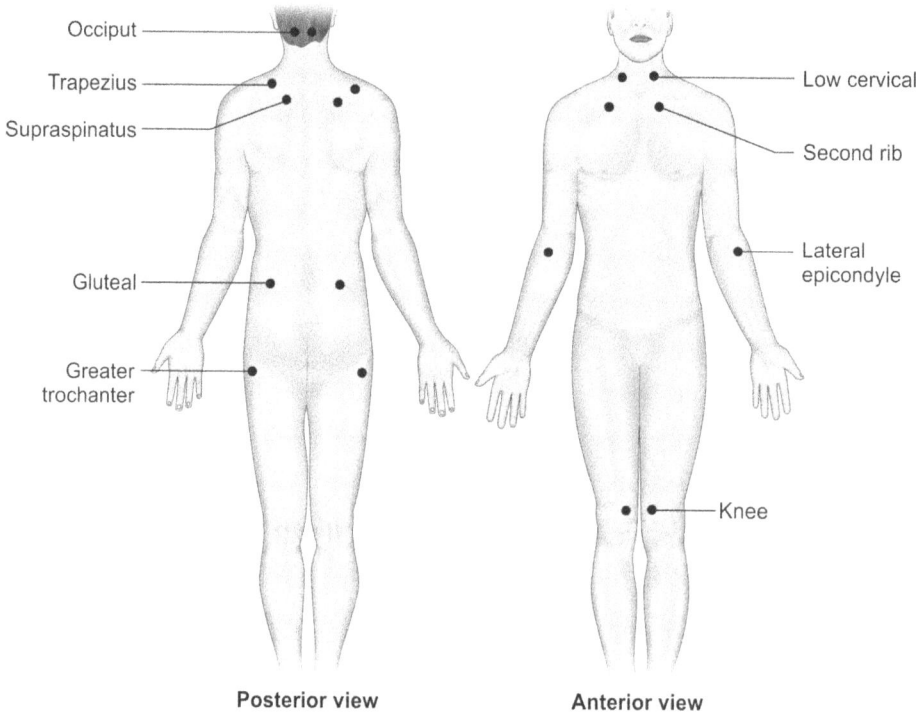

Fig. 3: Location of tender points of fibromyalgia.

- **Painful tender points (Fig. 3):** Painful tender points are present bilaterally over the particular regions on the body. There are 18 tender points.
  1. **Occiput:** At suboccipital muscle insertion.
  2. **Low cervical:** At the anterior aspect of intertransverse spaces at C5-C7.
  3. **Trapezius:** At the midpoint of upper trapezius.
  4. **Supraspinatus:** At the origin above the scapular spine near the medial border of scapula.
  5. **Second rib; at second costochondral junction**—just lateral to the junction.
  6. **Lateral epicondyle:** 2 cm distal to the epicondyle.
  7. **Gluteal:** In the upper and outer quadrant of buttock.
  8. **Greater trochanter:** Posterior to trochanteric prominence.
  9. **Knee:** Proximal to medial joint line.

Symptoms are often exacerbated by:
- Stress
- Overloading physical activities
- Change in weather
- Sudden change in barometric pressure
- Any traumatic event or illness
- Overstretching.

Diagnosis

American College of Rheumatology Diagnostic Criteria (2016) for Fibromyalgia

1. Widespread Pain Index (WPI) is more than or equals to 7 and Symptom Severity Scale (SSS) score is more than or equals to 5.
   OR
   Widespread Pain Index (WPI) is 4 to 6 and Symptom Severity Scale (SSS) score is more than or equals to 9.
2. Generalized pain, defined as pain in at least 4 of 5 regions (left upper, right upper, left lower, right lower, axial), must be present.

Jaw, chest and abdominal pain are not included in generalized pain definition.
3. Symptoms have been generally present for at least 3 months.
4. A diagnosis of fibromyalgia is valid irrespective of other diagnosis. A diagnosis of fibromyalgia does not exclude the presence of other clinically important illnesses.

Management

Medications

- **Analgesics:** Analgesics are used to relieve pain and inflammation, e.g. tramadol, pregabalin, amitriptyline also improves sleep pattern.
- **Antidepressants:** It helps to ease pain, fatigue, depression, anxiety and treat mood disorders, e.g. selective serotonin reuptake inhibitors (SSRI), cymbalta.
- **Anticonvulsants:** Anticonvulsants are used to relieve pain and improve sleep disorders, e.g. lyrica.
- **Sedating medication:** May be used to improve sleep without having any effect on pain.

Physiotherapy Treatment

- **Pain relieving modalities:**
  - **Hot therapy:** It promotes the healing process by relaxing the muscles and improving the blood circulation to the affected area. Improved blood circulation relieves muscle spasm by delivering the oxygen and nutrients and removing the waste byproducts.
  - **Electrotherapeutic modalities, like interferential therapy (IFT), electrical muscle stimulation (EMS), ultrasound therapy or transcutaneous electrical nerve stimulations (TENS):** They helps to reduce pain, muscle spasm, swelling. They inhibit the pain signals from reaching the spinal cord, while also triggering the release of endorphins which naturally relieve pain.
  - **LASER:** Laser reduces the pain and inflammation by accelerating the healing in damaged tissues, relaxing the muscles, and stimulating the nerve regeneration.
- **Massage:** It assists in pain relief and muscle relaxation by improving the blood circulation, increasing serotonin level, decreasing circulatory stress hormone, decreasing level of substance P (a pain messenger), decrease tender point pain, improve sleep patterns and overall sense of well-being.
- **Stretching exercises:** Stretching helps to restore functional muscle length, reduce swelling in affected joints, increase the flexibility by regaining the ROM, and improves the quality of sleep by promoting general relaxation and stress relief. Stretching of all the major muscle groups should be included.
- **Strengthening exercises:** Strengthening exercises helps to break the chronic pain cycle in fibromyalgia by improving the fitness and functional level, relieving physical and emotional stress and boosting the confidence and self-esteem of the patient. The strength training should include at least one exercise for each of the major body areas (chest, shoulders, abdominals, back arms and legs). Exercises can be performed with free weights, machine, stretch bands, household items or weight of own body.
- **Aerobic exercises:** Exercises like walking, running, cycling and swimming. These exercises helps to improve the quality of life by cardiovascular conditioning, improving and maintaining the strength of muscles, tone of muscle and build coordination and endurance.
- **Hydrotherapy:** It helps to relieve pain, relax muscles and conditioning of the body without adding unnecessary stress. Warm water may be used to improve the quality of sleep.

CHAPTER 15

Approach to Orthopedic Physiotherapy Assessment

To diagnose a patient's symptoms and problems, a thorough assessment is very important. It is also very vital in planning a proper physiotherapy or exercise therapy treatment. The basic physiotherapy assessment of a patient is done under following headings:

■ SUBJECTIVE ASSESSMENT

Demographics: Name, age, gender, address of patient

Chief complaint: It is patient's problem documented in his own language. No medical terminology is used here.

History: History of a patient is further divided into following subheadings:
- **History of present illness:** Involve incidents of last 24–48 hours.
- **History of past illness:** Up to last some weeks.
- **Occupational history:** Job history, i.e. if present symptoms are due to patient's occupation.
- **Medical-surgical history:** Certain surgeries and medical conditions like diabetes have direct impact on patient's sensory system.
- **Personal history:** Habits like smoking or drinking.
- **Drug history:** Like BP medication leads to blood vessel thinning and thus giving heating modalities, will cause rapid vasodilation.

■ PAIN ASSESSMENT

Remember OPQRST mnemonic
- **O**nset of pain
- **P**rovoking/palliating/aggravating factors: Factors which increases pain.
- **Q**uality of pain/nature of pain: Sharp shooting pain indicates nerve injury.
  - Dull ache might be due to muscular injury.
  - Throbbing pain/palpitations might be due to any vascular injury.
- **R**egion of pain
  - Site of pain: Noted in medical terminology according to anatomical landmarks.
  - Side of pain: Right or left or central.
  - Type of pain: Localized or generalized.
  - Character of pain: Radiating or non-radiating.
- **S**everity/intensity of pain: Visual analogue scale (VAS) or numerical pain rating scale (NPR)
- **T**ime (duration): That the patient has been experiencing the pain.

■ OBJECTIVE ASSESSMENT

On observation: This part of assessment involves extracting all possible clinical information by observing the patient as he enters the department. It involves:
- **Facial expressions:** Observe if patient is sad, apprehensive, in pain, anxiously alert or paranoid by his facial expressions.
- **Posture assessment:** Usually fundamental postures are observed unless a detailed posture assessment is needed. The unusual findings are noted down while observing patients fundamental positions

like standing-sitting in all planes with help of a plumb line.
- **Gait assessment:** Pattern of walking-normal, antalgic, Trendelenburg, stooped, etc. Detailed foot print analysis (FPA) can be done to find out different kinetic and kinematic variants of gait like:
  - **Cadence:** Number of steps per minute.
  - **Step length:** Distance between two consecutive heel strikes.
  - **Stride length:** Distance between two same heel strikes.
- **Deformity** including asymmetry, angulation, shortening and rotation.
- **Use of assistive device** like stick, walker or any supportive brace.
- **Swelling** could be indicative of generalized or localized edema.

On inspection: Close observation of the affected part is done by uncovering it. Following things are noted:
- Skin coloration: Redness, bluishness or pallor
- Presence of wounds
- Anatomical deformity
- Swelling.

On palpation: This part of assessment involves extracting clinical information by palpating the soft tissues of different depths at affected site with bare hands exerting different amount of pressure. Following things are checked:
- **Temperature:** Affected and non-affected body sites are compared by mere hand touch and no pressure. For warmth or cold indicative of inflammation.
- **Swelling:** Type of edema that is pitting or non-pitting is to be noted down by putting hand pressure.
- **Pulse:** Superficial pulses like carotid at neck or radial at wrist is palpated for rhythmicity of flow, character of pulse, i.e. fast/slow/normal and pulse rate.
- **Tenderness:** It assesses the pain perceived by patient because of touch of therapist's hands. It is documented in grades 1 to 4.

Grade 1	Patient complains of pain when therapist palpates.
Grade 2	Patient complains pain while palpation and also winces along.
Grade 3	Patient winces and withdraws the part during palpation.
Grade 4	Patient will not allow therapist to even start palpation.

- **Tenderness can also be graded as** mild, moderate or severe according to patient's subjective perception.
- **Spasm:** It is a protective instantaneous response of muscle against any nociceptive stimuli. It is documented according to Penn Spasm Frequency Scale on following grades:

Grade 0	No spasm/normal muscle.
Grade 1	Mild spasm induced by stimulation.
Grade 2	Infrequent full spasm occurring less than once in some hours.
Grade 3	Spasm occurring more than once per hour.
Grade 4	Spasms occurring 10 times per hour.

- **Severity of spasm is explained in these 3 terms:**
  1. **Mild:** Functioning of patient is not affected by spasm.
  2. **Moderate:** Functioning of patient might get affected.
  3. **Severe:** Functioning of patient is completely affected.
- **Deformity:** The type of deformity, if it is fixed (bony) or functional (because of soft tissues) is tried to find out by palpation.

On examination: This assessment part is further divided into three headings:
1. **Sensory examination:** Different sensations are checked by various methods like
   - **Superficial sensations:** Touch, pain, temperature.
   - **Deep sensations:** Deep pain, proprioception, kinesthesia.
   - **Combined cortical sensation:** Two point discrimination, stereognosis, barognosis and graphesthesia.

- **MRC scale for grading sensory function of peripheral nerve:** It is used for grading of sensation. Dermatome chart (Fig. 1).

Grade	Clinical features
S0	No sensation
S1	Deep pain sensation
S2	Skin touch, pain and thermal sensation, i.e. protective sensation
S3	S2 also with accurate localization but deficient stereognosis. Cold sensitivity and hypersensitivity are often present
S3+	Object and texture recognition but not normal sensation. Good but not normal, two point discrimination
S4	Normal sensation

2. **Neuromuscular examination:** The spinomotor integrity is checked by different reflexes. A reflex is an involuntary response to sudden stimulus at different sites. Reflexes broadly are of two types:
   i. **Superficial reflexes:**

Reflex	Stimulus	Response
Corneal	Touch eye of patient with soft cotton	Eye blink is normal response
Abdominal	Lateral to medial (towards umbilicus) tactile stimulation	Clenching of abdomen
Plantar	Tactile stimulation from later border of foot towards great toe	Clenching of toes and fingers

   ii. **Deep jerks:** Different muscle tendons are stimulated by clinical hammer blow.

Biceps jerk (C5–C6)	With elbow held at slight flexion and completely relaxed, stimulus is given at biceps tendon in cubital fossa
Triceps jerk (C7–C8)	Shoulder in 90° abduction, elbow hanged relaxed, stimulus is given at olecranon process

Contd...

Contd...

Knee jerk (L3–L4)	For quadriceps, knee hanged at 90° flexion as in relaxed high chair sitting, stimulus is given above patella
	For hamstring, patient in prone and knee extended, stimulus is given at hamstring tendon each.
Brachioradialis jerk	With wrist relaxed at neutral, stimulus is given at brachioradialis tendon at base of radius

These jerks are documented according to deep tendon reflex grading system:

Grade 0	Absent jerk/no response
Grade 1	Diminished response
Grade 2	Normal
Grade 3	Exaggerated
Grade 4	Clonus (repeated response even after single stimulation)

3. **Motor examination:**
   Muscle tone: It is physiological tone present in a resting muscle which is checked by passively moving the affected joint throughout range. The quality and quantity of passive movement is checked by therapist and accordingly muscle tone can be estimated:

Normal	Patient at rest and therapist performs passive movement throughout range is observed.
Spastic	When therapist performs passive range, involuntary resistance is offered by the patient. The total range may or may not complete. Muscle tone is said to be increased.
Flaccid	When passive movement is over smooth and joint seems over flexible so much so that at times can go more than normal range. Muscle tone is said to be decreased.

Now spasticity is documented even further as follows:
- **Spasticity:** It is measured by Ashworth scale having 6 grades:

Approach to Orthopedic Physiotherapy Assessment

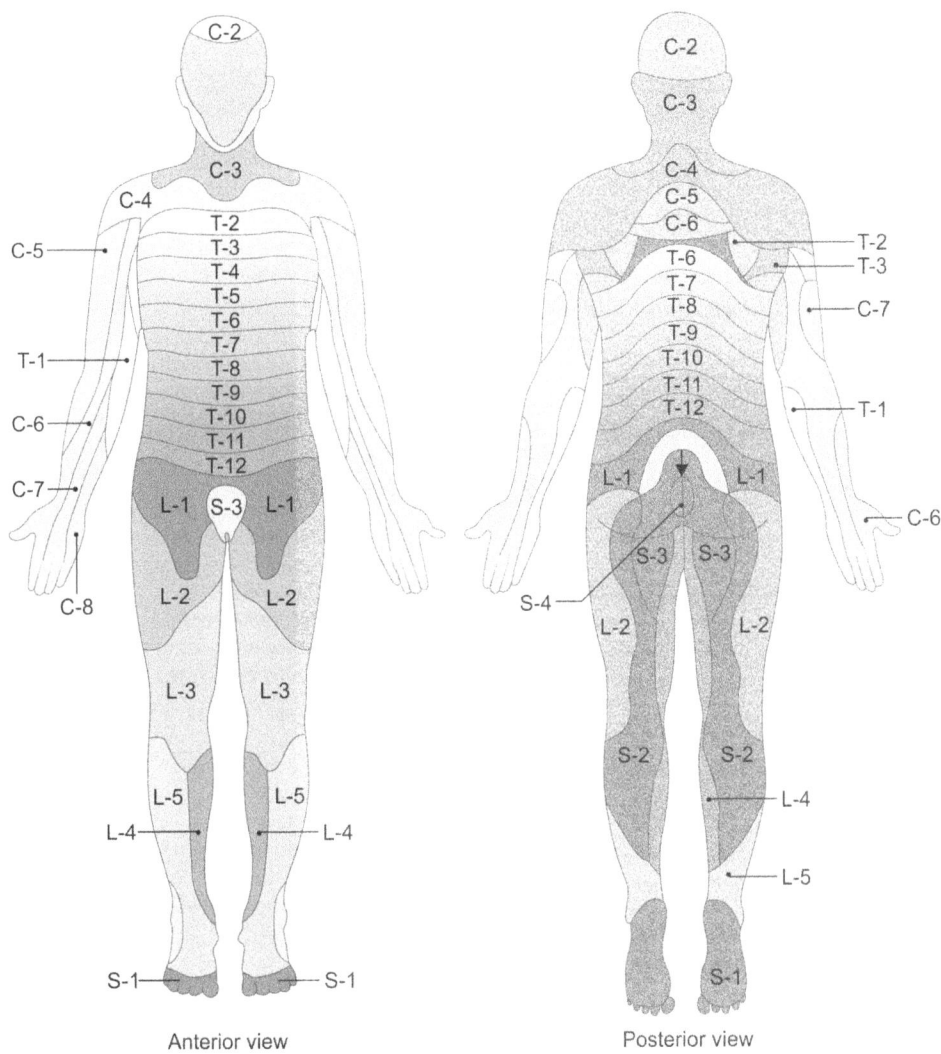

Fig. 1: Dermatome chart.

Grade 0	Normal muscle tone checked by passive movement (no spasticity)	**Grade 2**	More marked increase in muscle tone and resistance is felt throughout the ROM
Grade 1	Slight increase in muscle tone and minimum resistance is felt at end of passive	**Grade 3**	Considerate increase in muscle tone and passive movement is difficult to perform
Grade 1+	Slight increase in muscle tone with minimum resistance through less than half of passive range (initial or later)	**Grade 4**	Part is fixed and therapist cannot move it

Contd...

- **Range of motion:** With the help of goniometry, active and passive ranges of a joint are measured and documented.
AROM helps to understand the status of contractile tissue (muscle) function by voluntary doing ROM by patient.
PROM gives an idea about both contractile (muscle) and non-contractile (tendon, ligaments, capsule) tissue status while therapist move the affected joint through the range.

Date	Joint	Movement	AROM	PROM	End feel

End feel: At the end of PROM, feel of the limiting structure to range is known as end feel. It could be normal/abnormal end feel.

- **Normal (Physiological) End feels:**

Normal end feel	Description	Example
Soft	Soft tissue approximation	Knee flexion (contact between the soft tissue of posterior leg and thigh)
Firm	Muscular stretch	Hip flexion with knee straight (passive elastic tension of hamstring muscles)
	Capsular stretch	Extension of MCP joints (tension in anterior capsule)
	Ligamentous stretch	Forearm supination (tension in ligament in inferior radioulnar joint)
Hard	Bone contacting bone	Elbow extension (contact between the olecranon process of ulna and olecranon fossa of humerus)

- **Abnormal (Pathological) End feels:**

Abnormal end feel	Description	Examples
Soft	Occurs sooner or later in ROM than is usual or in a joint that normally has a firm or hard end feel. Feels boggy	Soft tissue edema, synovitis
Firm	Occurs sooner or later in ROM than is usual or in a joint that normally has a soft or hard end feel	Increased muscular tonus, capsular, muscular, ligamentous and fascial shortening
Hard	Occurs sooner or later in ROM than is usual or in a joint that normally has a soft or firm end feel. A bony grating or bony block is felt	Chondromalacia, osteoarthritis, loose bodies in joint, myositis ossificans, fracture
Empty	No real end feel because pain prevents reaching end of ROM. No resistance is felt except for patient's protective muscle splinting or muscle spasm	Acute joint inflammation, bursitis, abscess, fracture, psychogenic disorder

- **Muscle bulk:** The muscle bulk is measured by tape for both affected and non-affected sites in reference to certain anatomical landmarks and difference is documented to know any muscle wasting or atrophy.
- **Muscle power:** The muscle power or strength is checked with the help of manual muscle testing (MMT) on following grades:
Medical research council (MRC) Scale for muscle strength

Grade 0	No activity
Grade 1	Visible or palpable muscle contraction
Grade 2	Complete ROM in minimal gravity plane
Grade 3	Complete ROM against gravity

Contd...

Contd...

Grade 4 Complete ROM against gravity and moderate resistance

Grade 5 Complete ROM against gravity and maximal resistance

- **Myotome Chart:**

Upper limb myotome	
Neck flexion/extension	C1, C2
Neck side flexion	C3
Shoulder elevation	C4
Shoulder abduction	C5
Elbow flexion and wrist extension	C6
Elbow extension and wrist flexion	C7
Finger flexion, thumb extension and wrist ulnar deviation	C8
Finger abduction and adduction	T1
Lower limb myotome	
Hip flexion	L1, L2
Knee extension	L3
Ankle dorsiflexion	L4
1st metatarsal extension	L5
Ankle plantarflexion, eversion and hip extension	S1
Knee flexion	S2
Anal wink	S3, S4

- **Muscle endurance:** The maximum repetitions of resisted movement a person can do without getting fatigued documents his general endurance while same for a particular muscle and its movement documents muscle endurance.

Coordination and Balance Assessment

In this part of assessment, the coordination of patient is checked by various equilibrium and non-equilibrium tests while balance is checked by altering patients center of gravity (COG) as using wobble board or trampoline. Balance can also be checked by specific scales like Berg balance scale.

Functional Assessment

- Activities of Daily Life (ADLs) are assessed if they are affected by present symptoms
- Special tests for individual muscles, joint capsular stability or soft tissue mobility and stability as required are performed and results are documented.

Electrodiagnosis: Certain machines are used to check muscle or nerve's function like:

- Electromyography (EMG): To check muscle status.
- Nerve conduction velocity test: To check conduction speed in sensory or motor nerves.
- Strength duration (SD) curve: To check denervation or innervation extent of muscle fibers.

Note: From chief complains and history given by patient, some probable diagnosis is guessed by therapist. With further assessment and examination these probable diagnosis are narrowed down to one provisional diagnosis. With the help of next part of assessment that is on investigation, this provisional diagnosis is confirmed.

On investigation: The radiologists and technicians will provide with different images of body tissues and structure along with their conclusion as in:

- MRI
- CT scan
- X-Ray

The provisional diagnosis and these findings are clinically matched and a confirmed diagnosis is now formed.

Planning the treatment: To plan an effective physiotherapy treatment, first document the problem list of the patient. It could be for example—pain, stiffness or unable to reach at back pocket of trousers or unable to stand for long.

Now according to this, probable goals are set:

- **Short-term goals:** Which needs to be addresses immediately like pain or spasm.
- **Long-term goals:** Which can be addressed over a little later and needs time to be achieved like muscle strength or balance or coordination.

Index

Page numbers followed by *f* refer to figure, and *t* refer to table

A

Abductor contracture 151, 151*f*
Abductor digiti minimi, test for 194
Above elbow amputation 283, 289
Above knee amputation 283, 288, 289
Absorption 268*f*
AC joint, degeneration of 15
Acetabular
    component 275
    dysplasia 151
    liner 275
Acetaminophen 309
Achilles tendon 58*f*, 60
    ruptured 58*f*
Achondroplasia 177
Acromial fracture classification 76
Acrylic cement fixation, stem type with 276
Active exercise program 13
Active range of motion 76, 79, 81, 83, 85, 87, 95, 98, 104, 108, 110, 115, 124, 127, 129, 142, 145, 147, 149, 289
    exercise 240
Active-assisted range of motion 81, 83, 85, 87, 98, 104, 108, 110-113, 115, 118, 119, 124, 127, 145, 149, 275
Adam's forward bending test 169, 170*f*, 174, 174*f*
Adductor tightness 153*f*
Adson test 207, 208*f*
Aerobic exercises 233, 315
Alcohol 3, 181
    abuse 32
    avoidance of 261
Algodystrophy 71, 306
Allen and Ferguson classification 130, 130*t*
Allman classification 75*t*
Allograft 46, 50
American College of Rheumatology Diagnostic Criteria for Fibromyalgia 314
Amitriptyline 309
Amputation 282
    indications of 282
    level of 282
    selection of level of 282
    transfemoral 283, 294
    transhumeral 285
    transmetacarpal 283
    transmetatarsal 283
    transradial 285
    transtibial 283
Amputee prosthetic gait, analysis of 293
Amyloid disease 243
Amyloidosis 181
Analgesics 20, 225, 250, 256, 309, 315
Anderson D'Alonzo classification 128, 129*f*, 129*t*
Angiography 206
Angular displacement 68
Ankle
    and foot, postfracture stiffness of 125
    arthrodesis 280
    brace 219*f*
    deformities 255, 255f
    disarticulation 283
    injuries 56
    joint 281
        post-traumatic arthritis of 119
        stiffness 116
    sprain 56
        classification of 57
    Tinel's sign 218*f*
    trimalleolar fracture of 138
Ankylosing spondylitis 227, 227*f*
Annulus fibrosus 131, 235
Anterior cruciate ligament
    anatomy of 44*f*
    functions of 43
    injury 43, 44*f*, 114
    reconstruction surgeries 46
Anterior dislocation 139, 141, 144, 145, 145*f*
Anterior drawer test 45, 45*f*, 58, 58*f*
Anterior interosseous nerve syndrome 191, 202
Anterior scalene syndrome 200
Anterolisthesis 223*f*
Antibiotics 31, 56, 65
Antibody, antinuclear 256, 258
Anticonvulsants 309, 315
Ape thumb deformity 192
Apley's compression test 41, 41*f*
Apophyseal joint arthritis 221
Apprehension test 148, 148*f*
Arch
    supports 62
    taping 63*f*
Archer's elbow 18
Arms
    attitude of 143
    position of 168
Arsenic 181
Arterial thoracic outlet syndrome 205, 206
Artery, vertebral 206
Arthritic disease 279
Arthritis 29, 37, 246, 256, 257
    early post-traumatic 77
    infectious 279
    inflammatory 35
    post-traumatic 112, 119, 122, 146, 279
    septic 280
    subtalar 122
    symmetric 256
    tibiotalar 122
Arthrocentesis 260
Arthrodesis 134, 251, 278, 279
    combined 278
    extra-articular 278
    intra-articular 278
    triple 165, 280
Arthrofibrosis, post-traumatic 80
Arthrography 12, 12*f*
Arthropathies, neuropathic 272, 278
Arthroplasty 251, 272, 280
Arthroscopic lysis 14
Arthroscopy 40, 44, 48, 146
Arthrosis, patellofemoral 149
Articular fracture
    complete 110, 118
    partial 110, 118
Assistive device 186
    use of 317
Athletic activities 204
Atlas fracture 125, 126*f*, 127*t*
Atrophic phase 308
Atrophy 52, 148, 300
Attack, acute 260
Attitude and deformity 189, 192, 196
Autograft 46, 50
Autoimmune disorders 312
Avascular necrosis 71, 80, 95, 106, 119, 121, 146
Aviator fracture 137
Avulsion
    fracture 68, 122
    injury 123
Axial compression 130
Axial rotation assessment 167
Axillary border, superior half of 5
Axillary nerve 201
Axis fracture 127, 129*t*
Axon 182
Axonotmesis 182

B

Back pain 167, 173
    severe low 236
Backward walking 275
Backward weight shifting 291
Baker's cyst 54
Balance 300
    and coordination 287
    board 292, 292*f*
    exercises 54, 266
Banana fracture 137
Bandage wrapping technique 286*f*
Banjo splints 28, 28*f*
Bankart's fracture 137
Bankart's lesion 141
Bar, congenital 165
Barfly elbow 29
Barometric pressure 314
Barton's fracture 92, 93*f*, 137
    reverse 139
Basicervical fracture 103, 104
Below elbow amputation 283, 289
Below knee amputation 283, 288, 289
Benediction, hand of 192, 193*f*
Bennett fracture 137
    dislocation 98, 99*f*
Bernhardt-Roth syndrome 203
Bicruciate retaining design 273
Biologic disease modifying anti-rheumatic drugs 232, 256
Blood
    injection, autologous 20
    spinning therapy 24
    test 30, 55, 243, 256, 260
    vessel 70, 143

Body cast 134
Body perception awareness 310
Bone 155
　bruise 44
　diseases 246
　　metabolic 262
　dysplasia 246
　ends, alignment of 72
　healing time 103, 107
　infection 150
　loss
　　prevention medications 309
　　severe segmental 280
　normal 262f
　osteoporotic 262f
　tip of 285
Bony ankylosis 228, 251, 256
Bony erosion 227
Boston overlap brace, modified 226f
Bosworth fracture 137
Bouchard's node 249f
Boutonniere deformity 255
Bow legs 154, 154f
Bowing fracture 67, 67f, 89
Bowstring test 237, 237f
Boxer's fracture 99, 99f, 137
Braces 175, 178, 219
　action of 171
Brachial artery injury 82
Brachial plexus
　injury 80, 82
　palsy, post-traumatic 278
　paresis 75
Brachioradialis, test for 189
Bragard test 237
Breathing exercises 176, 233
Brudzinski sign 237
Bruises 2, 2f, 70
Bucket handle tear 40
Buckle fracture 67, 89
Budapest diagnostic criteria 309
Bumper fracture 137
Bursae 259
Bursectomy 18, 56, 65
Bursitis 1, 2, 2f
　aseptic 30
　infrapatellar 54
　prepatellar 54
　semimembranosus 54
　stages of 29, 29f
　subacromial 14, 14f
Burst fracture 131, 132f
　types of 132t

C

C bar splint 193f
Calcaneal fracture 120
　classification of 120f
Calcaneal osteotomy 165
Calcaneal pitch angle 160, 160f, 163, 163f
Calcaneus
　articular surfaces of 120f
　intra-articular fracture of 120
Calcitonin 265
Calcium 265
　deposition 15
Calf muscle 60
　stretching 219
　　exercises of 62f

Cancer 181, 253
Capitate fracture 97, 97f
Capsular stretching 13
Capsulitis
　adhesive 11, 11f
　idiopathic adhesive 10
　primary adhesive 10
　secondary adhesive 10
Card test 194, 195f
Caries spine 241
Carpal bones
　fracture, relative incidence of 94
　mobilization 213
Carpal compression test 212, 212f
Carpal fracture 94, 98t
Carpal ligament, transverse 213
Carpal tunnel
　release 214
　syndrome 93, 202, 210, 211f, 212, 279
Cartilage
　articular 248
　destruction 227
Cast 84, 86, 99, 119
　immobilization 90, 94, 109, 114, 117, 125
Causalgia 306
Celecoxib 309
Cement fixation, stem type without 276
Cementless fixation 272
Cerebral palsy 165, 166
Cervical
　collar 222f
　corset 222
　disc herniation 236
　lordosis, loss of 221
　rib syndrome 200
　spine 220, 230, 253
　spondylosis 220
　　X-ray findings of 221f
　traction 209
　vertebrae fracture, lower 129
Chance fracture 138
Chauffeur fracture 92, 93f, 138
Cheiralgia paresthetica 201
Chemical injury 282
Chemonucleolysis 239
Chemotherapy 245
Chest 269
　pain 313
　roentgenography 206
Chisel fracture 138
Chopart amputation 283
Chopart fracture 138
Chronic degenerative joint disease 246
Chymopapain injection 239
Clavicle fracture 74, 76t
　Allman classification of 75t
　classification of 74f
Claw
　foot 160f
　hand, partial 196
Clay Shoveller's fracture 138
Clergyman's knee 54
Closed fracture 66
Clostridium tetani 71
Cobb's angle 167f, 174, 175f
Cockup toes 256
Codman's exercises 7, 13

Cold
　abscess 242, 242f, 243
　compression 36
　laser 36
　pack 222
　therapy 56, 65, 256
Coleman block test 161
Colles' fracture 91, 92f, 138
Comminuted fracture 68, 96, 107, 112, 113, 117, 116
Common peroneal nerve 197, 198, 203
　anatomical course of 199f
Compartment syndrome 70, 82, 90, 111, 116, 123, 144
Complete fracture 67
　types of 68f
Complex regional pain syndrome 306, 306f
　symptoms of 308f
　types of 307
Compression 3, 31, 56, 59, 65, 131
　anteroposterior 102
　bandage 41
　force coupled with rotational forces 39f
　fracture 68, 130, 132f
　　subtypes of 132t
　non-mechanical 305
　potential sites of 200, 205f
Compressive flexion 130
Congenital disorders 159, 177
Continuous passive motion 275
Contracture 71, 144
Contrast bath 65, 305
Controlled environment therapy 286, 289
Contusions 1, 2
Coracoid fracture classification 76, 77f
Core muscle
　balance and coordination exercises of 240
　weakness 177
Corrective valgus derotation osteotomy 152
Corset 222
Cortical avulsion fracture 122
Corticosteroid 213, 256, 309
　drugs 232
　injection 33, 36, 41, 62
　intra-articular 250
Cortisone injection 20, 24
Cosmetic deformity 75
Costochondral junction, second 314
Costoclavicular compression syndrome 200
Costoclavicular space 204
Cotton fracture 138
Counterforce bracing 20, 24
Coxa valga 153, 153f, 154f
　acquired 153
　congenital 153
Coxa valgum 153
Coxa vara 150, 150f, 151f
　acquired 150
　classification of 150
　congenital 150
　X-ray findings of 152f
Cozen's test 19, 20f
　reverse 23, 23f

Cranial nerve injury 126
Craniotabes 270f
C-reactive protein 258
Crepitus 249
Cross finger test 195, 196f
Crush injury 180
Cryotherapy 17, 20, 41, 186, 219, 250, 261
Crystal deposition disorder 15
Cubital tunnel syndrome 202
Cuboid fracture 122
  Orthopedic Trauma Association
    classification of 123t
Curve
  location of 170
  severity 170
  types of 166, 170
Cyclic citrullinated peptide 258
Cyclist palsy 202
Cylinder cast 112
Cyriax release technique 207, 209, 209f
Cyst
  excision of 39
  popliteal 54
  removal of 39
  subchondral 249

D

Daily living, activity of 275, 280
Dancer fracture 123
Dashboard fracture 138
Dawbarn's sign test 17, 17f
De Quervain's tenosynovitis 34, 34f
Decompression
  spinal 245
  subacromial 18
  surgery 210
Deep friction massage 20, 24, 39
Deep vein thrombosis 275, 281, 302
Deformity 70, 150, 200, 243, 317
  congenital 282
  observation of 158
  spinal 165, 269
Denis classification 130, 131t
Denis system 130
Denis three column theory 130f
Dermatome chart 319f
Dermofasciectomy 34
Desensitization 187, 311
DEXA T-score 263f
Diabetes 11f, 181
  mellitus 11
Diaphyseal fracture 66, 89
Diaphysis 79
Die-punch fracture 92, 94f, 138
Diet 262, 271
Digits, amputation of 283
Digoxin 304
Dilantin 309
Diphtheria 181
Disarticulation 282
Disc
  herniation 235f, 236f
  types of 234
  surgical removal of 241
Disease-modifying antirheumatic drugs 232, 256
Dislocation 66, 139
  acute 146
  congenital 146

inferior 140, 141, 145
posterior 140, 141, 144, 145, 145f
subacromial 140
subclavicular 139
subcoracoid 139
subglenoid 139, 140
subspinous 140
superior 144
Displaced fracture 68, 112, 113
Displacement, 68
  lateral 68
Distal femoral fracture 109, 111t
  Muller's classification of 109, 110t
Distal humeral fracture 82, 85
  ASIF classification of 84f
Distal interphalangeal joint 255, 258, 279
Distal tarsal tunnel syndrome 217
Diuretics 213, 304
Dorsal Barton fracture 92
Dorsiflexion 115, 118, 119, 124, 127, 297
  eversion test 218, 218f
  external rotation stress test 59
Dowager's hump 172
Down's syndrome 162
Droopy shoulder syndrome 200
Drugs 181
Dual energy X-ray absorptiometry scan 263
Duchenne sign 196, 196f
Dupuytren's contracture 31, 32f
  stages of 32, 32f
Dupuytren's disease 10
Dupuytren's fracture 138
Duverney fracture 138
Dynamic exercises 25
Dynamic wrist and finger extension
  splint 190f
Dysmenorrhea 313
Dysplasia, patellar 148
Dystrophy, post-traumatic 306

E

Ear levels 168
Eburnation 248
Eccentric extension 275
Edema 186, 302, 303f, 309, 310
  complications of 303
  control 209, 285
  cycle 26f
  generalized 302
  localized 302
  non-pitting 302
Egawa test 194, 196f
Ehlers-Danlos syndrome 148, 162
Eichhoff maneuver 36
Elbow
  arthrodesis 279
  arthroplasty 279
  disarticulation 283
  dislocation 142, 145t
    classification of 143f
  joint 18, 253
    postfracture stiffness of 87
  movements 7, 8
  pad 31f
  protection of 31
  range of motion of 143
Electrical stimulation 28, 171, 256, 305
Electromyography 185

Electrotherapy modalities 31, 42, 186
Empty can test 5, 6f
Endocrine
  disease 246
  disorders 262
Endoneurium 180, 182
Endurance
  program 261
  training 60
Enthesopathy 227
Entrapment
  injury 181
  neuropathy 199
  site of 201, 203
Epicondyle, lateral 314
Epicondylectomy, medial 25
Epidural steroid injection 225, 238
Epineurium 180, 182
Epiphyseal fracture 66
Erector spinae muscles, lower 176
Erythema 52
Erythrocyte sedimentation rate 258
Essex-Lopresti fracture 90, 90f, 138
Evans classification 106, 106f, 107t
Exercises 7, 8, 42, 43, 47, 76, 264
  abdominal strengthening 176
  advance 293
  cardiovascular conditioning 240
  close chain 60, 266
  core strengthening 172, 240
  deep breathing 172
  diaphragmatic breathing 209
  endurance 43
  postural 266
  preprosthetic 291
  progressive resistance 76, 104, 149
  proprioception 17, 54, 60
Extensor carpi
  radialis
    brevis 189
    longus 189
  ulnaris 189
Extensor digitorum, test for 189
Extensor mechanism
  failure 113
  insufficiency 112
External fixation 74, 103, 109, 117, 119
External rotation 79, 85, 142, 147, 297
Extra-articular calcaneal fracture
  classification of 120, 120t
  types of 120f
Extra-articular manifestation 228, 229f, 252, 253f
Extracapsular fractures 103
Extremities 269
Extrinsic compression 181

F

Fabry's disease 181
Facet joint, degeneration of 220
Facial expressions 316
Fair test 216f
Faradic foot bath 164
Fasciectomy 34
Fasciotomy 34
Fat embolism 70, 109
  syndrome 114
Fatality 243
Fatigue 173

Femoral anteversion, excessive 154f
Femoral cutaneous nerve, lateral 203
Femoral fracture, proximal 103
Femoral head 275, 298
   basis of position of 144
   fracture 103
      classification of 104
      Pipkin classification of 105f
   prosthetic replacement of 107
Femoral intercondylar distance 155
Femoral neck
   fracture 103
      Garden classification of 105t
      orthopedic trauma association classification of 106t
      Pauwels classification of 105t
      types of 105f
   osteomyelitis of 150
Femoral nerve 199
   anatomical course of 199f
Femoral osteotomy 301
Femoral retroversion, excessive 152f
Femoral shaft fracture 107, 110t
   Winquist's classification of 108t
Femoral stem 275
Femoral stretch test 237, 237f
Femur
   head and neck of 298f
   intertrochanteric fracture of 106
   shaft of 108
Fenestration 241
Fibrillation 248
Fibromyalgia 312, 312f
   symptoms of 313f
   tender points of 314f
Fibrosis, stage of 236
Finger breadth 264
Finkelstein test 36, 36f
Fixation, percutaneous 81
Flap tear 40
Flat foot 163f, 255
   acquired 162
   complications of 162
   congenital 162
   inflammatory 162
   painful
      flexible 165
      rigid 165
   paralytic 162
   pathological 162
   physiological 162
   traumatic 162
Flesche test 231, 231f, 264
Flexibility 161
   exercises 187, 233, 265
Flexible flat foot 164
Flexion, adduction, internal rotation 216
Flexor carpi
   radialis 191
   ulnaris 191, 194
      test for 195
Flexor digitorum
   longus 198
   profundus 191, 194
   superficialis 191
Flexor hallucis longus 198
Flexor pollicis
   brevis 191

longus 191
   test 191, 193f
Flexor retinaculum, myofascial release of 213, 214f
Flowtron therapy 286, 289
Flu like symptoms 252
Fluid, aspiration of 31, 38, 56, 65
Foot
   amputation, partial 283, 285
   compartment syndrome 118, 121, 125
   deformities 159, 255, 255f
   injuries 56
   normal 159f, 160f, 162f, 163f
   plantar 48f
   pronation of 163f
Football 292
Footprint test 161, 161f, 163
Footwear modification 62, 65, 161, 164
Forearm
   compartment syndrome 86
   flexor pronator musculature, overuse of 22
   fracture 88, 91t
      classification of 88
      ipsilateral 82
   muscles, repetitive trauma of 18
   pronation 21
      resisted 23
   supination 21
Forward head posture 173
Fossa
   infraspinous 5
   subscapular 5
   supraspinous 5
Fracture 66, 141
   anatomical location of 116
   articular displacement 113
   bone, alignment of fragments of 68
   causes of 69, 69f
   classification of 66, 66f, 68f, 69f, 74, 82, 83
   combined mechanism 102
   comminution, basis of degree of 108
   complex 116
   complications of 70
   compound 66
   dislocation 14, 131, 133
      flexion distraction type 133, 133f
      flexion rotation type 133, 133f
      shear type of 133, 134f
   distal 82
      femur 45
      radius 91, 95t
      tibial 117, 119t
   extra-articular 110, 118, 120
   fifth metatarsal 124f, 125
   first metatarsal 125
   first to third metatarsal bone 125
   fourth metatarsal 125
   fragments 121f
      excision of 87
   general introduction of 66
   head of femur 104
   healing
      factors affecting 72
      stages of 71, 71f
      time 74, 77, 80, 82, 90, 109, 111, 112, 114, 115, 117, 119, 121-123, 125

high energy 116
impacted 68
intra-articular 73, 120
intracapsular 103
line, basis of
   angle of 68, 69f, 107
   extent of 66
   location of 66
location of 76, 82
longitudinal 112
mechanism of 85
middle 82
nomenclature 137
nondisplaced 68
parts, number of 79
pathological 69, 69f, 82
pattern, vasis of 116
proximal 82
segmental 67, 82, 107, 116, 117
simple 66, 116
single 67
subtrochanteric 106
symptoms of 70
third metatarsal 125
traumatic 122
types of 72
undisplaced 112
vertebral 125, 136
vertical 112
Fragments
   alignment of 68f
   displacement of 112
Freezing phase 12
Fregmentation 299
Freiberg test 216, 216f
Friedreich ataxia 165
Froment test 194, 195f
Frontal bossing 270f
Frozen
   phase 12
   shoulder 10, 11f, 12f, 80
      development, potential mechanism of 11f
Full weight bearing 108, 110, 111, 113, 115, 118, 119, 124, 127, 147, 149
Fusionless surgery 172

G

Gaenslens test 229, 231f
Gait 151, 156, 167, 244, 299, 300
   assessment 317
   deviation, identification of 294
   pattern 52, 237
   training 60, 292, 301
      techniques 292
Galeazzi dislocation 89, 90f
Galeazzi fracture 89, 90f, 138
Ganglion 37, 37f, 71
   common sites of 37
   sites of 38f
Garden classification 104, 105f, 105t
Gastrocsoleus complex, stretching of 60
Gastrointestinal disease 263
Gaucher's disease 246
General body relaxation techniques 171
Genitourinary complications 102
Gentle stretching 288
   exercises 33

Genu recurvatum 148
Genu valgum 154, 154f-156f, 157, 157f, 158, 158f, 159
Genu varum
  physiological 155
  resolve pathologic 156
Gerber's test 6, 7f
Gibbus deformity 173, 244f
Glenohumeral instability 15, 77
Glenohumeral joint mobilization 17
Glenoid fracture
  extra-articular 78
  intra-articular 77f, 78
Gluteal muscles, strengthening of 176
Glyceryl trinitrate 20
Glycosylation end-product, advanced 11
Golfer's elbow 22
  pain pattern 22f
  elbow brace for 24f
  taping for 24f
  test 23, 23f
Gosselin fracture 138
Gout 259
Gouty arthritis 258, 259f
  clinical presentation of 260f
Goyrand fracture 139
Gracaeu and Brahms procedure 161
Granulation tissue phase 251
Great toe 281
Greenstick fracture 66, 67f, 89, 89f
Growing system 172
Growth
  disturbance 71
  patterns, abnormal 299
  plate fracture 88, 88f
Guillain-Barre syndrome 181
Guyon's canal 202
  syndrome 202

H

Hairline fracture 67
Hallmark sign 13
Hallux valgus 255
Halo immobilization 128
Hamate fracture 97
  fragment, excision of 98
  Milch classification of 97, 97f, 97t
Hammer biceps curl 21
Hammer toe 255
Hamstring muscles, stretching of 176
Hand
  deformities 253
  extensor retinaculum of 35f
  injuries 31
  joints, arthritis of 256
  splinting of 257f
Handlebar palsy 202
Hangman's fracture 127, 138
  Levine and Edward classification of 128, 128f
Hard collar 128
Harrison's grove 269, 270f
Harrison's sulcus 269
Head 269
  on transfer technique 290, 290f
Healing
  delayed 125
  time, expected 128, 144, 146

Heart disease 252, 302
Heat 3, 28
  therapy 53, 250
Heberden's node 249f
Heel
  cord lengthening 165
  cups 63, 63f
  fat pad syndrome 121
  redness of 64f
  strike 291, 292f, 294
  swelling of 64f
Height, loss of 173
Hemarthrosis 70, 149
Hemi surface replacement 276
Hemi vertebra 165
Hemiarthroplasty 276
Hemilaminectomy 241
Hemipelvectomy 283
Hemiplegia, spastic 279
Herniation, types of 234f
Hilgenreiner epiphyseal angle 151, 151f
Hill-Sachs fracture 138
Hill-Sachs lesion 141
Hind foot pronation 255
Hip 169
  arthrodesis 280
  congenital dislocation of 298
  coxa vara of 151f
  deformities 150
  disarticulation 283, 289
  disease 246
    bilateral 280
  dislocation 144, 147t
  flexion 236
  flexors 240
  ipsilateral 280
  joint 255
    degenerative arthritis of 151
    replacement, types of 276
    subluxation 151
    surface replacement of 276
Hoffa fracture 138
Holdsworth fracture 138
Holstein-Lewis fracture 138
Hooter's elbow 18
Hormones 72
Hot pack 33, 36
Hot therapy 186, 256, 315
Housemaids knee 54
Hubscher's maneuver 164
Hueston tabletop test 33, 33f
Humeral head 79
Humeral shaft 79
  fracture 81, 83t
Hunched forward posture 173
Hutchinson fracture 138
Hyaluronic acid, intra-articular injection of 250
Hybrid fixation 272
  stem type with 276
Hydralazine 181
Hydrotherapy 233, 315
  exercises 240
Hyndman sign 237
Hyperabduction syndrome 200
Hyperextension injury 44f
Hyperflexion injury 44f
Hyperkyphosis, thoracic 176

Hyperparathyroidism 166
Hypersensitive area, desensitization of 311
Hypersensitivity 307
Hypophosphatemia rickets 267
Hypoplasia 148
  patellar 148
Hypothyroidism 181
Ibuprofen 309

I

Ice 3, 17, 23, 31, 59
  massage 62
Idiopathic scoliosis 165
  surgical interventions for 172
Iliotibial band 148
Immobilization 7, 73, 84, 86, 99, 144, 219
Impingement test 15
Implant
  components 275
  fixation 272
Incomplete fracture 66
  types of 66
Infection 29, 282, 303
  secondary 243
  systemic 272
Infectious diseases 312
Infrapatellar strap 53, 53f
Infraspinatus fossa, compartment syndrome of 77
Injury 77, 102, 126, 312
  acute 1, 5, 125
  chronic 5
  direct 29, 69, 76, 111
  electrical 282
  high
    impact 79, 81, 83
    ligament 57f
  indirect 69, 76, 112
  ipsilateral 117
  laceration 180
  level of 184
  ligamentous 121
  mechanism of 39, 43, 48, 56, 57f, 57t, 74, 79, 83, 86, 91, 95-98, 100, 104-107, 109, 111, 113, 115, 117, 120-123, 126f, 127-131, 142, 146
  severity of 184
  site of 190, 192, 195
  skeletal 103
  stretching 180
  surgical 306
  traumatic 180
  types of 184
  urogenital 103
  vertical shear 102
Interdigital nerve 203
Interferential therapy 315
Intermittent pneumatic compression pump 305
Internal fixation 85, 107
Internal rotation 79, 85, 142
Interossei, paralysis of 160
Interspinous gap change test 225, 226f
Intertrochanteric fracture 106, 150
  Evans classification of 106, 106f
Intervertebral disc
  anterior 2/3rd of 131
  degeneration of 220

herniation 234f
posterior 1/3rd of 131
space narrowing 221
Intervertebral disease, prolapsed 234
Intervertebral joints, fusion of 220
Intervertebral space, narrowing of 220
Intra-articular calcaneal fractures,
    Sanders classification of 121f, 121t
Intracompartmental pressure 27
Intramedullary nailing 82, 109, 115, 117
Intramuscular therapy 271
Intrathoracic dislocation 139
Intrinsic
    compression 181
    factors 10
    foot muscles, strengthening exercises
        of 62f
Iodine starch test 186
Iontophoresis 53
Irradiation 166
Irritable bowel syndrome 313
Ischemia 26f
Isoniazid 181

J

Jack test 164, 164f
Jefferson classification 125, 126t
Jefferson fracture 125, 126f, 138
    types of 126f
Jerks, deep 318
Joint 259, 283
    active infection in 272
    brace 250
    debridement 245
    deformity 259
    diseases 246
    dislocation 139
    disuse of 249
    fusion 251, 261, 278
        contralateral 278
        ipsilateral 278
        position of 279-281
    hyperlaxity 246
    hypermobile 165
    hypertrophy, uncovertebral 221
    instability 144
    margin of 249
    mobilization 4, 13, 21, 60, 65, 187, 209,
        233, 239
    movements, peripheral 232
    pain, distal radioulnar 279
    range of motion 187
    realigning of 251
    replacement 251, 261
    scoping 251
    sepsis 272
    space narrowing 249, 256
    stiffness 70, 144
    subtalar 281
    taping 250
Jones fracture 124, 138

K

Kidney 259
    failure 252, 302
Kilo-Nevin syndrome 202
Kinesiology taping 53f
Kleiger test 59, 59f

Knee 169, 314
    arthrodesis 280
    braces 41
    bursae 54f
    bursitis 54
    contour of 148
    deformities 154
    disarticulation amputation 283
    disease, bilateral 280
    flexion, delayed 275
    forced
        hyperextension of 43
        hyperflexion of 43
    immobilized 112
    injuries 39
    joint 255
        osteoarthritis of 246f
    osteoarthritis 109
        secondary 114
    pad 56f
        use of 56
    pain, anterior 149
    preservation 283
    replacement, types of 273
    stiffness 110
    support 41, 42
Knock knee 157, 157f
Knuckle bender splint 197, 197f
Knuckle deformity 244f
Krabbe's disease 181
Krukenburg's amputation 283
Kyphosis 172, 172f, 245
    Cobb's angle of 175f
    congenital 173
    mild 174
    moderate 174
    neuromuscular 173
    nutritional 173
    postural 173, 174f
    severe 174
    structural 173
    traumatic 173
    X-ray findings of 175f

L

Lachman's anterior test 45, 45f
Lachman's posterior test 49, 49f
Lambrinudi's operation 161
Laminectomy 241
Laminotomy 241
Lasegue test 237
Laser 315
    therapy 186
Lateral axial rotation opponens roll 215f
Lateral compression 102
    test 229, 231f
Lateral plantar nerve 198f
    entrapment 218
Lateral sliding board transfer 290
Latissimus dorsi 176
Le Fort
    ankle fracture 138
    facial fractures 138
Lead 181
    pipe fracture 138
Leg
    alignment 155f
    compartment syndrome of 114
    length discrepancy 299

Legg-Calvé-Perthes disease 150, 298,
    298f
    pathogenesis of 299f
    X-ray findings of 300f
Leprosy 181
Levator scapulae muscle 176
Levine and Edward classification 128,
    128f, 128t
Lidocaine 15
Lift off test 6, 7f
Ligament 57, 155
    destruction 253
    injury 114
        lateral 57f
        medial 57f
    posterior longitudinal 131, 235
Ligamentous laxity, generalized 148
Limb
    attitude of 141, 145
    elevation of 65, 304
    length
        discrepancy 109, 153
        measurement 156
        shortening of 117
    standing, single 292, 292f
Limp 299
Linder sign 237
Lisfranc amputation 283
Lisfranc fracture 138
Liver disease 181, 263, 302
Long flexors, paralysis of 160
Longitudinal ligament, anterior 131
Lordosis 176, 177f
Low energy
    fracture 115
    trauma 100
Low impact
    energy trauma 117
    injuries 79, 81, 83
Low midline sill sign test 225, 225f
Lower cross syndrome 173f, 177f, 266f
Lower extremity entrapment neuropathy,
    common 203t
Lower limb
    amputation 284f, 291
        levels of 283
    fractures 100
    nerve lesions 197
        clinical presentation of 199, 200t
    obesity for 272
Lower motor neuron disease 165
Lumbar corset 222, 222f
Lumbar disc herniation 236
    anatomy of 235f
    special tests for 236
Lumbar erector spinae 240
Lumbar hyper lordosis 177, 178f
Lumbar instability, interspinous gap
    change test for 225
Lumbar lordosis 178
    loss of 221
Lumbar lordotic curve 178, 178f
Lumbar scoliosis, left 167
Lumbar spine 220
Lumbosacral angle 178, 178f
Lumbrical, paralysis of 160
Lunate fracture 97, 97f
Lung function test 232

Index 329

Lymphatic drainage 304
Lymphocyte count 243
Lymphoma 253

M

Magnetic resonance
    imaging 12, 12f, 15, 19, 23, 38, 57, 65, 128, 207, 221, 236
    scan 5, 30, 40, 55
    neurography 185
Main en Griffe deformity 196
Maisonneuve fracture 138
Malalignment, rotational 109
Malgaigne fracture 138
Malunion 70, 75, 77, 80, 82, 83, 87, 90, 94, 99, 102, 107, 109, 114, 116, 125, 279
Mantoux test 243
Manual muscle test 174
Marble pick up exercise 62
March fracture 123, 138
Marfan's syndrome 162, 166
Marginal syndesmophyte formation 228
Mason classification, modified 87t
Massage 4, 28, 36, 53, 158, 217, 233, 315
    therapy 171, 257, 304
Masse's sign 196, 197f
Maudsley's test 19, 19f
Mayo classification 86t, 95, 95f
McMurray's test 40, 41f
Meary's angle 160, 160f, 163, 163f
Mechanical compression device 305
Medial capsular plication 148
Medial patellofemoral ligament repair 148
Medial plantar nerve 198f
    entrapment 217
Median nerve 202
    anatomical course of 191f
    clinical presentation of 192t
    examination of 191
    function 143
    gliding technique 213f
    injury 189
Meniscal allograft 43
Meniscal blood supply, zones of 40f
Meniscal injuries 39, 44, 114
Meniscal repair 42, 43
Meniscal tear 39f
    classification of 40f
Menisci, function of 39
Menisectomy 42
    partial 43
Mental status 287
Meralgia paresthetica 203
Metabolic disease 246
Metacarpal fracture 98, 100t
Metacarpophalangeal joint 253, 258
    stiffness 279
Metaphyseal fracture 66, 89
Metatarsal fracture 123
    second 125
Meyerding classification 223, 224f
Microdiscectomy 241
Milch classification 97, 97f, 97t
Mill's test 19, 19f
    reverse 24f
Milwaukee brace 175, 175f
Miner's elbow 29
Mirror visual feedback therapy 310, 310f

Mobility exercises 4, 232
Mobilization 222
Moist heat 13
Mononeuropathy 181
Monteggia dislocation 89, 90f
Monteggia fracture 89, 90f, 138
Moore's fracture 138
Morel-Lavalle lesion 102
Morning stiffness 251, 256
Morton neuroma 203
Motor dysfunction 308
Motor function 137, 185
Motor imagery program 310
Motor loss 200
Motor paralysis 190, 192, 195, 200
Motor supply 189, 191, 194, 197-199
Motor vehicle
    accidents 111, 127, 127f
    collision 145
Muller's classification 109, 110f, 110t
Multiorgan failure 181
Muscle 5, 155, 200
    abdominal 176
    atrophy 181
    bulk 185, 320
    contusions 2f
    endurance 321
    flaccid paresis of 181
    impairment, potential 173
    lumbosacral paraspinal 217
    manual 185
    power 320
    relaxants 216, 221, 250
    relaxation training 227
    repair 18
    strength 207, 249, 300
        Medical Research Council Scale for 320
    strengthen 289
    stretching 187, 240
    tightness 174, 207, 225
    tone 318
    wasting 181
    weakness 15, 22, 253
        marked 272
Muscular dystrophy 166
Muscular imbalance 206f
Muscular pain 313
Musculature around stump 285
Mutilans deformity 255
Mycobacterium tuberculosis 241
Myelin 182
    sheath 182
Myelography 236
Myeloma, multiple 263
Myositis ossificans 71
Myotome chart 321
Myxedema 302

N

Nachlas test 237
Navicular body fracture, Sangeorzan classification of 122, 122f
Neck 206
Necrosis 299
Needle aspiration 38
Neer's classification 79, 80f, 80t
Neer's test 16
Neoplasm 282

Neoplastic lesion 279
    stabilization after resection of 278
Nerve 5, 70, 200, 201, 203
    conduction velocity 185, 212
    damage 141
    gliding exercises 209, 213
    grafting 188
    injury 82, 93, 143, 144
        and anticipated recovery 184, 184t
        grade of 184
        management, principles of 188
        Seddon's classification of 182f
    lesion, classification of 181
    mobilization 239
    palsy 102
    roots 189, 191, 197-199
        impingement 235f
    stretching 187
    transfer 188
    transplant 188
    types of 184
Neural flossing 187
Neural glide 219
Neural stretch 25
Neurodystrophy 306
Neurofibromatosis 165
Neurogenic thoracic outlet syndrome 205, 206
Neurological disorders, nonprogressive 159
Neurolysis 188
Neuromuscular disorders, progressive 159
Neuropraxia 182
Neurorrhaphy 188
Neurovascular injury 58, 77, 87, 109, 114, 116, 117, 125, 279
Night splint 63, 63f, 213
Nightstick fracture 90, 90f, 138
Ninhydrin print test 186
Nodules 249, 252
Nonoperative anterior cruciate ligament injury, physiotherapy protocol for 45
Nonsteroidal anti-inflammatory drugs 20, 24, 31, 41, 53, 56, 65, 213, 216, 221, 225, 232, 250, 256, 309
Nonunion 70, 75, 77, 80, 82, 87, 90, 96, 102, 107, 116, 118, 125, 279
Non-weight bearing 127, 297
Nucleus
    degeneration 235
    extrusion 235
    prolapsed 235
    protrusion 235
    pulposus 235
Numbness pattern 218f
Numerical pain rating scale 316
Nursemaid fracture 138
Nutcracker fracture 122
Nutrition 72, 262, 264, 265

O

O'Donoghue's triad, presence of 42
Obesity 162, 177, 247, 272
Oblique fracture 68, 107, 116
Odontoid fracture 128
    Anderson D'Alonzo classification of 128, 129f
Okay test 143, 191, 192f

Olecranon bursitis 29, 29f, 30f
 types of 29
Olecranon fracture, classification of 86f
One level injury 133
Open fractures 66, 82, 113
Open mouth odontoid view 128
Open reduction 85, 146
 and internal fixation 73, 81-87, 91, 98, 100, 109, 111, 119, 124, 125, 146
 and posterior spine fusion 129
Opioids 309
Opponens splint 194f
Oral analgesics 13
Oral medication 17
Oral steroids 13
Oral therapy 271
Organophosphates 181
Orthopedic physiotherapy assessment 316
Orthopedic Trauma Association Classification 105, 106t
Orthosis 256
 thoracolumbosacral 175
Orthotics 41, 62, 63f, 65, 134, 186
Oschner's clasping test 192, 193f
Osgood-Schlatter disease 51, 52f
 X-ray findings for 52f
Osgood-Schlatter syndrome 52
Ossification, heterotrophic 93, 144
Osteoarthritis 246f, 249, 258t, 259, 278
 idiopathic 246
 pathophysiology of 247f
 predisposing factors of 247f
 primary 246
 secondary 149, 246
 spinal 220
 stages of 248, 248f
 X-ray finding of 249f
Osteochondral fracture 45, 112, 148
Osteochondritis 246
Osteoclasis 159
Osteomalacia 166, 267, 271
 clinical presentation of 269
 pathophysiology of 268f
Osteomyelitis 71, 117, 150
Osteonecrosis 71, 112, 121, 278
Osteophytes 249
 development of 249
 formation 220
 presence of 221
Osteoporosis 246, 253, 256, 262
 basic prevention of 265f
 severe 272
 transient migratory 306
 types of 262
Osteoporotic bone, severe 82
Osteotomy 159, 251
Overuse injuries 1

P

Paget's disease 137, 150, 246
Paget-Schroetter syndrome 200
Pain 27, 30, 35, 60, 159, 218f, 243, 249, 251, 299, 300, 307, 312
 assessment 316
 centralize 239
 chronic 112
 control 7, 13, 209
 limits of 222
 management 265
 nature of 12
 pattern 6f, 211f
 reduce 56, 213, 232, 301
 relieving modalities 4, 62, 179, 219, 222, 250, 261, 315
 site of 12
 syndrome, post-traumatic 306
Painful arc sign 16, 16f
Painful tender points 314
Palmar cutaneous nerve 191
Palmar digital branch 191
Paradiscal lesion 242
Paralytic disorder 278
Paramedial bulge 234
Paraneoplastic syndrome 181
Paraplegia 243
Paraproteinemias 181
Paraproteinemic syndrome 181
Parrot beak tear 40
Pars interarticularis 223
Passive range of motion 81, 98, 104, 118, 124, 127, 129, 142, 145, 147, 149
 exercises 28
Patella
 alta 148
 dislocated 147f
 high riding 148
 sleeve fractures 113
Patellar dislocation 146, 149t
 apprehension test for 148f
 habitual 146
 recurrent 148
 types of 146
Patellar fracture 111, 113t, 149
 classification of 112f
Patellectomy
 partial 113
 total 113
Pauwels classification 104, 105f, 105t
Peace sign 195, 196f
Pectoralis muscles, stretching of 176
Pedicle, displacement of 167
Pellegrini-Stieda disease 139
Pelvic
 fracture 100
  modified tile classification of 101f, 101t
  Young-Burgess classification for 102f, 102t
 osteotomy 301
 rotation 291, 291f
 stable fractures 104t
 tilt exercises 172, 240
Pelvis 169
Pen touching test 191, 192f
Percutaneous pinning 84, 99, 125
Perineurium 180, 182
Peripheral nerve 180, 318
 anatomy of 180f
 injury 182
  factors affecting prognosis of 184
 lesion 180
  causes of 180
  general introduction of 180
  mechanical causes of 180
 regeneration 182, 183f
Peripheral neuropathy 253
 non-mechanical causes of 181

Peripheral test 263
Peroneus longus, chronic dysfunction of 123
Perthes disease 246
Pes anserine bursitis 54
Pes cavus 159, 159f
 causes of acquired 159
 footprint test of 161f
Pes planus 162, 162f
 footprint test of 164f
Phalen test 212, 212f
 reverse 212, 212f
Phenytoin 181
Phonophoresis 36
Physeal fracture 66
Physiotherapy
 management 245, 281
 treatment 24, 27, 53, 56, 59, 62, 65, 73, 78, 186, 208, 226, 239, 309
 protocol 7
 postoperative 76, 81, 82, 88, 91, 94, 98, 100, 107, 111, 113, 115, 117, 119, 123, 127, 129, 134, 141, 144, 146
Piedmont fracture 138
Pigeon chest 269
Pilon fracture 117
Pipkin classification 105
Pipkin fracture dislocation 139
Piriformis muscle
 anatomy of 215f
 muscle energy technique of 217
 spasm of 215
Piriformis syndrome 203, 214, 215, 215f
Pitting edema 302, 302f
 grades of 304
Pivot transfer technique 290
Plantar arch taping 219
Plantar fascia 60, 161
 stretching exercises of 62f
Plantar fasciitis 60, 60f, 61f
 X-ray findings of 61f
Plantar fasciotomy 63
Plantar flexion 115, 118, 124, 127, 297
Platelet rich plasma 24
 injection of 61
Plexus injuries, neurologic 80
Plumber's elbow 29
Pneumothorax 75
Pointing index 192
Poliomyelitis 165
Pollock's sign 196
Polyarteritis nodosa 181
Poor playing techniques 22, 22f
Pope's blessing 192
Porphyria 181
Posadas' fracture 139
Positive coracoid pain test 13
Posterior arch
 complete disruption of 101
 incomplete disruption of 101
 intact 101
Posterior cruciate ligament injury 47
Posterior cruciate
 ligament
  anatomy of 48f
  functions of 47
  tear 47f
 retaining design 273
 substituting design 273

Index

Posterior drawer test 49, 49f
Posterior interosseous nerve 201
   injury 90
Posterolateral bulge 234
Postfracture joint stiffness 82, 83, 85, 99, 112
Postoperative rehabilitation protocol 42
Postsurgical rehabilitation protocol 8, 46
Posttraumatic subtalar joint
   arthritis 121
   stiffness 116
Postural awareness 208, 222, 238
Posture 177, 244
   assessment 316
Pott's fracture 139
Pott's spine 241
   pathophysiology of 242
Pouteau fracture 138
Pre-gait training techniques 291
Pressure
   prolonged 29
   sore 71
PRICE
   regime 3, 3f
   therapy 53
Progression, stages of 308
Pronator syndrome 202
Proprioceptive neuromuscular facilitation 17, 187
Prosthetic arthroplasty 81
Prosthetic fitting, optimal length for 282
Proteoglycans, loss of 248
Protrusio acetabula 255
Proximal femur fracture 108t
   classification of 103, 104f
Proximal fragment, osteonecrosis of 112
Proximal humeral fracture 14, 78, 81f
   Neer's classification of 79, 80f, 80t
Proximal humerus, parts of 79f
Proximal interphalangeal joint 254, 279
Proximal tarsal tunnel syndrome 217
Proximal tibial
   fracture 113, 115t
   nerve 203
   swelling 52
Pseudogout 30
Psoriasis 272
Pulley exercises 14
Pulse 317
Pump handle test 230, 231f
Pyridoxine 181, 213

Q

Q angle 155, 158
Quadratus lumborum 240
Quadriceps weakness 52
Quadrilateral space syndrome 201
Question mark deformity 232

R

Rachitic rosary 269, 270f
Racket sports 18
Radial artery injury 90
Radial deviation 95
Radial head fracture 86, 88t
   classification of 86, 87f
Radial nerve 201
   anatomical course of 189f
   deep 188
   function 143
   injury 188
      clinical presentation of 190t
      special test for examination of 189
   superficial 188
   branch of 201
Radial shaft fractures, Orthopedic Trauma Association classification of 89t
Radial tunnel syndrome 201
Radiocarpal osteoarthritis, post-traumatic 93
Radiography, conventional 263
Radioulnar synostosis, post-traumatic 90
Range of motion 28, 58, 76, 79, 87, 95, 98, 108, 110, 118, 119, 124, 127, 142, 145, 147, 149, 174, 214, 221, 224, 250, 272, 281, 289, 299, 300, 320
   examination of 35
   exercises 13, 33, 42, 65, 79, 81, 83, 91, 95, 98, 100, 104, 108, 110, 115, 124, 127, 129, 134, 142, 149, 187, 261, 265
   gentle pendulum 17
Raynaud's syndrome 313
Rectus femoris 52
Red-red zone 40
Red-white zone 40
Reflex
   superficial 318
   sympathetic
      dystrophy 279, 306
      syndrome 94
Refsum's disease 181
Regional anesthesia technique 309
Relieve acute pain 17
Renal disease 263
Residual limb, positioning of 287, 288, 288f
Resisted muscle strength, measurement of 35
Retrocalcaneal bursitis 63, 64f
Rheumatoid
   arthritis 30, 181, 251, 253, 254f, 255f, 258, 258t, 278, 279, 312
      diagnostic criterion of 256
      juvenile 166
      stages of 251, 252f
   factor, serum 256
   nodules 252f, 256
Rheumatologic disorders 263
Rib
   hump 169
   pelvic distance 264
Rice therapy 31, 41, 55, 56, 59, 304
Rickets 150, 166, 267, 267f, 269, 270f
   clinical presentation of 268
   nutritional 267
   pathophysiology of 268f
   renal 267
   stages of 269
   types of 267
Risser grades 168f, 168t
Robert Jones fracture 138
Rolando fracture 98, 99f, 139
   reverse 99
Roos test 207, 207f
Rotator cuff
   endurance of 14
   four muscles of 5
   injury 4, 15, 141
   muscles 5f, 5t, 14
   strengthening exercises 17
   tear 4f
      massive unreconstructable 278
      pain pattern of 6f
      types of 4
Rule of three 188
Runner's fracture 139

S

Sacral inclination 178, 178f
Sacroiliac joint 228
   test for 229
Sag sign, posterior 49, 49f
Salter-Harris fracture 139
Salvage operation 245
Sanders classification 121f, 121t
Sangeorzan classification 122, 122t
Sarcoidosis 181
Saturday night palsy 201
Scalene triangle 200
Scalenus anticus syndrome 200
Scaphocapitate syndrome 97
Scaphoid
   fracture 94
      Mayo classification of 95, 95f
   mechanism of injury of 95f
Scapholunate instability 37
Scapula
   glenoid and neck fracture of 78t
   neck fracture of 77f
Scapular
   exercises 17
   fracture 76, 79t
   level 168
   stabilizers 14
Scar 285
Schatzker classification 114, 114f, 114t
Scheuermann's disease 173
Scheuermann's kyphosis 174f
Schwann cells 180
Sciatic nerve 197, 203
   anatomical course of 197f
   injury 146
Sciatic scoliosis 165
Sclerosis, subchondral 249
Scoliometer 170, 170f
Scoliosis 165
   adolescent 165
   compensatory 165
   congenital 165
   double major 167
   functional 165, 170
   infantile 165
   juvenile 165
   neuromuscular 165
   nonstructural 165
   permanent 165
   postural 165
   structural 165, 170
   symptoms of 169f
   temporary 165
   thoracic 169f
   traumatic 166
Scottish rite brace 300, 301f
Scotty dog appearance 224, 224f
Screening test 263
Scrubbing 311

Seat belt 131
　fracture 138
　type injury 131, 133f
Seddon's classification 182, 182f, 182t
Segond fracture 45, 139
Sensation 287
　combined cortical 317
　deep 317
　superficial 317
Sensory 309
　changes 181
　disturbances 307, 313
　examination 38, 317
　function 143, 185
　　Medical Research Council
　　　classification of 185t
　integration training 310
　loss 190, 192, 195, 200
　re-education 187
　retraining 186
　supply 189, 191, 194, 197-199
Sepsis 181, 272
Septic olecranon bursitis 31
Septicemia 71
Sequestration, stage of 235
Sexual dysfunction 102
Shepherd fracture 139
Shock 108
　hypovolemic 70, 108
Shoe modifications 219
Short muscles, stretching of 179
Shortwave diathermy 222
Shoulder 206
　arthrodesis 278
　athroplasty 278
　contour of 141
　disarticulation 283, 285, 289
　dislocation 14, 139, 142t
　　classification of 139, 140f
　elevation exercises 13
　exercises, active 14f
　hand syndrome 306
　injuries 4
　joint 253
　　recurrent dislocation of 141
　level 168
　movement 7
　　progressive loss of 12
　normal 11f, 12f
　pain 11
　paralysis 278
　surgery 12
　wheel exercises 14
Shrinker socks 286
Sicard test 237
Sickle cell anemia 298
Sideswipe injury 142
Sideward walking 291
Silhouette appearance 52
Simian hand 192, 193f
Sinuses 243
Sir Robert Jones method 28f
Sitting posture 209, 238
Skeletal maturity 167, 170
Skin
　and soft tissue, basis of integrity of 66
　care 186
　color, asymmetry of 307
　over stump 285

problems 252
resistance test 186
temperature, asymmetry of 307
Sleeping posture 208, 238
Sliding board transfer amputee 289, 289f
Sling 87
　immobilization 78, 80
Slipped capital femoral epiphysis 298
Smith's fracture 91, 92f, 139
Soft tissue 70
　injury 1, 103
　　common overuse 2
　　types of 1
　massage 17, 20, 24
　mobilization 219
　reconstruction 161
　techniques 222
Soleal sling syndrome 203
Soto-Hall test 237
Sound leg step
　backward 293
　forward 292
Spasm 215, 317
Spasticity 318
Speed's test 16, 16f
Spinal brace 171
Spinal cord 135
　exact relation of 135
　implantation 309
　injury 137t
　relation of 135, 136f
Spinal disorders 220
Spinal flexion exercise program 227
Spinal fusion 172, 245
Spinal hyperextension test 174
Spinal instability 245
Spinal instrumentation 172
Spinal ligaments, degeneration of 220
Spinal mobility exercise 179, 240
Spinal range of motion 169
Spinal roots 194
Spinal segment 135f, 137
Spinal trauma
　Denis classification of 130, 131t
　major injuries of 131t
Spine 229, 243
　active range of motion of 171
　fracture of 166
　lordosis of 177f
　normal 166f, 177f
　rotation 170
　scoliotic 166f
　stiffness in 173
　X-ray findings of 230f
Spiral fracture 69, 107, 116
Splay foot 255
Splinting 28, 33, 34f, 86, 186, 257f
Spondyloarthropathy, tuberculous 241
Spondylolisthesis 177, 222
　congenital 223
　degenerative 223
　dysplastic 223
　isthmic 223
　pathological 223
　traumatic 223
Spondyloptosis 223
Spondylosis 220
　lumbar 221

Sports
　activity 142
　injuries 145
Sprain 1
　classification of 1f
　mild 1, 37, 57
　moderate 1, 57
　severe 1, 57
Squeeze test 59, 59f
Stable fracture 107
Stahl index 161, 163
Standing posture 238
Standing tip toe test 164, 165f
Static wrist cock up splint 190f
Steindler stripping 161
Stellate fracture 112
Steroid 225
　injection 31, 56, 65
　　intra-articular 13
　　intrabursal 17
　prolonged use of 298
Stieda fracture 139
Stiffness 173, 243, 249, 313
　post-fracture 114
　post-traumatic 80
Straddle fracture 139
Straight leg raising 110, 275
　test 236, 237f
Strain 1
　classification of 2f
Strength 287
　duration curve 185
Strengthening 60, 222
　exercises 4, 21, 21f, 25, 36, 46, 53, 60,
　　62f, 79, 81, 95, 98, 104, 108, 110,
　　118, 124, 127, 134, 142, 149, 154,
　　156, 164, 171, 175, 179, 187, 209,
　　214, 226, 240, 250, 261, 266, 315
Stress 314
　emotional 312
　fracture 67, 69, 122, 123
　loading program 311
　psychological 312
　repetitive 22
Stretching exercises 17, 21, 21f, 24, 29, 36,
　53, 62, 65, 154, 156, 158, 164, 171,
　176, 209, 214, 226, 240, 261, 315
Strokes, deep 304
Student's elbow 29
Stump
　bandaging 286
　　principles of 286
　edema, control 286, 288
　exercises 289
　hygiene 287
　length, ideal 283
　management 285
Subacromial bursa, function of 14
Subacromion bursitis pain pattern 15f
Subacromion impingement syndrome 77
Subaxial spine injuries 130t
　Allen and Ferguson classification of
　　130
Subcapital fracture 103, 104
Subchondral bone 248
　cyst 248
　exposure of 248
Subcoracoid space 204

Index

Subluxation 139
Subscapularis 6
Sudeck's atrophy 71
Sudeck's reflex neurovascular dystrophy 306
Sudomotor 309
Sunderland classification 182, 182t
Sunlight 271
Superficial peroneal tunnel syndrome 203
Supinator syndrome 201
Supplementation 271
Supraclavicular pressure 207, 207f
Supracondylar fracture 109
Suprapatellar bursitis 54
Suprascapular nerve 201
  syndrome 201
Supraspinatus 314
  fossa, compartment syndrome of 77
  tendinitis 5, 15
Surgery 31, 172, 184
  delayed 188
Suture line 285
Swan neck deformity 254
Sweating, asymmetry of 308
Swelling 30, 30f, 55f, 56, 60, 64f, 70, 249, 251, 256, 307, 317
Syme's amputation 283, 289
Sympathectomy 309
Syndesmosis injury, tests for 59
Syndesmotic sprain 60
Synovectomy 245
Synovitis 227, 248, 254, 268f
Syringomyelia 165
Systemic inflammatory disease 280
Systemic lupus erythematosus 30, 181, 312

T

Talar 1st metatarsal angle, lateral 160, 163
Talar tilt test 59, 59f
Talus fracture 121
Tarsal fracture 119, 124t
Tarsal tunnel
  anatomy of 217
  release 219
  syndrome 203, 217, 217f, 218f
  types of 217
Taylor brace 175, 175f
Tear
  displaced 40
  full thickness 4
  horizontal 40
  longitudinal 40
  partial thickness 4
  radial 40
  serious ligament 148
Temporomandibular joint 253
Tenderness 30, 35, 70, 173, 317
  over tibial tubercle 52, 53f
Tendinitis 1, 2, 2f
  infraspinatus 6
Tendon 18
  adhesions 279
  covering of 2
  debridement surgery 21, 25
  glide exercises 33, 34f, 213, 214f
  injury 37, 117, 121
  release 21

rupture 94, 279
sheaths 259
transfer 161
transplant 188
Tennis elbow 18, 18f
  elbow brace for 20f
  pain pattern 18f
  taping 21, 21f
Teres minor 6
Tetanus 71
Thallium 181
Thenar abduction with extension 215f
Therapeutic exercise 17, 31, 175, 209, 239, 257, 261, 305
Therapeutic modalities 20, 24, 161, 305
Thermal injury 282
Thigh, compartment syndrome of 108
Thompson's test 58
Thoracic erector spinae muscle, strengthening of 176
Thoracic outlet syndrome 200, 204f, 205
  clinical presentation of 206t
Thoracic scoliosis, right 166
Thoracic spine 220
Thoracolumbar scoliosis, right 166
Thoracolumbar vertebrae fracture 130, 134t
Thoracoplasty 166
Thromboembolism 70
Thumb
  deformity 255
  spica
    cast immobilization 96
    splint 36, 36f
  up test 189, 190f
Thyroid disease 11
Tibial component 273
Tibial fracture, bilateral 117
Tibial nerve 197
  anatomical course of 198f
  posterior 203
Tibial osteotomy 156
Tibial plafond fracture 117
  Orthopedic Trauma Association classification of 117, 118f, 118t
Tibial plateau fracture, Schatzker classification of 114, 114t
Tibial shaft fracture 115, 118t
  Orthopedic Trauma Association classification of 89f, 116, 116f, 116t
Tibial tuberosity
  elevation of 52
  medialization of 148
Tibialis posterior dysfunction syndrome, test for 163
Tight muscles, stretching of 179
Tile classification, modified 101f, 101t
Tillaux fracture 139
Tinel's sign 185
  positive 218
  supraclavicular 207, 208f
Tissue
  mobilization technique 33
  viability of 282
Toddler's fracture 139
Toe sign 164, 164f
Toe touch weight bearing 108, 110, 111, 115, 118, 119, 147

Tophi
  removal of 261
  X-ray findings of 260f
Torus fracture 67, 89, 139
Total hip replacement 275, 275f
  implant components of 276f
Total joint
  arthroplasty 279
  replacement 84
Total knee replacement 273, 273f
  surfaces replaced in 273
  surgeries 157
Tourniquet test 212
Toxins 181
Traction 111, 222, 288
  injury 76, 180
Tragus to wall test 230, 231f
Transcervical fracture 103, 104
Transcutaneous electrical nerve stimulations 315
Transtibial gait deviations 296
Transverse fracture 68, 89, 107, 112, 116
Trapezius 314
Trauma 282, 306
  degree of 72
  direct 298
  high energy 100, 117
  multiple 82, 117
Trendelenburg gait 151, 153
Trepezium fracture 96
Triangular fibrocartilage complex, disruption of 92
Trigger point release therapy 217
Triquentrum fracture 96, 96f, 106
Trochanter, greater 314
Trochanteric fracture, classification of 106f
Trochlear dysplasia 148
Trochleoplasty 148
Trough fracture 139
Trough sign 139
Trunk muscle 289
Trunk rotation
  angle of 170
  asymmetrical 170
  measuring angle of 170f
T-score 263
Tubercle
  greater 5
  lesser 5
Tuberculin skin test 243
Tuberculosis 280
  musculoskeletal 241
  spine 241
    X-ray finding of 244f
  spondylitis 241
Tuberosity
  avulsion fracture 122
  greater 79
  lesser 79
Tumor, malignant 272

U

Ulnar deviation 95
Ulnar nerve 202
  anatomical course of 194f
  function 143
  injury 85, 193
    clinical presentation of 195t

release 25
special test for examination of 194
Ulnar olecranon fracture 85, 87t
Ultrasonic therapy 36
Ultrasound 5, 13, 17, 19, 23, 30, 33, 39, 40, 55, 61, 65, 186, 222, 250
therapy 315
Unicompartmental implants design 273, 274f
Union, delayed 70, 82, 118, 279
Unstable fracture 96, 107
Upper cross syndrome 173f, 266f
Upper extremity 129, 142, 145, 206
entrapment neuropathy, common 201t
Upper limb
activity 292
amputation 285f
levels of 283
fractures 74
muscle weakness of 15
nerve lesions 188
Upper trapezius 176
Uremia 181
Urinary bladder irritability 313

V

Varus derotation osteotomy 154
Vascular disease, severe 272
Vascular injury 80, 82, 144, 184
Vasculitis 181, 253
Vasomotor 309
disturbances 181
Vastus lateralis 148
Vastus medialis
oblique 275
weakness 148
Venous thoracic outlet syndrome 205, 206
Vertebra
congenital deformities of 166f
distortion of 169f

Vertebral basilar artery injury 126
Vertebral body
anterior 2/3rd of 131
posterior 1/3rd of 131
Vertebral canal diameter 221
Vertebral lesions, types of 242, 242f
Vertebral rotation, measurement of degree of 168f
Vertebral segments 135, 135f, 136f
Vessels injury, subclavin 75
Villonodular synovitis, pigmented 30
Vincristine 181
Viscera 70
Visual analogue scale 316
Vitamin
B12 deficiency 181
B6 213
D
deficiency 177, 268
metabolism 268, 268f
supplements 265
therapy 271
Volar Barton fracture 92
Volkmann's ischemia 70, 83
Volkmann's ischemic contracture 25, 25f, 26f
mild 26, 26f, 27
moderate 26, 26f, 27
severe 27, 27f

W

Waddling gait 151
Wagon wheel fracture 139
Wagstaffe-Le Fort fracture 138
Waist fracture, non-displaced 96
Waistline, position of 168
Wallerian degeneration 182
Walther's fracture 139
Wand exercises 13
Wartenberg's syndrome 201
Washing out joint 251
Wax therapy 33

Wedge
fractures 116
vertebra 165
Weight bearing 59, 103, 110, 113, 119, 124, 127, 134, 147, 149, 297
exercises 265
normal 118
partial 104, 108, 110, 111, 115, 118, 119, 124, 127, 147
Wheelchair propulsion 287, 290
White-white zone 40
Winquist's classification 108, 108f, 108t
Wound infection 70, 279
Wright test 207, 208f
Wrist
and ankle, widening of 270f
and hand
deformities 254f
paralysis 279
arthrodesis 279
brace 38
disarticulation 283
drop 189
extension 25
extensor, test for 189
flexion 23
isometric 25
fracture 91, 95t
injuries 31
joint 253, 279
postfracture stiffness of 94
splinting of 257f

Y

Yoga 233
Young-Burgess classification 101, 102f, 102t

Z

Ziehl-Neelsen staining 243
Z-score 264

www.ingramcontent.com/pod-product-compliance
Ingram Content Group UK Ltd.
Pitfield, Milton Keynes, MK11 3LW, UK
UKHW031323150525
2007IPUK00011B/34